LEADERS

IN

HOMOEOPATHIC THERAEUTICS

WITH

GROUPING AND CLASSIFICATION

By

E. B. NASH, *M.D.*

Author of
"Leaders in Typhoid", "Regional Leaders",
"Leaders in Sulphur", "How to Take the Case",
"Leaders in Respiratory Organs"
&
"Testimony of the Clinic"

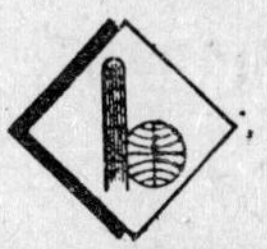

B. JAIN PUBLISHERS PVT. LTD.
NEW DELHI - 110 055

Price : Rs. 25.00

Reprint Edition : 1989

Published by :
B. Jain Publishers Pvt. Ltd.
1921, Street No. 10, Chuna Mandi
Paharganj, New Delhi - 110 055 (INDIA)
Printed at :
J. J. Offset Printers
Kishan Kunj, Delhi - 110 092

ISBN 81—7021—012—7

BOOK CODE B-2389

To My Wife,
My Loving and Faithful Co-Laborer,
Sympathizing with Me in Trial,
Rejoicing with Me in Success,
I Gratefully Dedicate
this Book.

E. B. NASH.

PREFACE

For offering this book to the profession, I have no apology to make, for I claim my right to do so; and if anyone finds imperfections in it, remember I lay no claim to perfection. I can offer severe criticism myself.

I will, however, state in brief my object in writing as I have:

First.—To fasten upon the mind of the reader the strongest points in each remedy. Good off-hand prescribing can be done in simple uncomplicated cases if we have fixed in our minds, for ready use, the *characteristic* symptoms.

The elder Lippe was remarkable for such ability.

Second.—To try to discourage the disposition to quarrel over Symptomatology and Pathology. Neither can be ruled out, and it is foolish for our school to divide on such a bone of contention. Every symptom has its pathological significance, but we cannot always give it in words; but the fact that it *has* such meaning is sufficient reason for prescribing on the *Symptom* or *Symptoms* without insisting on, or trying to give, the explanation.

Third.—To insist on the fact that the question of dose is still an open one, and so I have taken pains to give the dose I have found best, not insisting that anyone is bound to give the same; but it is fair to say that if they use a different one and fail, they must blame themselves, not me.

Fourth.—To condemn the abuse of drugs, both in the old school and ours.

If there is any one point in the Homœopathic system of Therapeutics that recommends it before that of the old school, it is that we have discovered a law by which we are able to apply remedies for the curing of the sick without entailing upon them drug effects, often more serious than the original disease.

No honest man of either school ought to object to such an improvement in the science of therapeutics.

FIFTH.—I have hoped to so write as to induce any old school physician, who could overcome prejudice so far as to read any or all of this book, to experiment along the lines I have indicated, believing that any such physician, of sound head and honest heart, will be irresistibly led to give Homœopathy a large, and perhaps finally, the largest place in his confidence and practice.

Finally to express, after nearly forty years of conscientious experimentation, my firm and confirmed belief in the Simillimum, the single remedy and the minimum dose.

Thanking the profession in general for their help to me, I reciprocate by offering my humble contribution to an already valuable homœopathic literature.

E. B. NASH.

Cortland, N. Y., November 5, 1898.

PREFACE TO SECOND EDITION

THE call for a Second Edition of this work, and in so short time after its first appearance, is, indeed, very gratifying to me, and I have endeavored to make it even more acceptable than at first by valuable additions in the way of new remedies, and further comparisons. I have tried to avoid increasing the size of the work at the expense of its reliability, which is an error into which many authors have fallen.

This is an age of speculation, and "fads" of all kinds are in order, but disappointment and failure is the sure outcome. I believe in the Homœopathy taught by Hahnemann, and that is what I purpose to proclaim.

Thanking my colleagues for their appreciation of the first edition, as evidenced by the many letters received and the rapid sale of the same, I offer the second with increasing confidence and gratitude.

E. B. NASH.

Cortland, N. Y., July, 1900.

PREFACE TO THIRD EDITION

NOT much by way of preface need be said for this third edition of "LEADERS." The demand for it is evidence that the work has, among other popular works, taken its place to stay. That this is very gratifying to the author is quite reasonable to suppose, because of the appreciation of his efforts by his professional brethren.

E. B. NASH.

Cortland, N. Y., June, 1907.

PREFACE TO FOURTH EDITION

THE call for the Fourth Edition of this work is cause for increased gratification to the author.

In addition I have received congratulatory letters from many physicians in different countries and languages. To my professional brethren, who have so kindly received the fruit of my efforts, I return sincere thanks.

I have tried in this edition to improve it by prefixing to each remedy a few of the leading symptoms, the text of the former editions following as a commentary with comparisons. It is hoped by this double arrangement to impress the remedies more firmly in the mind for practical off-hand prescribing.

I anticipate the charge that this is repetition. and answer, that it is only by repetition oft repeated, that the average mind can retain for ready use the salient points in our vast Materia Medica.

I do not believe that this arrangement will lessen the usefulness of "Regional Leaders," which contains over two thousand characteristics in self-quiz style, which is very popular with students. To my good wife, who has done the clerical work under my dictation, is due much praise. This on account of my blindness. As I draw near the end of my earthly career I hope to leave an influence for good that will live many years.

May the spirit of pure Homœopathy formulated in the words, "Similia Similibus Curantur," by the Master, possess all those who believe this to be the only law of truly scientific medical therapeutics.

DR. E. B. NASH.

Cortland, N. Y., July, 1913.

INTRODUCTION

To My Colleagues, Young and Old:

I desire in this form to put on record things new and old in the practice of medicine, as I have found them, in a professional career of over thirty years.

In my younger days I found great pleasure and profit in reading the writings of Hering, Dunham, Wells, Lippe and others, who have now ceased from their labors and gone to their well-earned rest.

I have carefully tested their teachings, and now that my own hair begins to grow frosty, I desire to leave some testimonial to the truth of those teachings. My aim is not to write a complete Materia Medica, nor yet an exclusive work on practice, though it may partake of the character of both, but rather facts and observations in practice and principles, which I have abundant reasons for believing true and reliable.

While I may not hope always to instruct those of my professional brethren who are contemporaries and abreast with me in professional attainments and experience, I do hope not to tire, but rather to entertain them, at least, a part of the time; and still more do I hope to be a real help to the beginner, even as I myself was helped.

I do not propose to adopt the usual way by beginning with *Aconite* and ending with *Zincum,* but to follow the bent of my inclinations, or, as it is sometimes expressed, the movings of the spirit, and may I not here invoke the aid of the spirits of the immortal Hahnemann, Bœnninghausen and the galaxy of bright names that adorn the fair page of the history of Homœopathy to help me.

Finally, I desire in every chapter to write something useful to somebody, and if in any part of this work I should give expression to anything wrong I here declare once for all my entire willingness to be *forgiven.*

E. B. NASH, M. D.

Cortland, N. Y.

LEADERS IN

Homœopathic Therapeutics

NUX VOMICA.

For very particular, careful, zealous persons, inclined to get excited or angry, spiteful, malicious disposition, mental workers or those having sedentary occupations.

Over-sensitiveness, easily offended; very little noise frightens, cannot bear the least even suitable medicine; faints easily from odors, etc.

Twitchings, spasms, convulsion, < slightest touch.

Chilliness, even during high fever; least uncovering brings on chilliness. Very red face.

Persons addicted to stimulants, narcotics, patent medicines, nostrums, debauchees, etc.

Frequent and ineffectual desire for stool or passes little at a time, > after stool.

Modalities: < uncovering, mental work, after eating, cold air, dry weather, stimulants, 9 A. M.; > wet weather, warm room, on covering, after stool.

Spasm (from simple twitchings to the clonic form); *sensitiveness, nervous* and *chilliness* are three general characteristics of this remedy.

Anxiety with irritability and inclination to commit suicide, but is afraid to die.

Sleepy in the evening, hours before bedtime; lies awake for an hour or two, at 3 or 4 A. M., then wants to sleep late in morning.

Awakens tired and weak and generally worse, with many complaints.

Stomach: Pressure an *hour* or *two* after eating as from a stone (immediately after, *Kali bi., Nux m.).*

Convulsions with consciousness *(Strych.);* < anger, emotion, touch, moving, alternate constipation and diarrhœa *(Ant. crud.).*

Menses: Too early, profuse and lasting too long, with aggravation of all other complaints during their continuance.

Nux vomica acts best when given at night, during repose of mind and body; *Sulph.* in the morning.

* * * * *

Among the symptoms called characteristic, as given by Constantine Hering, are these:

"After aromatics in food or as medicine, particularly ginger, pepper, etc., and after almost any kind of so-called 'hot' medicines (Goullon)." Also, "will also benefit persons who have been drugged by mixtures, bitters, herbs and so-called vegetable pills, etc.—(B.)"

This is putting it in too wholesale a fashion. It would be true if said that *Nux vomica* will *often* benefit such cases. The fact is that it will benefit those cases in which the use of such drugs, aromatics, pills, etc., has brought about a condition that simulates the symptoms produced in the provings of *Nux vomica,* or in cases to which it is homœopathic, and no others. Another fact is that these things often *do* produce such a condition, and that is one reason why so many physicians are almost invariably prescribing *Nux vomica* the first thing, in cases coming from allopathic hands, without even examining the case. But it is unscientific. We have a law of cure, and there are cases in which the *Nux vomica* condition is *not* present but another more similar remedy must be given. It does not alter the case to say, "Well, I did not know what had been given," for *Nux vomica* will neither antidote the effects of the drug poison nor cure the disease condition unless it is homœopathically indicated, especially if given in the dynamic form.

Here are two more of Hering's card symptoms, in which are given the temperaments that are most susceptible to the action of *Nux:*

"Over-sensitiveness, every harmless word offends, every little noise frightens, anxious and beside themselves, they cannot bear the least even suitable medicines.—(B.)" And, "For very particular, careful, zealous persons, inclined to get excited and angry, or of a spiteful, malicious disposition."

This is a graphic picture of what is called the "Nervous temperament," and practice corroborates the truth of the value of these temperamatic indications for this remedy; but there are a number of remedies that have as markedly this so-called nervous temperament, such as *Chamomilla, Ignatia, Staphisagria,* and others.

So no physician would be justified in prescribing *Nux vomica* on temperament alone, be the indication ever so clear. The *whole case* must come in. There seems to be another kind of condition belonging to this nervous group of *Nux vomica* that has not so much of the excitable in it. "Hypochondriasis, with studious men, sitting too much at home, with abdominal complaints and costiveness."

Now, if you take a second look at these cases, you will find that a very little irritation will arouse this kind out of their hypochondriac gloom and make them angry or irritable similar to the first condition, so that on the whole the first proves to be the predominant one.

If the gloomy or hypochondriac condition of mind persists, we will more likely have to look to such remedies as *Aurum, Nat. mur.*, etc., to find the true simillimum. These nervous symptoms of mind and body are wonderful leaders to the selection of the right remedy.

"Frequent and ineffectual desire to defæcate or passing but small quantities of fæces at each attempt."

This symptom is pure gold. There are a few other remedies that have it, but none so positively and persistently.

It is the guiding symptom in the constipation to which *Nux vomica* is homœopathic, and in my experience will then, and then only, cure.

Carrol Dunham wrote over twenty-five years ago on this symptom. He said, in effect—while *Nux vomica* or *Bryonia* are equal remedies for constipation there was never any reason for confounding them, or alternating them, as they were so different. The *Nux vomica* constipation was caused by irregular peristaltic action of the intestines, hence the frequent ineffectual desire; but the *Bryonia* constipation was caused by lack of secretion in the intestines There was with *Bryonia* absolutely no desire, and the stools were dry and hard as if burnt.

And the above symptom is found not in constipation alone. It is always present in dysentery. The stools, though very frequently consisting of slimy mucus and blood, are small and very unsatisfactory. Dr. P. P. Wells pointed out the very reliable additional symptom for *Nux vomica* in dysentery—that the *pains were very greatly relieved for a short time after every stool.* This is not so with *Mercury*, but the pain and tenesmus continue *after* the stool, as it is sometimes well expressed as "a never-get-done" feeling. But it makes little difference whether the patient is afflicted with constipation, dysentery, diarrhœa or other diseases, if we have this frequent ineffectual desire for stool present we always think of *Nux vomica* first, and give it unless other symptoms contra-indicate it.

"Catamenia a few days before time, and rather too copious, or keeping on several days longer with complaints at the onset, which remain until after it is over."

This is also an oft-verified symptom of *Nux vomica.* Of course there are many other remedies for too early or too copious menstruation. *Calcarea ostrearum* is one of them, but the temperament of the *Calcarea* patient is not at all like *Nux vomica.* I have found that patients that required *Nux vomica* for this condition could hardly ever take *Pulsatilla* for anything. For instance, if the patients had a green, bland, thick discharge and you gave them *Pulsatilla* it would often bring on too early and profuse menstruation. In such cases I had to give *Sepia,* which would act like a charm on the catarrh and not aggravate the menses.

These cases calling for *Nux vomica* often occur in young girls or women at the climacteric. We often have the characteristic rectal troubles also present. *(Lilium tig.)* The pains are pressing down and extend to the rectum and sometimes also to the neck of the bladder. Inefficient *labor pains,* extending to rectum, with desire for stool or frequent urination, are quickly relieved, and become efficient, after the administration of a dose of *Nux vomica* 200.

If, in addition, your menorrhagic patient is costive, has gastric troubles, and especially if generally < in the morning, we have an almost sure remedy in *Nux vomica.*

"Feels worse in the morning soon after awaking (Lach and *Nat. mur.), also after mental exertion (Nat. carb.,* vertigo; *Calc. ost., Silicea,* occipital); *after eating (Anacard.,* reverse), *and in cold air (Puls.,* reverse)." If Bœnninghausen had never done anything but give us his incomparable chapter on aggravations and ameliorations, this alone would have immortalized him.

It seems to me, after profiting by them in a practice of over thirty years, it is impossible to over-estimate them.

But some one will say, perhaps—there are twenty-eight remedies in Allen's *Bœnninghausen,* in large caps, that are worse in the morning. That does not seem like coming very close to a choice of the single remedy.

But, when we look at those that are worse in the evening, we find thirty-eight remedies, and only eight of them occurring under *both* morning and evening, and these eight are worse not *generally,* but rather in some *especial* symptoms. For instance, in *Rhus* the loose cough is worse in the morning, the tight, dry one in the evening.

So you see we are quite on the way to making a choice after all. But now take all the aggravations of *Nux vomica* as regards time, mind, gastric (symptoms), temperature, etc., where can you find the combination so prominently under any other remedy? Of course those physicians who are not able to appreciate anything but pathological symptoms have not much use for these modalities. But one thing is certain, they cannot do as good homœopathic work without as with them.

"Great heat, whole body burning hot, especially face red and hot, yet the patient cannot move or uncover in the least without feeling chilly." This condition of

feverishness is of common occurrence and yields to *Nux vomica* with a promptness that would delight the heart of a Lippe. It makes no difference what the name of the fever, whether inflammatory, remittent, or fever accompanying sore throat, rheumatism, or any other local trouble, if we have these indications, we may confidently give this remedy and will not often be disappointed in the result. It took me years to learn the value of this symptom, because I was a routinist and thought that *Aconite, Belladonna,* or both in alternation, must be given in all cases where high fever was present. So I have some sympathy for young physicians now, who from false teachings have been led into the same error. But let me say here, for the benefit of all such, that there is a much better way: namely—to closely individualize, which is not always difficult; give the single remedy in the potentized form, giving it time to act, and wait for reaction before repeating.

Of course low potencies will often cure, and that in spite of alternation, over-dosing, and frequent repetition. But they will often fail, and, in the great majority of cases, will not accomplish anything like the satisfactory results of the true simillimum, the single remedy, and the minimum dose.

"After eating: (Kali bich., Nux moschata) sour taste, pressure in the stomach an hour or two afterward, with hypochondriacal mood, pyrosis, tightness about waist; must loosen clothing (Lachesis, Calcarea and Lycopodium), confused, cannot use mind two or three hours after a meal, epigastrium bloated, with pressure as from a stone in the stomach."

This is a group of symptoms as given in "Guiding

Symptoms." There are so many symptoms given under the digestive organs that it shows that *Nux vomica* has really a very wide range of action in gastric troubles. And there are no really characteristic and peculiar symptoms to mention, unless it be the peculiar aggravation of stomach symptoms *"an hour or two after eating,"* instead of immediately after, as is the case with *Nux moschata* and *Kali bichromicum.* The pressure as from a stone occurs also under *Bryonia* and *Pulsatilla.*

More stress may be placed upon the cause of the stomach, liver, and abdominal complaints for which *Nux vomica* is the remedy. For instance, coffee, alcoholic drinks, debauchery, abuse of drugs, business anxiety, sedentary habits, broken rest from long night watching *(Cocc., Cup. met., Nit. ac.),* too high living, etc. So we find that *Nux vomica* is adapted to complaints arising from these causes, which is abundantly verified in practice.

One thing is very apt to be present in these cases: namely—the very characteristic rectal symptoms already noticed.

We ought not to leave *Nux vomica* without speaking of its great efficiency in headaches and backaches.

The headaches often occur in conjunction with the gastric, hepatic, abdominal and hæmorrhoidal affections. Here also the modalities, more than the character of the pain, decide the choice. The aggravations are: from mental exertion, chagrin or anger; in open air (opposite *Pulsatilla),* on awaking in the morning, after eating, from abuse of coffee or spirits, sour stomach, in the sunshine, on stooping, from light and noise, when moving or opening the eyes *(Bryonia),* from coughing, high living or highly seasoned food, in stormy weather, after drugging, from masturbation, from constipation or hæmorrhoids.

These headaches may or may not localize in any particular part of the head.

The patient is just as apt to say in one part of the head as another, and will often say, in no particular part, "it feels badly and aches all over."

The pains in the back are more peculiar. The patient is apt to have the backache in bed, and must sit up to turn over; as turning or twisting the body, aggravates when standing *(Sulphur)* (worse when sitting, *Kobalt, Pulsatilla, Rhus toxicod., Zincum)*, or sitting is especially painful. The pain is mostly located in the lumbar region, though it may be in the dorsa, and is often in connection (like *Æsculus hipp.)* with hæmorrhoids. *Æsculus* is especially < from walking or stooping. Backache, caused by masturbation *(Kobalt,* < sitting; *Staphisagria,* lying at night) finds one of its best remedies in *Nux vomica.* We might here launch out into a description of the general action of *Nux vomica* upon the spinal cord, including the motor and sensory centers, etc., but that can all be found in other works. So now we will leave *Nux,* except as we refer to it in comparison while writing of other remedies. In reviewing what we have written, we are impressed that some may be led to think that we have narrowed down the sphere of this truly great remedy too much. Let us say here, that it is not our aim in this work to write exhaustively upon any remedy, but to point out a few of the chief virtues and characteristic symptoms, around which all the rest revolve.

To write exhaustively would be to write a complete Materia Medica.

In actual practice there are two kinds of cases that come to every physician. One is the case that may be prescribed for with great certainty of success on the symptoms that are styled *characteristic* and *peculiar*. (Organon, § 153.) The other is where in all the case there are no such symptoms appearing; then there is only one way, viz., to hunt for the remedy that, in its pathogenesis, contains what is called the "*tout ensemble*" of the case. The majority of the cases, however, do have, standing out like beacon lights, some characteristic or keynote symptoms which guide to the study of the remedy that has the whole case in its pathogenesis.

PULSATILLA.

Mild, gentle, yielding disposition; sad and despondent, weeps easily, sandy hair, blue eyes, pale face, muscles soft and flabby.

Changeable remedy, pains travel from one joint to another; hæmorrhages flow and stop and flow again, no two stools alike, no two chills alike, no head nor tail to the case—mixed.

Bad taste in the mouth, < mornings, with great dryness, but *no thirst*.

Stomach easily disturbed, especially by cakes, pastry or rich fat foods.

Thick bland discharges from all mucous membranes.

Catamenia too late, scanty or suppressed, particularly by wetting the feet.

Modalities: < in warm room, warm applications, abuse of Iron, chilliness with the pains, > by *cool open air*, walking slowly around, cold food or drink, tying up tightly > the headache.

Pains accompanied with constant chilliness, and the more severe the pain the harder the chill (with profuse sweating, *Cham.*; with fainting, *Hepar sulph.*; with frequent micturition, *Thuja*; with delirium, *Verat. alb.*).

* * * * *

The disposition of *Pulsatilla* is almost the opposite of that of *Nux vomica*. *Nux vomica* is called the man's remedy and *Pulsatilla* the woman's remedy. This means simply that the complaints of one are found oftener with men, while those of the other are found oftener with women.

Now to call attention to another of Hering's characteristics, and I know of no one who has expressed them better, we have—*"Mild, gentle and yielding disposition; cries at everything; is sad and desponding; weeps about everything; can hardly give her symptoms on account of weeping."* And again: *"Sandy hair, blue eyes, pale face, inclined to silent grief with submissiveness."* (*Silicea* is its chronic.) Here we have a description of the *Pulsatilla* temperament as near as words can express it, and it is a fact that when you find it in a patient, no matter what the pathological condition, *Pulsatilla* will almost surely help. There are few exceptions. So we learn not to put too much stress on pathological states to the neglect of symptomological conditions.

Pulsatilla is a remedy of wide range of action. Farrington mentioned its use in seventy-three different affections, and has not by any means exhausted them all; and if you study *Pulsatilla* in Hughes' *Pharmacodynamics* you will notice that, although he recommends it in many diseases, he does not, and evidently is not able to, talk as much from a pathological standpoint especially from the provings of the drug as he does of many other remedies. It seems to me like folly to undertake to pose as either an exclusive pathologist or symptomatologist. Both pathology and symptomatology are valuable and inseparable; neither can be excluded. Pathology is what the *doctor* can tell (sometimes); symptomatology is what the *patient* can tell.

There is another condition of *Pulsatilla* which may be considered characteristic, and which Hering does not mention in his cards, viz., *changeableness of symptoms* (*Ignat., Nux mosch.*). All that Hering said was "*wandering pains shift rapidly from one part to another, also with swelling and redness of the joints.*" Now if this occurs in rheumatism *(Manganum acet., Lac caninum, Kali bichrom., Kalmia lat.)*, and especially if in the *Pulsatilla* temperament we may perform a miracle of curing with this remedy. But this shifting or changeableness is not confined to the pains, which may be either rheumatic or neuralgic, but is found in the disposition. The patient is now irritable, then tearful again, or mild and pleasant; but, even with the irritableness, is easily made to cry The hæmorrhages flow, and stop, and flow again; continually changing. The stools in diarrhœa constantly change in color; they are green, yellow, white, watery or slimy; as Guernsey expresses it—"no two stools alike." *(Sanicula.)* This is often found in the so-called cholera-infantum or entero-colitis of children in hot weather.

We sometimes have patients come into the office, and find, in trying to take their case, no "head or tail" to it. It is mixed. The suffering and pain is now here, now there. The symptoms are contradictory, as we term them. This condition should always call attention to

Pulsatilla and it will often clear up and cure the case. *Ignatia* also has these ever-changing, hysterical and contradictory symptoms, both pre-eminently woman remedies.

Pulsatilla like *Nux vomica* is a great remedy for disorders of digestion. Symptoms—"*Bad taste in the mouth, especially early in the morning, or nothing tastes good, or no taste at all.*" (*Bryonia,* bad taste with coated tongue and thirst; *Pulsat.,* no thirst.)

"*Great dryness of the mouth in the morning, without thirst. Stomach disordered from cakes, pastry, rich food; particularly fat pork.*" (I would say—fat meats generally.) These are reliable symptoms, as given in Hering's cards, and are not very much like the symptoms of *Nux vomica,* which is not disturbed by fats, but on the contrary likes them and they agree. With *Nux vomica* warm food agrees best; with *Pulsatilla,* cold things.

The bad taste in the mouth is persistent and the *loss* of taste is frequent, as is also the loss of smell. How peculiar that *Pulsatilla* should have dry mouth and no thirst, while *Mercurius* should have characteristically moist mouth with intense thirst. There is no accounting for taste, as the man said when he saw a fellow kiss his mother-in-law.

I do not know that I could give a satisfactory pathological reason for this. Is it not a good thing that we do not have to give the pathological explanation for such a symptom before we can use it to cure our patients? To be sure there is always a reason for these things, but we do not need to know what it is before we can utilize the symptom.

The merest tyro in prescribing could hardly mistake

the symptoms of *Pulsatilla* for those of *Nux vomica,* and yet I have found physicians prescribing these remedies in alternation, at intervals of two or three hours.

Having called attention to the action of *Pulsatilla* on the digestive organs, which are lined with mucous membranes, we now wish to notice that it has a peculiar action on mucous surfaces generally. This peculiarity consists in the character of the *discharges* from them. They are *thick, bland* and yellowish green. These are found in nasal catarrh; leucorrhœa; expectoration; gonorrhœa; in ulcers; from the ears and eyes; in short, from every mucous outlet of the body.

The expectoration of *Pulsatilla,* which is thick, green and bland, tastes bitter, while that of *Stannum* is sweet and that of *Kali hydroiodicum* and *Sepia* salty. One of Schuessler's tissue remedies *(Kali sulphuricum)* greatly resembles *Pulsatilla* in the character of its discharges, and not only that, but also in its wandering pains, evening aggravations and ameliorations in cool, open air. *Kali hydroiodicum* is also ameliorated in open air and worse in a warm room. Now that we are on the subject of greenish discharges, especially the expectoration, we will mention also *Carbo veg., Lycopodium, Paris, Phosphorus* and *Sulphur.* Of course, the other symptoms must decide the choice between several remedies having one symptom in common.

A certain physician in Albany, N. Y., was called in consultation on a so-called case of phthisis pulmonalis. The case was in allopathic hands. After carefully examining the case, he was asked: "What is your diagnosis, doctor?" *"Stannum,"* said the doctor. "What!" *"Stannum,"* replied the doctor. *Stannum* was the diagnosis of tne *remedy*, not the disease. It was given and *cured the patient.*

Now we come to the curative action of *Pulsatilla* in affections of the female genital organs. The fact that it has such a decided action upon these, added to the womanish disposition of this remedy, is additional reason why it is called the woman's remedy, as we said when writing upon the disposition and temperament. *"Catamenia too late and scanty, or suppressed, particularly by getting feet wet,"* and "Painful menstruation with great restlessness, tossing in every possible direction," and we have already mentioned the changeable characteristics in the flow of the menses, viz., they stop, and flow, stop and flow again, etc. So, also, the menorrhagia.

In these menstrual troubles of *Pulsatilla* the wetting or chilling of the feet is of prime importance and, acting upon it, you may save your patient from consumption as a result of such exposure and suppression. Now don't pour down mother tincture of *Pulsatilla* by the ten-drop doses, as is the manner of those who do not believe in potentized remedies. You may give *Pulsatilla* in the high, higher, and highest potencies, and confidently expect the best results. I have often seen the delayed menses of young girls of *Pulsatilla* temperament appear promptly and naturally under the M. M. of Swan and C. M. of Fincke (also with *Kali carbonicum, Tuberculinum,* and others). So also have I seen them restored after suppression, by the same. Now if you should try one of these very high potencies in a case of menstrual difficulty, and it should not succeed, don't jump to the conclusion that I have been mistaken, for *Pulsatilla* is not the only remedy for such cases. Homœopathy is too often blamed when the blame lies in the stupidity of the prescriber. *Magnesia phos.* will relieve more cases of painful menstruation than *Pulsatilla,* and that is not a cure-all, either. *Study up your case.*

But after all, the prime characteristic of this wonderful remedy lies in its modality. *"Better in cold air and from cold applications."* The patient is not only better generally in the open, cool air and worse in a warm, closed room, but local affections also, as, for instance, the vertigo; pain in head, eyes, ears; itching of eyelids; roaring; coryza; pain in face; toothache; colic; labor pains; sciatica; ulcers, are all better in open air. These affections that are > in cold air are also especially > while walking or moving slowly about *(Ferrum)* in open or cool air. Remember that *Pulsatilla* as well as *Rhus toxicodendron* is ameliorated by motion, but *Pulsatilla* in cold or cool open air, while *Rhus tox.* wants motion in warm dry air.

With *Pulsatilla* warm applications aggravate, warm room oppresses; heat of bed aggravates itching *(Mercurius)* and chilblains; cold drinks retained, warm vomited.

Other remedies have aggravations from heat; but *Pulsatilla* leads them all. The relief from cold and cool, open air is as positive as that of warmth or heat is for *Arsenicum.*

Now to close our remarks on *Pulsatilla* we will give a few choice symptoms without any particular comments upon them.

"Affections consequent on the abuse of *Iron.*" "Chronic affections following cases of badly managed measles." "Pressure, or tying up tightly, relieves the headaches." *(Argentum nit., Apis mellifica.)* "Increased inclination to micturate, < *when lying.*" "Metastasis of gonorrhœa to testicles." "Chilliness, with pains, yet wants cool room." "One-sided sweats." "Inflamed parts bluish." *(Lachesis, Tarantula Cub.)* "Pulsations through the whole body." "Metastasis of mumps to mammæ or testicles." In any of these local affections we should expect to find the mind and modality of this remedy present or not be very confident of a brilliant cure.

BRYONIA ALBA.

All complaints < *on motion.*

Dryness of *mucous membranes* generally (lips, mouth, stomach, wants drink in large quantities, at long intervals; intestines, dry hard stools as if burnt).

Effusions in *serous membranes* (meninges, pleura, peritoneum, etc.).

Constipation (no desire) or diarrhœa, < mornings on beginning to move.

Stitching pains, especially in serous membranes and joints.

Sitting up causes nausea and faintness.

Modalities: < from motions, warm weather after cold. > from quiet, lying on painful side.

Suitable to dry, spare, nervous, slender persons, of irritable disposition; rheumatic tendency. Complaints in hot weather, or exposure to dry, cold air, in wet weather *(Rhus tox.).*

Cough, dry, hard, racking, with scanty expectoration; with splitting headache; delirium, about the business of the day; (typhoid) headache; < stooping; ironing; hot weather; coughing; motion, vertigo; with nausea, and faintness; < from sitting up after lying down. Pres-

sure, as from a stone, at pit of stomach, relieved **by eructation.**

Vicarious menstruation; nose bleeds when menses should appear *(Phos.)*.

Mammæ heavy, of a stony hardness; pale, but hard; hot and painful.

Rheumatism of joints; with pale swelling, great pain, worse on touch or least motion.

* * * * *

As in *Pulsatilla*, so in *Bryonia*, the leading characteristic lies in its "modality." Three words express it—*aggravation from motion.*

What is aggravated on motion? Sufferings of almost any and every kind. We will not undertake to enumerate them. All that Hering says in his cards on that line is—"*Joints red, swelling, stiff, with stiching pain from slightest motion,*" and this so far as it goes is genuine, but it is only the beginning of all the ailments that are < on motion.

Look in "Guiding Symptoms," under "Motion," and see the long list of symptoms aggravated by motion, and even these do not cover all. Now we begin to realize the value of this modality.

It makes no difference what the name of the disease, if the patient feels greatly > by lying still and suffers greatly on the slightest motion, and the more and longer he moves the more he suffers, *Bryonia* is the first remedy to be thought of, and there must be very strong counter-indications along other lines that will rule it out.

Nor does it make much difference what organ or tissue is the seat of the disease, mucous, serous or muscular, the same rule applies.

Another very valuable modality of *Bryonia* is again expressed in three words—*amelioration from pressure.* This is the reason the patient, much to the astonishment of the nurse, wants to *lie on the painful side* or part. (Opposite *Belladonna, Kali carbonicum.)*

No one can realize the value of these two modalities until he has often met them at the sick bed and witnessed the prompt relief from the use of *Bryonia.*

When writing upon *Pulsatilla,* we noticed the characteristic action of that remedy upon the mucous surfaces. Here *Bryonia* acts just as characteristically, but it is so different. With *Bryonia* it is *excessive dryness* or lack of secretion in them. It begins in the lips, which are *parched, dry and cracked,* and only ends with the rectum and stools, which are *hard and dry as if burnt.* The same condition is undoubtedly present in the stomach, which is evidenced by the excessive thirst; which can only be satisfied by *large draughts of water;* a little does not satisfy.

The same condition obtains in the lungs and bronchia, which causes *hard, dry cough* with little or no expectoration, and with *soreness and pain in the chest* when the patient coughs. *(Natrum sulphuricum* has loose cough with *soreness.)* The urine is scanty and only exceptionally (or as I would express it reactionally) copious. We must remember that every remedy has a dual action. These two actions are termed primary and secondary. I think that the so-called secondary action is only the reaction of the organism against the first or primary (so-called) action of the drug. For instance—the real action of *Opium* is to produce sleep or stupor, the reaction is wakefulness; of *Podophyllum, Aloes,* etc., catharsis; the reaction constipation, and I think that the truly homœopathic curative must be in accord with the primary (so-called) effects of every drug in order to get the best and most radical cure, but if given for the secondary (so-called) symptoms, the primary ones having passed by, we should carefully inquire for all the symptoms which have preceded those which are present; and taking both past and present, let them all enter into the picture whose counterpart is to be found in the drug which is to cure. Any other method is only palliative and not curative.

Bryonia has also a very decided effect upon the *serous membranes.* It is very useful in the second stage of inflammation, after the stage of serous effusion has set in. In most of these cases the first stage has been attended by symptoms calling for the exhibition of such remedies as *Aconite, Belladonna, Ferrum phos.*, etc., but not always; and right here let me call attention to the most characteristic *pains* of this remedy. They are *stitching pains.* Now observe, the characteristic pains of inflammatory affections of the serous membranes *are stitching pains;* this is the reason why *Bryonia* comes to be such a regal remedy in pleuritis, meningitis, peritonitis, pericarditis, etc. The subjective symptoms corresponding to the remedy must go down before it, and the objectives must as surely follow. Only one remedy can equal *Bryonia* for stitching pains, viz., *Kali carbonicum.* (Stitching pains in chest are particularly found under *Bryonia, Kali carb., Natrum mur., Squilla* and *Mercur. viv.)* And there is this difference between them: The *Bryonia* stitches come on or are aggravated by the least motion, while those of *Kali carbonicum* will occur whether the patient moves or not. *(Bryonia* > by pressure, *Kali carb.*, not.) But in both remedies they cry out sharply with the pains. *Apis* has pains which cause the patient to cry out sharply, but they are stinging pains—*like a bee sting.* All these three are great remedies for effusions into serous cavities, and *Sulphur* precedes and follows equally well anyone of them.

A word right here in regard to interpolating *Sulphur,* when, as we express it, "the seemingly indicated remedy does not act." Some would stumble over that, and ask —as they would have a right to do—how about your similia, etc., in such a use of *Sulphur?* I answer—*Sulphur* is a remedy of wide range of action, and covers more perfectly those conditions and symptoms which are the outgrowth of psora than any other remedy; so it does meet the case complicated by psora very often, and either cures it or removes the complication so that the other remedies may act. But remember it will not always do it, and other antipsoric remedies must be chosen. It must be the simillimum for the psoric condition.

Bryonia stands alongside of *Nux vomica* and *Pulsatilla* for disorders of alimentation. All three remedies have a sensation as of a stone in the stomach, *Bryonia* and *Nux vomica* more so than *Pulsatilla. Bryonia* leads in thirst, *Nux vomica* less, and *Pulsatilla* little or none. All have bad taste in the mouth; *Bryonia* and *Pulsatilla* bitter and *Nux vomica* sour. All have nausea and vomiting; *Bryonia* worse on motion, as rising up, *Nux vomica* in the A. M. and after eating, *Pulsatilla* in the evening and also after eating.

The gastric derangements of *Bryonia* often occur as a result of dietetic errors, especially when warm weather sets in after cold. Those of *Nux vomica* more from continued over-eating and inactivity, the abuse of drugs, coffee, tobacco or alcoholics; *Pulsatilla* from too rich foods, pastries, fat foods and ice cream (in excess); a little ice cream feels good in the *Pulsatilla* stomach, but much overdoes the matter, because it is *too rich.*

All three remedies have attacks of diarrhœa, although constipation is most characteristic of *Bryonia* and *Nux vomica,* and is only exceptionally found under *Pulsatilla.*

Bryonia diarrhœa is worse in the morning, on movement, and often occurs as an effect of over-eating in the heat of summer. *Nux vomica* diarrhœa is also apt to be worse in the morning, is mostly caused by over-eating and is apt to put on the dysenteric type. The *Pulsatilla* diarrhœa is more apt to occur in the night, from causes above mentioned, and is attended with great rumbling of the bowels.

All have white, sometimes very thickly-coated tongue, but taking into account the *causes* of these gastric and bowel troubles, temperament and modalities there should not be much difficulty in choosing the right remedy for any case.

So far as temperament is concerned, *Bryonia* is like *Nux vomica,* but *Bryonia* has much more of the "rheumatic diathesis." Both are easily irritated or angered, and are oftenest found indicated in spare, dark-complexioned subjects. Both are aggravated generally on motion, but *Bryonia* very much the more so, while *Pulsatilla* is sometimes like *Rhus toxicodendron* relieved by motion.

Now a few special indications for *Bryonia* and we will leave it:

"Bursting headache, as if it would split the head open, aggravated by stooping; coughing; ironing; opening or moving the eyes; moving any way; in hot weather. Nausea and faintness when rising up, relieved when lying still.

"Epistaxis instead of menses (vicarious menstruation), also blood spitting.

"Mastitis; breasts pale, hot, hard, heavy and painful.

"Suppression of lochia with bursting headache.

"Suppression of milk, menses, measles or rash of scarlatina, or where all these are slow in appearing; of course the other *Bryonia* symptoms must be present.

"Frequent desire to take long breath; *must* expand the lungs. *(Cactus, Ignatia, Nat. sulph.)*

"Cough dry, < *after eating, sometimes with vomiting;* < moving; < *coming from open air into warm room. (Nat. carb.)*

"Cough hurts head and chest, holds them with hands." *(Eupatorium perf., Natrum sulph.)*

These are some of the peculiar symptoms which cannot be ranged under any general head, and are excellent leaders to the consideration of *Bryonia,* all and each of which will be found associated with the more general characteristics already noticed.

The dominant school do not know what they have lost in not being acquainted with the virtues of this remedy, as developed in our provings and clinical use, but we know what we have gained.

ANTIMONIUM CRUDUM.

Thick, milky white coating on tongue (in many complaints).

Derangements from overloading the stomach, especially fat food; nausea.

Crushed finger-nails: grow in splits like warts and with horny spots.

Corns and callosities on soles, with excessive tenderness; can only walk with pain and suffering.

Alternate constipation and diarrhœa in old people, especially with the characteristic tongue.

Child cannot bear to be touched or looked at, fretful, cross.

Feverish conditions at night.

Headache; after river bathing; from taking cold; alcoholic drinks; deranged digestion; acids, fat, fruit; suppressed eruptions. Mucus; from anus, ichorous, oozing, staining yellow; mucous piles. Cannot bear heat of sun; < from exertion in sun; exhausted in warm weather.

* * * * *

This remedy, like the three of which we have been writing, has a strong affinity for the alimentary canal. Its leading characteristic is in its *thickly-coated, white, very white, white as milk, tongue.*

Many remedies have white tongue, but this one leads them all. It is also a great stomach remedy, and in disorders of this organ arising from over-eating, where there is much nausea, distress, and especially the characteristic tongue, it is to be thought of before any of the three of which we have written. It is especially to be considered if the gastric derangement is of recent date. The process of digestion is hardly under way; the eructations taste of the food as he ate it, and the sufferer feels as if he must "throw up" before there will be any relief. In such a case a few pellets of *Antimonium crudum* on the tongue will often settle the business, save the loss of a meal, and all further suffering.

Diarrhœa may often follow these dietetic errors, especially during the heat of the summer season, and then the stools are peculiar in that they are partly solid and partly fluid, showing that digestion has been only partially performed in the whole length of the canal. *Antimonium crudum* and *Bryonia* sometimes present about equal claims in a case of summer complaint; but the case in its entirety must decide the choice between them.

There is a form of diarrhœa which alternates with constipation, oftenest found with old people, where *Antimonium crudum* is the only remedy. Then it is also one of the best remedies for mucous piles; there is a *continuous oozing* of mucus staining the linen. very disagreeable to the patient.

There are some mind symptoms that are very peculiar, "the greatest sadness and woeful mood with intermittent fever;" again, "sentimental mood in moonlight, ecstatic love," and again, *"child cannot bear to be touched or looked at."*

Of the first two symptoms I can say nothing from experience or observation, but of the last, that it is a gem. Many times in cases of gastric or remittent fever, for which *Antimonium crudum* is a very excellent remedy, I have been led to its use by this very condition of the mind: the child is cross, but not like *Chamomilla* wants to be carried and soothed, but will scream and cry, and show temper at every little attention. Another thing that I have noticed in many of these cases is, that the fever runs higher at night and is accompanied with great thirst; the white tongue is almost always present. Such children are quite apt, even when around the house, to have *"sore, cracked and crusty nostrils, and corners of the mouth,"* and so this may appear when sick.

There is a peculiar constitutional condition found in some people which calls for this remedy. It is found in the extremities; *finger-nails grow in splits,* like warts, with horny spots (*Silicea* nails crippled, on fingers and toes; *Graphites* nails become *thick,* crippled; *Thuja* nails brittle, crumbling, distorted), and if by accident one becomes injured or split, it does not repair as it should, but grows out of shape. Then the toe-nails are brittle and grow out of shape also, or shrivel up and do not grow at all. The feet are covered on the soles with *corns and callosities which are* VERY TENDER, can hardly walk on them on account of this tenderness. Some of the worst cases of chronic rheumatism have been cured by this remedy, guided by the excessive tenderness of the soles of the feet. (*Baryta* soles get sore from foot sweat; *Pulsatilla* soles pain and are tender; *Ledum* heels and soles tender when walking; *Medorrhinum* couldn't walk except on knees; *Lycopod.* soles swollen and painful.) Horny excrescences anywhere on the skin make one think of *Antimonium crudum.* The remedy is oftenest found indicated in the extremes of life, in children and old people.

Now the peculiar modalities which deserve particular mention are: First, the troubles are often caused or aggravated by heat, and especially by the *heat of the sun.* (*Bryonia, Glonoine, Gelsem., Nat. carb.*) The patient feels exhausted during warm weather; the gastric troubles come on, or are worse, such as nausea, vomiting and diarrhœa. The cough is worse, and, like *Bryonia,* is worse on coming into a warm room from cold air. These affections are particularly worse in sunshine, but also from radiate heat of the fire, so that *Antimonium crudum* takes a high rank as a hot weather remedy. Second, *cold bathing aggravates or causes trouble. (Rhus tox., Sulphur.)* "Child cries when washed or bathed in cold water." Cold bathing causes headache, cold in the head, gastric catarrh, diarrhœa, suppressed menses, toothache, etc. When any case of long standing comes to us, and the patient dates the beginning of the trouble to going in swimming or falling into the water, we think of *Antimonium crudum* and examine for further indications for the drug.

Now a few scattering symptoms that have found their remedy in *Antimonium crudum:* "Copious hæmorrhage from the bowels, mixed with solid fæces; chronic redness of the eyelids; toothache in *decayed teeth,* worse at night; gastric trouble after acids, sour wine, vinegar," etc.

MERCURIUS.

Swollen, flabby tongue, taking imprint of the teeth; gums also swollen, spongy or bleeding; breath very offensive.

Sweats day and night without relief in many complaints.

Creeping chilliness in the beginning of a cold, or threatened suppuration.

Sliminess of mucous membranes.

Moist tongue, with intense thirst.

Glandular swellings, cold, inclined to suppurate; ulcers with lardaceous base.

Modalities: < at night in warmth of bed, while sweating, lying on right side.

Bone diseases; pains worse at night.

Dysentery: stools slimy, bloody, colic, fainting; great

tenesmus during and after, followed by chilliness, and a "cannot finish sensation."

The more blood and pain the better indicated.

Affects lower lobe of right lung; stitches through to back *(Chel., Kali c.)*.

Intense thirst, although the tongue looks moist and the saliva is profuse.

In low potencies, hastens suppuration; in high, aborts suppuration, as in quinsy.

* * * * *

As in *Antimonium crudum,* so in *Mercurius,* the leading characteristic is found in the mouth, or, I might rather say, characteristics, for the *gums are swollen, spongy, sometimes bleeding;* the tongue is also *swollen, flabby, taking the imprint of the teeth (Arsenicum, Chelidonium, Podophyllum, Rhus tox.* and *Stramonium),* generally moist, yet with intense thirst; the whole mouth is moist with salivation which is soapy or stringy, and the odor from the mouth is *very offensive;* you can smell it all over the room. No remedy has this condition of mouth in any degree equal to *Mercury.* It is found in very many complaints, and if anything corroborative of the truth of "similia," etc., were desired the curative power of *Mercury,* when indicated by these symptoms, ought to be satisfactory. Many a time have I given great relief to my patient, and great credit to Homœopathy, by brilliant cures of that painful affection, quinsy, guided by these symptoms. Of course, in addition to the above symptoms the tonsils were greatly swollen and often apparently on the verge of suppuration. Right here let me warn against giving *Mercurius too low,* for if you do, it will hasten suppuration instead of aborting it. If anyone is skeptical as to the efficiency of the very high potencies, I invite him to a test in just such a case. Give a single dose, dry upon the tongue, or if you must seem to do more, dissolve a powder in four tablespoonfuls of water and give in half-hourly doses. Then *wait*. I have done it many times and am convinced. If the patient has that other strong characteristic of *Mercurius,* viz., *profuse perspiration, without relief* of the suffering, success is doubly sure. (Sweat relieves, *Arsenicum, Natrum mur., Psorinum.)*

I wish right here, as perhaps the most appropriate place, to disclaim being an exclusive high-potentist. The question of dose is, and I believe must remain, an open one as long as different degrees of susceptibility are found in different diseases and persons. I have experimented along the whole line and know that both the high and the low are efficacious in certain cases. The preponderance of evidence, however, is greatly in favor of the high and the highest. This is my opinion. You may differ, and are welcome to do so.

The fever symptoms of *Mercurius* are notable, especially in the sweats. The chill also is peculiar as I have observed it. It is not a shaking chill, but is simply *creeping chilliness.* Often when this creeping chilliness is felt it is the first symptom of a cold that has been taken, and, if left alone, the coryza, sore throat, bronchitis or even pneumonia may follow; but, if taken early, a dose of *Mercurius* may prevent all such troubles. The chilliness is felt most generally in the evening and increases into the night if not removed by *Mercury*. It also alternates with flashes of heat; first chilly, then hot, then chilly, etc., like *Arsenicum.* It is often felt in single parts.

Then again it is felt in abscesses and is the harbinger of pus formation. If pus has already formed, especially much of it, the only thing *Mercury* can do is to hasten its discharge; but if little or none is actually formed a dose of *Mercury* high will often check the formation and a profuse sweat often follows with a subsidence of the swelling and a rapid cure of the disease.

Now the sweats. They are very profuse and do not relieve like the sweats of inflammatory diseases generally do, but on the contrary the complaints *increase with the sweat.* (*Tilia.*) In what diseases is this condition found? It may be found in almost every disease: In sore throat, bronchitis, pneumonia, pleuritis, peritonitis, abscesses, rheumatism, etc., to the end of a long list. In short in any disease in which this profuse and persistent sweating without relief is present *Mercurius* is the first remedy to be thought of.

Worse at night, and especially in the *warmth of* the bed, is another strong characteristic of *Mercurius.* *(Ledum pal.)* There is a long list of remedies that have aggravations at night, but not so many from warmth of the bed. I have cured many skin diseases of various names guided by this modality. The glands and bones also come strongly under the influence of this remedy. The glandular swellings are cold, inclined to suppurate, having these chilly creepings aforementioned. These with the bone-pains in the exostoses and caries are all *aggravated* at night in the warmth of the bed.

The mucous membranes are everywhere affected; the discharges from them are at first thin and excoriating, even from the catarrh of the nose to the diarrhœic, or dysenteric, discharges. Afterwards they become thicker, or more bland, like the *Pulsatilla* discharges. These are worse at night also, even the leucorrhœa.

Hahnemann ranked *Mercury* (first) for syphilis, as he did *Sulphur* for psora and *Thuja* for sycosis, and no doubt justly so, for *Mercury* in its various forms symptomologically covers more cases of that disease than any other remedy. But it must be remembered that *Mercury* is no more a panacea for syphilis than is *Sulphur* for psora or *Thuja* for sycosis, else there would be no truth in similia similibus. The case in hand must simulate *Mercury,* or that remedy is not "in it," but some other remedy is. Experience abundantly corroborates this and proves the truth of the law, *Similia Similibus Curantur.*

MERCURIUS CORROSIVUS.

Most persistent and terrible tenesmus before, during and after stool; stool scanty, mucus tinged with blood.

Tenesmus of the bladder and rectum at the same time; urine passed in drops with much pain.

Throat intensely inflamed, swollen, burning, with swollen gums, which bleed easily.

* * * * *

While we are on the subject of mercury we may as well notice the various combinations of the drug. *Mercurius solubilis* and *vivus* are so nearly alike that with the same indications some use one and some the other preparation. It is claimed by some that the *vivus* is better adapted to men and *solubilis* to women. I have not observed it, but do think that the *solubilis* works better in skin troubles. Of *Mercurius corrosivus* we have to say that it leads all other remedies for *tenesmus of the rectum.* This tenesmus is incessant. Stool does not relieve it, and this is what decides between it and *Nux vomica* in dysentery. It has also severe tenesmus of the bladder, and may here vie with *Cantharis, Capsicum* and *Nux vomica,* especially in dysentery.

Other symptoms must decide the choice.

This severe tenesmus may begin in the rectum and extend to the bladder or vice versa.

It is a very efficient remedy in gonorrhœa, in the second stage, when the greenish discharge has set in and the burning and tenesmus *continues.* It seems to have gained some reputation in Bright's disease. I have no experience with it here, but would expect it to do good *if it were indicated.*

It seems, according to the testimony of others, to be a useful remedy for catarrhal affections of the eyes and nose. Here also I have no testimony to offer, but would not cast doubt upon it for that reason. I do not desire to place my own experience ahead of that of others. We are co-laborers. Let each add to the general store of medical knowledge, that all may draw freely from it as occasion demands.

MERCURIUS CYANATUS.

Dr. Beck, of Monthey, in Switzerland (I think it was), first brought this remedy to notice as of great value in that much-dreaded disease, diphtheria. Von Villiers claimed to have had astonishing success with it in Germany, losing only two per cent. (if I remember correctly) of the cases treated with it. He recommended the 30th potency, but others have used the 6th and claim equally good results. There are, so far as I can find, no very marked characteristic symptoms by which to choose it.

It seems to spread its action all over the buccal cavity. Dr. T. F. Allen published a good cure with it, and then claimed that he chose this preparation of *Mercury* on account *of the remarkable prostration,* which he attributed to the cyanogen element in it. This looks reasonable. But I think we must investigate further to bring out its true characteristics. There is a chronic condition of the throat in which I have found it very efficacious. It is in cases of public speakers. The throat feels raw and sore, and examination reveals a broken down appearance of the mucous membrane bordering on ulceration. It is not granulated, but looks raw in spots, as if denuded of membrane. I have helped this kind of throat, so that the patient wanted me to remember what it was I gave him so that I could repeat the prescription if the trouble returned. I forgot to state that it hurt the patient to speak, and there was also hoarseness. This is all I know of this remedy, but I believe it well worth proving and study.

MERCURIUS PROTOIODIDE.

Tongue coated thickly yellow at the base; tip and edges red or pale; takes the imprint of the teeth.

Swelling of the throat; begins on the right side (diphtheria) (left, *Lachesis*).

Genuine Hunterian chancre (1,000th clinical).

* * * * *

It is a preparation that has a *very* reliable and prominent characteristic. It is: *"Tongue coated thickly, yellow at the base."* The tip and edges may be red or pale and take the imprint of the teeth, like the other *Mercuries.* Of course, other remedies have a yellow-coated base of the tongue like *Kali bichromicum, Natrum phos.* and *Chelidonium,* so that this symptom would not indicate *Mercurius protoiodide* to the exclusion of all others, but I think I am safe in saying that this remedy has it in the greatest degree.

In diphtheria the swelling of the throat and the formation of membrane begins on the right side, like *Lycopodium,* and the fœtid breath and flabby tongue, showing imprint of teeth, are generally present. Now if you have the thick yellow coating at the base of the tongue you need not hesitate to give this remedy. In regard to dose, I have seen good results from the 3d trituration to the C. M. potency. For myself I prefer the high, and have had abundant opportunity to test all the different potencies. If you are so prejudiced that you cannot give anything above the 12th because you cannot discover the drug with the microscope, don't give it too long; withdraw it after a few doses and give the powers of reaction a chance.

But diphtheria is not the only disease in which the yellow base of the tongue is an indication for the use of this remedy. Stomach and liver troubles often produce this appearance of the tongue. It is also a good remedy for Hunterian chancre, and no secondary symptoms follow its proper use. Here it must be given high.

CINCHONA OFFICINALIS.

Debility and other complaints after excessive loss of fluids, blood-letting, etc.

Hæmorrhages profuse, with faintness, loss of sight and ringing in the ears.

Great flatulence, with sensation as if the abdomen were packed full; not > by eructation or passing flatus.

Painless diarrhœa (yellow, watery, brownish, undigested).

Periodical affections, especially every other day.

Excessive sensitiveness, especially to light touch, draft of air; hard pressure relieves.

Modalities: < from slight touch, least draft of air, every other day. > by hard pressure on painful part.

Dropsy following excessive loss of fluids; great debility, trembling, aversion to exercise; nervous; sensitive to touch, to pain, to drafts of air; unrefreshing sleep after 3 A. M.

Face pale, hippocratic; eyes sunken and surrounded by blue margins; pale, sickly expression, as after excesses.

Hæmorrhages; from all outlets *(Crotalus, Sulphuric acid, Ferrum)*. Blood dark, or dark and clotted, with ringing in the ears, loss of sight, general coldness and sometimes convulsions *(Fer. phos.)*.

General shaking chill over whole body.

Sweat, with great thirst; sweating during sleep, on being covered.

* * * * *

This remedy is used by both schools of medicine for conditions of great weakness and debility. The old school, as they always do, prescribe it for all cases of debility, on general principles, under the name of tonic. It remained for Homœopathy to indicate its exact place here. Hahnemann expresses it: *"Debility and other complaints after loss of blood or other fluids, particularly by nursing or salivation, bleeding, cupping, etc., or whites, seminal emissions, etc."* I would add profuse suppuration and long continued diarrhœa. If the depletion has been sudden, as from a hæmorrhage from the womb, lungs, bowels or nose, there will be *faintness, loss of sight, ringing in the ears,* etc. For this state of things we have a "friend indeed" in *China,* and it should be given in frequently repeated doses, not too low, until reaction is established; then at longer intervals, as occasion demands. If the debility is the effect of a slow and long-continued drain the symptoms that might indicate it must be sought in the Materia Medica; our space forbids trying to note them here, but prominent among them are *pale, sallow face, sunken eyes with dark rings around, throbbing headaches, night sweats, and sweats easily on least motion or labor.* It is always well when a patient comes to us in a very debilitated condition to think of *China,* and to make careful inquiry for some debilitating waste that would account for it; for if it is a woman she may be suffering from a very profuse leucorrhœa, which from delicacy she will not mention, or if a young or even married man, he may be suffering from seminal losses, of which he would not speak if not encouraged to do so.

Again this remedy has its sphere of usefulness in disorders of the alimentary canal. It has loss of appetite, but *canine hunger* is more characteristic. It is a great flatulent remedy, the choice often remaining between it, *Carbo veg.* and *Lycopodium.* H. N. Guernsey expresses it about right in these words—*"Uncomfortable distention of the abdomen, with a wish to belch up, or a sensation as if the abdomen were packed full, not in the least relieved by eructation."* Such patients are troubled with slow digestion, and as they express it: sometimes it seems as if the food all turned to gas. They feel so full and oppressed they can hardly breathe and still will feel hungry at meal-time.

That the process of digestion is seriously impaired is

shown by a tendency to diarrhœa, especially from eating fruit. The stools are watery, yellow, brownish, or light colored and *undigested,* and what is not generally found under other remedies they are *painless.* The stools are also accompanied with large discharge of *flatulence.* *(Calcarea phos.)* This is in accord with the windy condition of the bowels generally. This condition of abdomen with attending diarrhœa is often found in children, and the child is weak, pale, with dark rings around the eyes. Here *China* is the remedy, not *Cina* on the theory of "worrums," and it is astonishing what improvement follows in a short time.

Now as to this remedy as an anti-periodic. The popular use of it by the old school, and the laity under their instruction in this sense, or as a panacea for all so-called malarious diseases, is a curse to the race. That it is a great remedy, when indicated by the symptoms, for periodical affections, whether of malarial origin or not, is true, and so it is true of *Eupatorium perfoliatum, Ipecacuanha, Natrum muriaticum, Arsenicum album,* and a host of other remedies. Affections that do not come strictly under the head of malarial, if they are *worse every other day,* should call attention to *Cinchona.*

I remember a bad case of inflammatory rheumatism, which had been treated by an eclectic physician with local applications until the disease had been driven to the heart, which I quickly relieved by *China,* being led to its choice by this every-other-day aggravation of the symptoms. Of course, there were other indications for the remedy, but this was the key that helped to unlock the case.

Those who depend on *China* or its alkaloid as a general

cure-all for intermittents will meet with disappointments all along the way, for while it may have the power to suppress the paroxysms in many cases it has the power to *cure* in comparatively few. I have seen a case suppressed time and again with it, return as often, for over a year and a half that I cured with a single prescription of *Eupatorium perfoliatum.* And so with *Natrum muriaticum* and *Arsenicum album.* With all its vaunted power over malarial affections, especially intermittent fever, the indications for its use are not so clear cut as for many other remedies.

I once had three cases of intermittent fever in one family, living in the same house and exposed to the same influences. Quinine failed to cure any one of them, and a different remedy, as indicated by the symptoms according to the homœopathic law of cure, was required for each case and promptly cured it. The respective remedies were *Eupatorium perfoliatum, Ignatia* and *Capsicum.* Now any good homœopath can tell you the leading symptoms for all three remedies.

That is science.

I once knew a druggist who told me that he had at last discovered one thing that mothers-in-law were good for. Of course I asked him what it was. I wanted to *know.* He answered, to try patent medicines on. She died (the mother-in-law) shortly after. Well, there is one thing that quinine in the hands of the average old school physician is good for, and that is to make patients for homœopaths, for we find more patients to treat coming from its abuse than we find calling for its use as a curative, and from a purely business standpoint we are greatly indebted to them (the allopaths) for a good bit of practice.

But how in the name of gratitude we can ever pay them out of the poisonous results of our little pill practice I don't know.

Now what are the best remedies for what is called the *Quinine* cachexia? Here, as ever, we must answer, the *indicated* one. *Ipecac.*, *Arsenicum*, *Natrum mur.*, *Pulsatilla* and *Ferrum* are often indicated, but they do not cover all cases any more than do *Hepar sulph.*, *Nitric acid* or *Kali hydroiodicum,* all cases of chronic mercurial poisoning. It is nonsense—worse than nonsense—it is old-schoolism to say I gave *Nux vomica* because the patient had taken pepper tea, or *Pulsatilla* for *Quinine,* or *Kali hydroiod.* for *Mercury.* We do not prescribe *Aconite* because the patient has fever (the old school does), but because the patient has with the fever other symptoms which enable us to choose between *Aconite* and many other remedies that have fever also, and this to the exclusion of all the rest. *This is science again.*

China is one of the best remedies in chronic liver troubles. There is pain in the right hypochondria, and often the liver may be felt below the ribs, enlarged, hard and sensitive to touch. The skin and sclerotica are yellow, the urine dark colored and stools light, lacking the color due to a proper secretion of bile. Now if in addition to all this we have in part or whole the abdominal symptoms so characteristic of this remedy *China* will do excellent service. It is equally good in splenic diseases which closely resemble the splenic troubles resulting from the abuse of *Quinine.* I have found the 200th do better than lower potencies in these troubles.

I wish to say in addition to what has already been said of *China* for hæmorrhages, that the bleeding may come from any or every outlet or orifice of the body. *Carbo veg.*, *Ferrum*, *Crotalus horridus*, *Phosphorus* and *Sulphuric acid* also claim attention here.

China has excessive sensitiveness of the nervous system. The special senses seem too acute; the mind is unpleasantly affected, and nothing is more characteristic of this remedy than its extreme *sensitiveness to touch.* (*Asafœtida*, *Hepar* and *Lachesis.*) It affects the skin all over the body, even the hair feels sore (so says the patient), because moving the hair hurts the sensitive scalp, and in addition to this, one peculiar thing is that while the *lightest touch will increase to an extreme degree the pains of the diseased part, hard pressure relieves.* That seems impossible, but is true nevertheless. The sensitiveness is so extreme that a current of air blowing on the part will cause great pain and suffering.

Plumbum also has this excessive hyperæsthesia, and I once cured a very obstinate case of post-diphtheritic paralysis, being led to its administration by this symptom. *Capsicum* also has it. The patient can hardly bear to be shaved on account of it.

CARBO VEGETABILIS.

Vital force nearly exhausted; complete collapse.

Blood stagnates in the capillaries; venous turgescence; surface cold and blue.

Hæmorrhages (nose, stomach, gums, bowels, bladder or any mucous surface), with indescribable *paleness* of the surface of the body.

Mucous membranes break down, become spongy, bleed, ulcerate and become putrid.

Excessive flatulence, pressing upward, stomach and abdomen.

Hunger for oxygen, decarbonized blood; cries, "fan me, fan me hard!"

Anæmic, especially after acute diseases, which have greatly depleted the patients; chronic effects.

Persons who have never fully recovered from the exhausting effects of some previous illness; has never recovered from effects of typhoid, weak digestion; the simplest food disagrees; eructations give temporary relief.

Bad effects from loss of vital fluids *(Caust.)*; hæmorrhage from any broken-down condition of mucous membrane.

Looseness of teeth, easily bleeding gums.

In the last stages of disease, with copious cold sweat, cold breath, cold tongue, voice lost, this remedy may save a life.

Coldness of the knees, even in bed *(Apis)*; of left arm and left leg; very cold hands and feet; finger-nails blue.

Persons who have never recovered from effects of some previous illness or injury; suppression by *Quinine* or drugging; typhoid or yellow fever.

China is its great complementary.

* * * * *

In our remarks upon *China* we said that for flatulent conditions the choice lay often between it, *Carbo veg.* and *Lycopodium. Carbo vegetabilis* also ranges alongside *China* for debilitated states. The weakness of *Carbo vegetabilis* is not surpassed by any other remedy. This, with *Arsenicum* and *Muriatic acid* form a trio of remedies which according to well-known indications has snatched many a patient from the very jaws of death. Picture of *Carbo veg.*: *Vital forces nearly exhausted, cold surface, especially from knees down to feet; lies motionless, as if dead; breath cold; pulse intermittent, thready; cold sweat on limbs.* This is truly a desperate condition. Then add to these symptoms, *blood stagnates in the capillaries, causing blueness, coldness and ecchymoses;* the patient so weak he cannot breathe without being constantly fanned. Gasps: "Fan me! Fan me!" *Carbo veg.* has saved such cases. This is a picture of a case of typhoid fever, and in one case we saw added still to this, hæmorrhage of dark, decomposed, unclotted blood; could not clot on account of its broken down condition; blood oozing from gums and nostrils, and an indescribable *paleness,* not only of the hippocratic face, but also of the skin of the whole body, yet *Carbo veg.* restored to health, and in an aged woman at that. I have here, as faithfully as I can, portrayed the wonderful power of this remedy in such a desperate case. Of course no remedy can raise the dead, no matter how strong the indications before death; but no remedy can come nearer than this and the dominant school know little or nothing about it, and never can until they will consent to use it in the homœopathic form and according to homœopathic indications.

The sphere of this remedy is not by any means limited to low or weakening states in connection with acute diseases. To give an idea of its use when indicated by the symptoms in chronic ailments, I can do no better than quote from Henry N. Guernsey: "No truer remark was ever written than that *Carbo vegetabilis* is especially adapted to cachectic individuals whose vital powers have become weakened. This remark is made particularly clear when considered in the light of those cases in which disease seems to be engrafted upon the system by reason of the depressing influence of some prior derangement. *(Psorinum.)* Thus, for instance, the patient tells us that asthma has troubled him ever since he had the whooping cough in childhood; he has dyspepsia ever since a drunken debauch which occurred some years ago; he has never been well since the time he strained himself so badly (*Rhus tox., Calcarea ost.*); the strain itself does not now seem to be the matter, but his present ailments have all appeared since it happened; he sustained an injury some years ago, no traces of which are now apparent, and yet he dates his present complaints from the time of the occurrence of that accident; or again, he was injured by exposure to damp, hot air and his present ailments result from it. It will be well for the physician to think of *Carbo vegetabilis* in similar cases which are numerous and may present very dissimilar phenomena, as these circumstances being suggestive of *Carbo veg.* it in all probability will be found to be the appropriate remedy, which the agreement of the other symptoms of the case with those of the drug will serve to corroborate." This is from the pen of one of the best prescribers that ever lived, and I feel justified in quoting it entire.

This remedy seems to affect deeply the whole alimentary tract, and the same broken down, weakened condition appears. The *gums break down, become spongy, bleed on touching or sucking them, or become retracted from the teeth, lower incisors,* and are painfully sensitive or sore on chewing or even pressing the teeth hard together. The stomach also becomes weak. Acidity and pyrosis is frequent; the plainest food disagrees, fat foods especially. Here *Carbo vegetabilis* succeeds when *Pulsatilla* fails.

The most marked and valuable place for this remedy is in its power to relieve complaints from *excessive flatulence in the stomach.* "Great accumulations of flatulence in the stomach." "Stomach feels full and tense from flatulence." Great pain in stomach on account of flatulence, worse especially on *lying down,* should always call attention to this remedy. All this may occur in different affections ranging from a simple dyspepsia to incurable cancer of the stomach. In the latter case, and even in cases not so serious, we may have added *burning in stomach.* This flatulence is also generated in the abdomen, but, in the *Carbo vegetabilis* cases, is most troublesome in upper part; yet may extend so far as to cause great meteoristic distention, especially in typhoid fevers, dysenteries, etc. It is a remedy of inestimable value in hæmorrhage from any broken down condition of mucous membranes. This action upon the mucous membranes does not stop with the alimentary tract, but attacks those of the respiratory tract also. Beginning with the larynx, it causes and cures great hoarseness, which is characteristically *worse in the damp air, especially of evening.* It may be very bad even (if the air is damp) in the morning; but morning hoarseness is oftener reached by *Causticum.* This condition may go on extending and increasing until it reaches the bronchia. This is particularly true in case of elderly people of broken down constitutions, venous system predominating. It is a great remedy for the bronchitis of old people; also for asthma of the same, in very desperate cases where the patient appears as if dying. Here the choice must be sometimes made between this remedy and *China.*

In the chest there is sometimes *"burning as from glow-*

ing coal," and again, "weak, fatigued feeling in chest," where the choice may fall between it and *Phosphoric acid, Stannum* and *Sulphur.* It has been found very efficacious in desperate cases of pneumonia, and comes in quite naturally after *Tartar emetic* has failed to assist the patient to clear his lungs of the great quantities of loosened mucus, when cyanosis and paralysis threaten from weakness. Its sputa then is apt to be fœtid with cold sweat and breath and the characteristic *wanted-to-be-fanned condition.*

Before we leave this remedy I want to emphasize its power over hæmorrhages, which may occur from lungs, nose, stomach, bowels, bladder or any mucous surface. No remedy can take its place in broken down, greatly debilitated constitutions where the surfaces from which the blood oozes seem too weak and spongy to hold the blood in them. Their vitality is gone with the patient's nervous vitality. The patient's face and skin is *very pale,* even before the hæmorrhage has occurred. *China* and *Carbo vegetabilis* are decidedly complementary.

LYCOPODIUM.

Depression of mind and sensorium, stupid; lower jaw drops; chronic conditions, memory fails; uses wrong words to express himself; mixes up things; failing brain power.

Right-sided complaints, or begins on right and travels leftward; throat, ovaries, uterine region, kidney and skin troubles; hernia.

Sense of satiety, or hunger, but soon fills up.

Great flatulence with rumbling, mostly intestinal and pressing downward.

Lithic acid diathesis; red sand in clear urine; > pains in back or kidneys after passing.

Dark-complexioned people; emaciated in face and upper parts, bloated or swollen in lower; keen intellectual, but feeble muscular development.

Modalities: < 4 to 8 P. M., after eating, in warm room; > in cool open air, on motion.

Irritable; peevish and cross on waking; ugly, kick and scream; easily angered; cannot endure opposition or contradiction; seeks disputes; is beside himself.

Complexion: pale, dirty, unhealthy; sallow; looks older than he is.

One foot hot and the other cold.

Great thirst after the sweat.

Chill on left side of the body *(Caust., Carbo v.)*.

Sour vomiting between chill and heat; must uncover *(Lach.)*.

Perspiration immediately after the chill. Thirst after sweating stage.

In intermittents, the flatulence, sour eructations, sour taste, sour sweat, sour vomiting.

* * * * *

This remedy with *Sulphur* and *Calcarea* forms the leading trio of Hahnemann's anti-psoric remedies. This makes a good starting point, as the boy said when he set a pin in a vacant chair. They all act very deeply. Each finds its affinity in a certain class of people or temperament. *Lycopodium* acts favorably in all ages, but particularly upon old people and children. It acts upon persons of keen intellect, but feeble muscular development; lean people, leaning towards lung and liver troubles. Such people are apt to suffer from lithic acid diathesis, for which this is also a great remedy. The *Lycopodium* subject is sallow, sunken, with premature lines in the face; looks older than he is. Children are weak with well-developed heads, but puny, sickly bodies. They are irritable, and when sick awake out of sleep ugly and kick and scream and push away the nurse or parents. These temperament remedies are not always appreciated by those who do not understand the true spirit of our own art of healing; but when appreciated the skillful observer can often see the picture of the right remedy in the face and build of his patient before he speaks a word. A remedy must not only be well proven, but extended clinical use and observation is necessary to develop it and indicate its true sphere of usefulness. I have known temperaments so intensely *Aconite* or *Belladonna* that they could not take these remedies except in the high and highest potencies, and then only in single doses at long intervals. Why should this be thought incredible? Carpenter, in his Physiology, tells of a person who was so susceptible to *Mercury* that she was salivated by sleeping with her husband, who had taken *Mercury*.

This is one of the leading trio of flatulent remedies, *Carbo veg.* and *China* being the other two. With *Lycopodium* there seems to be an almost constant fermentation of gas going on in the abdomen, which produces a loud croaking and rumbling. Remember, while *China* bloats the whole abdomen *Carbo veg.* prefers the upper and *Lycopodium* the lower parts. With *Lycopodium* this flatulent condition is very apt to occur in connection with chronic liver trouble. Again this rumbling of flatulence is often found particularly in the region of the splenic flexure of the colon or left hypochondria.

A feeling of satiety is found under this remedy which alternates with a feeling of hunger of a peculiar kind. The patient sits down to the table *very hungry,* but the first few mouthfuls fill him right up and he feels *distressingly* full; in a Pickwickian sense "too full for utterance." This alternation of hunger and satiety is not markedly found under any other remedy.

Constipation predominates under *Lycopodium,* and like *Nux vomica* there may be frequent and ineffectual desire for stool, but while that of *Nux vomica* is caused by irregular peristaltic action that of *Lycopodium* seems to be caused by a spasmodic contraction of the anus, which prevents the stool and causes great pain.

Lycopodium should be thought of in anal troubles associated with chronic liver troubles, especially if with much flatulence.

Lycopodium is of use in right-sided hernia. It has cured cases of long standing without the aid of a truss.

The liver troubles of *Lycopodium* are more apt to be of the atrophic variety, while those of *China* are hypertrophic, both being equally useful in their sphere.

Lycopodium has almost, if not quite, as marked action upon the urinary organs as upon the liver. It is the chief remedy for *"red sand in the urine."* This not simply the reddish sediment which is generally termed "brick-dust sediment," and which is found under many remedies, but is an actual sandy, gritty sediment that settles at the bottom of the otherwise perfectly clear urine. Unless this condition is removed we have sooner or later renal calculi, or gravel forming, and terrible attacks of renal colic. In children this sand is sometimes found in the diaper after severe crying spells, and in adults much pain in the back in region of kidneys, which is relieved after the discharge of urine containing the sand. (See *Borax, Sarsaparilla* and *Sanicula.*) No one remedy helps these cases more promptly or permanently than *Lycopodium.*

Lycopodium is also one of our best remedies for impotence. *(Agnus castus.)* An old man marries his second or third wife and finds himself not "equal to the occasion." It is very embarrassing for the whole family. A dose of *Lycopodium* sets the thing all right and makes the doctor a warm friend on both sides of the house.

Young men from onanism or sexual excess become impotent. The penis becomes small, cold and relaxed. The desire is as strong as ever, and perhaps more so, but he can't perform. *(Selenium, Caladium.)* I have known apparently hopeless cases of this kind cured by the use of this remedy, high single doses at intervals of a week or more. Give it low, however, if you want to, but do not blame me if you don't succeed.

Lycopodium affects the right side most, or at least the troubles begin on the right side. Swelling and suppuration of the tonsils I have aborted more than once in old quinsy subjects by an early dose of this remedy. In fact, I have had such success with *Lachesis, Lycopodium, Lac caninum* and *Phytolacca* that some who employ me for nothing else come for those powders that *"break up quinsy"* so quick. In diphtheria, if the disease begins in the nose or right tonsil and extends to the left, you will think of *Lycopodium,* but remember that *Mercurius protoiodide* also begins on the right side, but there is no difficulty in choosing between the two. *(Bromine* diphtheria begins below and comes upward, just the reverse of *Lycopodium.)* Pains in the abdomen, ovarian and uterine regions also begin in right side, *running from right* to left; right foot gets cold while the other remains warm, eruptions begin on right and travel across to left side. Sciatica the same; any complaint that begins on right and goes to left makes me think of *Lycopodium.* The "sides of the body" subject is of more account than some imagine. Drugs have an affinity for particular parts, organs and even sides of the body.

Upon the respiratory organs this remedy also has a strong influence. It is one of our best remedies for chronic dry catarrh of the nose, which becomes completely closed, so that the patient has to breathe through the open mouth, especially at night. Here the choice often lies between this remedy, *Ammonium carb.* and *Hepar sulphur.*, other symptoms, of course, deciding the choice. In infants *Sambucus* comes in for a share of attention.

Lycopodium has often saved neglected, *mal-treated or imperfectly cured cases of pneumonia* from running into consumption. It may even come into the later stages of the acute attack itself, and here as usual the disease is apt to be in the right lung, and especially if liver complications arise. The disease has passed the first or congestive stage, and generally the stage of hepatization, or is in the last part of this stage, and is trying hard to take a favorable turn into the breaking-up or third stage, the stage of resolution. Just here is where many cases die, neither free expectoration, nor perfect absorption of the disease product taking place. There is extreme dyspnœa, the cough sounds as if the entire parenchyma of the lung were softened; even raising whole mouthfuls of mucus does not afford relief, the breath is short and the wings of the nose expand to their utmost with a fan-like motion. Now is the time when *Lycopodium* does wonders. Again, even when this stage is imperfectly passed, and the patient still coughs and expectorates much thick, yellow, purulent or greyish-yellow, purulent (sometimes fœtid) matter, tasting salty, with much rattling in the chest, *Lycopodium* is indispensable. Here the choice may have to be made between this remedy and *Sulphur, Kali hydroiod.* or *Silicea.* The characteristic aggravation as to time, of this remedy, is from *4 to 8 o'clock* P. M. *Colocynth* has 4 to 9 aggravation of abdominal pains, and *Helleborus niger,* of the headache, with coryza; but the 4 to 8 aggravations of *Lycopodium* are general, not confined to any one, or one *set* of symptoms.

Lycopodium profoundly impresses the sensorium. We see by studying its pathogenesis that it *depresses.* This is found particularly in typhoid. The patient lies stupid, eyes do not re-act to light; lower jaw drops; apparent impending paralysis of the brain.

This condition may also be found in the advanced stage of many different acute diseases, such as cerebro-spinal meningitis, typhoid fever, pneumonia, etc. Now if you get the 4 to 8 P. M. aggravation this remedy surely comes in. But this depression of the sensorium is also found in chronic form. You remember what was said of this remedy in the impotence of old men. If you find corresponding failure in the sensorium of old men, the memory fails, they use wrong words to express themselves, mix things up generally in writing, spelling, and are, in short, unable to do ordinary mental work on account of failing brain power, remember *Lycopodium.* Here again *Anacardium, Phosphorus, Baryta* or *Opium* may come in for comparison. Also *Picric acid* and *Agnus castus.*

Many more things might be written of this wonderful polychrest, but I have given the most important. Its strongest curative powers are not developed below the 12th potency, hence neither the old school nor the homœopaths who confine themselves exclusively to the low preparations know much about it. Like *Carbo vegetabilis, Silicea* and *Sulphur* its best powers are only developed by Hahnemann's peculiar process of potentization; "prove all things; hold fast that which is good."

SULPHUR.

Hahnemann's king of anti-psorics; combating all psoric manifestations, as described in Hahnemann's chronic diseases.

Itching eruptions on the skin everywhere; scratching is followed by burning.

Burning everywhere, general and local, especially feet; has to stick them out of bed to cool them.

Redness of all orifices, as if pressed full of blood (lips, ears, nostrils, eyelids, anus, urethra, etc.).

Exudations into serous sacs following acute inflammations.

Weak, faint, after hot flashes, followed by sweat, especially at 11 A. M.

Modalities: < 5 A. M. (diarrhœa), standing; 11 A. M., close room, open air, *bathing,* cold damp weather; > doors and windows open, sitting or lying.

* * * * *

I now come to an attempt to give some idea of the curative sphere of Hahnemann's king of anti-psorics. I do not in this place feel it incumbent upon me to enter into a defense of Hahnemann's psora theory against those who discard it because they do not understand it. With those who do understand and profit by it there is no need of such defense. The truth stands confirmed (with those who have put to the test Hahnemann's rules for the use of *Sulphur)* that it has power to meet and overcome certain obstacles to the usual action of drugs when indicated by the symptoms, or least seemingly so. That is the reason why the indication as laid down in the books reads: "When seemingly indicated drugs do not cure, use *Sulphur,*" because psora is the obstacle to be overcome. If you now ask me, what is psora? I answer in true Yankee style, what is scrofula? Perhaps psora is scrofula, or scrofula is psora. Call it either or neither. Yet it is present, a something named or unnamed which must be recognized and complicates so-called acute diseases. Now there is nothing so very remarkable about this. Syphilis does the same. Once contracted or inherited, no matter what ordinary acute disease appears, we are at times obliged to turn aside from its treatment to give a quietus to the old enemy before we can overcome the acute affection. So it is with *Sulphur* and psora. Theorizing and philosophizing, no matter how wise they sound, must go down when facts oppose them. (See case of gastralgia under *Arsenicum* and neuralgia under *Causticum.)*

Now upon this symptom—"When carefully selected remedies fail to act favorably, etc.," as we said when writing of a certain group under *Nux vomica*—this is putting it in too wholesale a fashion. Let no one understand that *Sulphur* is the only remedy capable of removing psoric complications, but simply that *Sulphur* will be likely to be oftener indicated here, because it oftener covers the usual manifestations of psora in its pathogenesis than any other remedy. There are anti-psorics, like *Psorinum, Causticum, Graphites,* etc., which may have to be used instead of *Sulphur.* And we know which one by the same law which guides us in the selection of the right remedy any time. Another thing must not be forgotten. All the anti-psoric remedies have their own individual sphere of action outside their anti-psoric powers; and often a close study of the case in hand, where other remedies have failed, as we had supposed, on account of psora, will reveal that the anti-psoric remedy was the true similli-mum from the start, independent of any psoric element.

To undertake to go over the whole range of action of *Sulphur* would be simply to give its whole symptomatology. That is not the object of these notes, but we can notice only the *red line* indications which lead the careful prescriber to its further study in the Materia Medica.

One of the chief characteristics of this remedy is found under the head or rubric of sensation, viz., that of **Burning.** Burning on vertex (outer and inner head); burning in eyes, painful smarting; burning water from nose; burning in face without redness; burning pain in tongue; burning vesicles in mouth; sore throat with great burning and dryness, first right, then left; burning in stomach; burning and pressure in rectum; burning and itching in hæmorrhoids; burning in anus; burning in urethra; burning in vagina, scarcely able to keep still; nipples burn like fire; burning in chest, rising to face; burning between scapulæ *(Phos.* and *Lycop.);* burning of hands; burning of feet; puts them out of bed to cool them; hot flushes and burning all over; burning skin of whole body; itching eruptions burn after scratching.

After reading such a list of burning in the cured and characteristic symptoms of *Sulphur* one does not wonder that hell is represented as being heated by this substance, for it seems by its pathogenesis as though it were *eternally burning. Arsenicum album, Phosphorus* and *Sulphur* lead the list in our Materia Medica for *burners*. These burning sensations are found in both acute and chronic diseases. Of course there are several other remedies that have this symptom in an intense degree, and must be chosen if the other symptoms come in to complete the picture of similarity. Among these of first importance may be named *Aconite, Agaricus, Apis, Belladonna, Cantharis, Capsicum, Carbo animalis* and *Phosphoric acid*. I think *Arsenicum* leads in all acute diseases, while *Sulphur* leads in chronic affections. We, as homœopathists, do not yet fully appreciate the value of *sensations*.

The action of *Sulphur* upon the circulation is to cause and cure local congestions and a chronic tendency thereto. In other words, it seems to have the power of equalizing the circulation in persons subject to such local congestions and inflammations. These, either acute or chronic congestions, may manifest themselves in boils, swellings, felons, abdominal or portal congestions and inflammations, and here it is especially indicated if caused by suppressed hæmorrhoids; congestions to the head may result from the same cause; the chest becomes congested, when there is great difficulty of breathing; *feels so oppressed that he wants doors and windows open*. This rush of blood seems to fill the whole chest, the heart feels as if "too full," palpitates and labors, as if trying to rid itself of a burden.

The orifices of the body are red, as if pressed full of

blood. *The lips are red as vermilion; ears very red; eyelids red, anus red, urethra red.* All these are manifest indications for *Sulphur.* Especially is this true if these symptoms follow, or are consequent upon, the suppression or retrocession of some eruption or skin trouble. If inward affections work outward towards the surface there is not usually cause for alarm, but if they go the other way look out for breakers, there is shipwreck ahead. No one need tell me that there is no relation of skin to internal troubles. I have seen too much of it, and have cured many cases of that character, where a restoration of the skin disease relieved the internal which had followed its retrocession or suppression.

There is one thing about *Sulphur* that is often underestimated by the profession in general, viz., its power of absorption. It is after the stage of effusion has set in or even later when this stage is passed and the results of the inflammatory process are to be gotten rid of; like the enlargement of the joints in rheumatism, *exudations into serous sacs, pleura, meningeal membranes,* peritoneum, etc. *Bryonia* is one of the remedies first thought of in these cases, and we have another remedy that is making a record for itself here, viz., *Kali muriaticum;* but when the case is complicated by psora and, especially, when the characteristic *burnings* stand out prominently *Sulphur* is almost sure to be needed before the case is finished. *Bryonia* and *Sulphur* complement each other; but, of course, the symptoms must decide and may decide in favor of neither of them. Right here it may be well to speak of that power possessed by *Sulphur* of arousing or exciting defective reaction. Your former remedy was well chosen and seemed to help the patient in a measure, but the case *relapses,* lingers or progresses slowly to perfect recovery. It is on account of a depression of the *vital force,* as Hahnemann would call it. It may be on account of psora or not. Now give a dose of *Sulphur* and let it act a few hours if in an acute case, or a number of days if chronic. Then you may return to your former remedy and get results which you could not before the *Sulphur* was given. It clears up the case and prevents its becoming chronic or a lingering unsatisfactory convalescence.

No remedy has more general, positive and persistent action upon the skin than *Sulphur.* With or without eruption, itching and *burning,* are the characteristic sensations attending the skin symptoms. If any one doubts the itch-producing power of *Sulphur,* let him work a day or two in the bleaching room of a broom factory. I have tried the experiment, and we all remember the fact that our mothers and grandmothers used to cure or rather over-cure itch with it.

So strong is this affinity of *Sulphur* for the skin that it seems bent on pushing everything internal out on the surface. Especially is this true if it is something that naturally belongs there. Over twenty-five years ago I had a case that illustrates this. A lady (maiden) had been an invalid for fourteen years. Her trouble seemed to center in her stomach. So that for all that long period of time she could eat nothing but a little Graham bread and milk, hardly enough to sustain life, and in the earlier part of her sickness for a long time was able only to take a teaspoonful of milk at a time. She was an almost literal walking skeleton. I found, after much questioning and several failures to relieve her much, that about fifteen years before she had with an ointment suppressed an eczema of the nape and occiput. She boasted that she had never seen a vestige of it since. I gave that lady *Sulphur* 200th and in three weeks from that time had that eruption fully restored and her stomach trouble completely relieved The deacon of her (Presbyterian) church exclaimed as she came walking up a long hill to service, "Here comes Susan F——, who has been dying for the last fourteen years and lo and behold, she is the biggest, fattest one among us!" Now how about the relation of skin to internal trouble? I can report a number of as convincing cases in my own practice cured with *Sulphur, Arsenicum, Causticum* or other remedies. One thing must be recognized and never lost sight of, viz., that *symptoms weigh* whether we can give the pathological interpretation of them or not. Here are a few of that kind from the pathogenesis of *Sulphur:*

"Particularly efficacious with lean, stoop-shouldered persons, who walk or sit stooped; standing is the most uncomfortable position."

"Dirty, filthy people, prone to skin affections."

"Children cannot bear to be washed or bathed."

"Voluptuous itching; scratching relieves; after it *burning.*"

"Complaints continually relapsing."

"Congestion to single parts."

"Pain in heart, extending to back."

"Scrofulous (psoric) chronic diseases that result from suppressed eruptions."

"Discharges from every outlet acrid, excoriating and reddening."

"Offensive odor of body despite frequent bathing."

"Hot flushes with spells of faintness, or debility passing off with a little moisture, faintness or debility."

"Weak, faint spells frequently during the day."

"Burning in feet, wants to find a cool place for them; puts them out of bed to cool them off." *(Chamomilla, Medorrhinum, Sanicula.)*

"Feels suffocated; wants doors and windows open, particularly at night."

"Diarrhœa after midnight; painless, driving out of bed early in the morning, as if the bowels were too weak to retain their contents."

"Weak, empty, gone or faint feeling in stomach about 11 A. M."

"White tongue with very red tip and borders."

"Bright redness of lips as if the blood would burst through." *(Tuberculinum.)*

"Heat on crown of head; cold feet; frequent flushing."

Every true homœopath knows the value of these and many more symptoms of this remedy. No one else appreciates them. Again, none but those who use the potentized *Sulphur* can ever know what it is capable of curing.

CALCAREA OSTREARUM.

Deficient or irregular bone development. (Fontanelles open, crooked spine, deformed extremities.)

Leucophlegmatic temperament.

Fair, fat, flabby, obesic.

Coldness, general and local, subjective and objective, especially as if had on cold, damp stockings. Affections from working in cold water.

Sweats general (night sweats and on exertion). Local; head (children), axillæ, hands, feet, etc.

Digestive tract sour (sour taste, eructations, vomiting, sour curds, diarrhœa).

Great debility; cannot walk far or *go upstairs* for short breath; easily strained.

Modalities: < cold air, *ascending,* or exertion; straining from *lifting.*

* * * * *

This is another of Hahnemann's constitutional remedies which, as Farrington says, "may come into use, in almost any form of disease." We may say come into use because it may be on account of certain idiosyncrasies which come under the remedial power of *Calcarea* that the disease, whatever it is, is made less amenable to ordinary treatment.

The temperament of *Calcarea* is altogether different from that of *Sulphur.* You remember the lean, stoop-shouldered *Sulphur* subject. *Calcarea* is on the contrary what cannot be better expressed than in the term used by Henry N. Guernsey, viz., **Leucophlegmatic temperament.**

The *Calcarea* patient is constitutionally fat, over-fat or strongly inclined to obesity. The color of the skin is white, watery or chalky pale. Of torpid disposition (especially children), sluggish or slow in its movements. The *Sulphur* is almost the exact opposite, quick, wiry, nervous, active. There is none of the bilious, swarthy, yellowish appearance in *Calcarea* that we find in *Lycopodium.* These three remedies, *Calcarea, Sulphur, Lycopodium,* are a trio that find each their counterpart in many persons the world over. Of course we find the tendency to obesity under other remedies, as, for instance, under *Graphites,* but with this obesity we almost always find accompanying it the peculiar skin troubles of *Graphites.* Sometimes we seem to find a condition that seems to simulate each remedy in some one feature; for instance, the obesic temperament of *Calcarea* and the eruptive tendency of *Sulphur.* This may combine so as to make a case that will be covered by *Hepar sulph.* Such cases are more difficult to cover with a perfect simillimum. But when we do find a purely *Calcarea, Sulphur* or *Lycopodium* subject the fact is inestimable as a help to a brilliant result in many cases.

Malnutrition is one of the disorders calling for the exhibition of this remedy.

"Tardy development of the bony tissues with lymphatic enlargements."

"Curvature of the bones, especially spine and long bones."

"Extremities deformed, crooked."

"Softening of the bones; *fontanelles remain open too long* and skull very large."

These symptoms are quoted from "Hering's Guiding Symptoms," and show the lack of, or imperfect, nutrition of bones. They are nourished irregularly, or unevenly. One part of a bone, the vertebræ for instance, is nourished, while the other is starved. While all this irregular bone development is going on the soft parts are suffering from over-nutrition. Thus we have recorded in the pathogenesis: "Tendency to obesity, especially in children and young people."

"Nutrition impaired with tendency to glandular enlargements."

"Granular vegetations; polypus (in nose, ear, bladder, uterus, etc.)."

This is a fair picture of the general or constitutional use of *Calcarea ost.*, and it remains to give some of the characteristic or peculiar symptoms guiding to its selection.

When writing of *Sulphur* we called particular attention to the sensation of burning under that remedy. *Calcarea* has characteristically the opposite, viz., **Coldness.** *(Cistus.)*

"Cold, damp feet."

"Sensation in feet and legs as if she had on cold, damp stockings."

"Coldness of legs with night-sweats."

"Internal and external sensation of coldness of various parts of head as if a piece of ice were lying against it; with pale puffed face."

"She feels a sort of inward coldness."

"Aversion to open air, the least cold air goes right through her."

All this is so directly opposite to *Sulphur* that any confusion between them seems impossible.

Sensations of coldness in single parts should always call to mind *Calcarea*, as well as general coldness. *(Cistus* and *Heloderma.)*

If *Calcarea* has one symptom that not only leads all the rest, but also all other remedies, it is found in the **profuse sweats on the head of large-headed, open fontanelled children.** The sweat is so profuse that during sleep it rolls down the head and face wetting the pillow far around. Many a little child has been saved from dying of hydrocephalus, dentition, rachitis, marasmus, eclampsia, cholera infantum, etc., where this sweating symptom was the guiding symptom to the use of *Calcarea.* It is also especially indicated, other symptoms agreeing, in sweats of male organs, nape of neck, chest, axilla, hands, knees, feet, etc. *Partial sweats.* It is also a remedy for night sweats generally when they occur in connection with consumption or other debilitating diseases.

In all these sweatings of *Calcarea* the surface is characteristically cold at the same time, and especially would we find the lower extremities cold.

Calcarea has characteristic symptoms in the digestive tract. One is that everything in the whole length of the tract seems **sour.** Eructations sour; sour vomiting of large curds *(Æthusa);* sour diarrhœa. And then there is a sour smell of the whole body. This is not like the offensive odor of the body that *Sulphur* has.

Then there is a peculiar symptom of the appetite that has often been verified—"Longing for eggs, particularly in children, in sickness or during convalescence, even before they are able to swallow. The stomach externally is swollen or seems distended, standing right out like an inverted saucer. Abdomen is also much distended from hard and swollen mesentery, even when the rest of the body is emaciated."

The diarrhœa, which may vary as to color and consistence, instead of being aggravated in the morning, like *Sulphur,* is *worse in the afternoon.* The patient is **generally better** when constipated.

Calcarea has not so positive and unvarying action upon the skin as *Sulphur,* but is indispensable in skin affections which seem to depend upon some constitutional dyscrasia that it covers in its general action, for instance, in eczema capitis or milk crusts in children of the *Calcarea* type. Here, of course, no remedy can take its place. Indeed all skin troubles in *Calcarea* subjects disappear when through its action the system is set right, showing that the skin troubles after all were only secondary. The skin of the *Calcarea* subject is generally cold, soft and flabby.

We must not omit to notice the action of *Calcarea ost.* on the respiratory organs, for the reason that it is of great importance in its use in that dread disease, pulmonary consumption. Whether, as Professor Bennet believes, this disease be essentially one of faulty nutrition, or as Virchow believes, one of inflammation, or if Professor Rindflesch's theory, relegating it to the class of diseases known as infectious, be true, or whatever its primary cause may be, we know that *Calcarea ost.* is one of the most effective agents, if indicated by the temperament and symptoms, in the cure of this malady, and if applied at a stage when a cure is at all possible.

Very many cases in the incipient stage come within range of *Sulphur* or *Calcarea.* As we have already given the leading indications of *Sulphur,* we will now give some of them for *Calcarea:*

"Leucophlegmatic temperament."

"Middle and upper portion of right lung." *(Sulph.,* upper left.)

"Chest painfully sensitive to touch and on inspiration."

"Shortness of breath on walking, especially on ascending."

"Painless hoarseness, < in the morning."

"Especially in women who have always been too early and profuse in menstruation, and who have habitually cold feet to the knees."

"Tendency to looseness of the bowels, < afternoons."

"Appetite failing and emaciation progressing."

Here are a few of the prominent indications, and on them many a case has been cured. Of course there is generally cough, and it may be tight or loose, yet the case rests mainly on the symptoms outside the cough. This remedy in this disease and the success attending its use is one of the illustrations of the soundness of Hering's advice when he says "treat the patient, not the disease."

CALCAREA PHOSPHORICA.

Tardy closing or re-opening fontanelles in slim, emaciated children, with sweaty heads.

Diarrhœa or entero-colitis; stool passes with much flatulence and spluttering noise.

Rheumatic troubles, which are < in fall or spring, when the air is full of melting snow.

* * * * *

While on the subject of *Calcarea* we may as well notice this other combination.

The *Phosphorus* element in this preparation seems to change the temperament, for while it retains its wonderful remedial power over tardy bone development it acts best in spare subjects instead of fat. So that if we find a sickly child with fontanelles remaining open too long or re-opening after once closed, the child being spare and anæmic, we think of this remedy.

We would also think of *Silicea* in one of these poor subjects, but in the *Calcarea phos.* the sweaty head is not a prominent symptom, while with *Silicea* it is markedly so. *Calcarea phos.* also has a very peculiar desire, the little patient instead of wanting eggs wants "ham rind," a very queer symptom, but a genuine one. *(Magnesia carb.* craves meat in scrofulous children.)

Diarrhœa is very prominent, and the stools are green and "spluttering;" that is the flatulence (of which there is much) with the stool makes a loud spluttering noise when the stool passes. I have made some very fine cures in such cases where there seemed little hope for the child and hydrocephaloid seemed impending. The little patients were shrunken, emaciated and very anæmic. *Marasmus.*

(Calcarea phos. is an excellent remedy in rheumatic troubles < spring and fall, especially when the air is cold and damp from *melting snow.)*

Calcarea phos. is an excellent remedy for broken bones where the bones refuse to knit. (Also *Symphytum.)*

I have found *Calcarea phos.* very useful in the headaches of anæmic school girls. Here we sometimes have to choose between it and *Natrum mur.*

Feels complaints more when thinking of them *(Oxalic acid, Helonias).*

SILICEA.

Weak, puny children; not from want of nourishment taken, but defective assimilation.

Inflammations tending to end suppuration or refusing to heal; becoming chronic.

Coldness, lack of vital warmth, even when taking exercise; must be wrapped up, especially the head, which >.

Suppressed sweat, especially of feet, which is profuse and offensive.

Weak, nervous, easily irritated, faint-hearted; yielding, giving up disposition, "grit all gone."

Constipation; stool protrudes and then slips back again, again and again; weak expulsive power.

Modalities: < from cold or draft, motion, open air, at new moon; > in warm room, *wrapping up head;* magnetism and electricity.

Scrofulous, rachitic children with large heads; open fontanelles and sutures; much sweating about the head, which must be kept warm by external covering; large bellies; weak ankles, slow in learning to walk.

Diseases, caused by suppressed foot-sweat; exposing the head or back to any slight draft of air; from vaccination *(Thuja);* dust complaints of stone cutters, with total loss of strength.

Vertigo; spinal headache ascending from nape of neck to head, as if one would fall forward; worse looking upward.

Unhealthy skin; every little injury suppurates.

Promotes expulsion of foreign bodies from the tissues, fish bones, needles, bone splinters.

* * * * *

Silicea is another of our invaluable constitutional remedies, and also one which is of little or no use except as developed by Hahnemann's process of potentization. Like *Calcarea,* it is especially useful in sweaty-headed children *(Sanicula)* with defective assimilation. It is not in the fat, torpid, obesic patients, over-nourished in one part and insufficiently so in another, like *Calcarea,* that *Silicea* is indicated, but in the over-sensitive, imperfectly nourished (generally), not from want of food, but from imperfect assimilation. The *Silicea* child is not larger than natural anywhere except in its "big belly," which is due to diseased mesentery. Its limbs are shrunken, its eyes sunken and its face pinched and old looking. It does not increase in size or strength, learns to walk late; in short, if not actually sick in bed, everything seems to have come to a standstill so far as growth or development is concerned. Now if this state of things continues the bowels become very constipated, and a peculiar constipation it is, too. The little fellow strains and strains, *the stool partly protruding and then slipping back (Sanicula* and *Thuja),* as though the general weakness of the patient affected the expulsive power of the rectum, or else the bowels become very persistently loose, especially during dentition or the hot weather of summer. The stools are changeable, but *Pulsatilla* does no good, almost every kind and color of loose stool appearing. The child takes nourishment enough, but, whether vomited or retained, goes on emaciating and growing weaker and weaker until it dies of inanition, unless *Silicea* checks this process. Many such cases have I saved with this remedy and made them healthy children. I have always used the 30th and upwards, hence cannot speak of the lower preparations. (*Silicea* also has constipation < before and during menstruation.)

Silicea ranks among the first of our remedies for inflammations ending in suppuration. It seems to make no particular difference whether the suppuration takes place in the soft or hard parts, for it is equally efficacious in glandular or bony ulcerations. It seems to come in at a later stage than *Hepar sulph.* or *Calcarea sulphide* which expedite the discharge of pus already formed, while *Silicea* comes in for healing after the discharge has taken place. Cellular tissues with deep-seated suppurations, including tendons and ligaments, also come within the range of its healing powers. In these cases the constitution of the patient has an important bearing in the selection of this remedy. The *Silicea* subject is weakly, with fine skin, pale face, lax muscles. Even the mind and nervous symptoms come into the general picture of "weakness." He is nervous and irritable, weak, faint-hearted, yielding, giving up disposition, "grit all gone." *(Pulsatilla.)* In such a case *Silicea* is grand. I hate to use the term, but as the old school would say, "it builds them up," and so it seems, for under its action the patient's spirits rise, hope revives, the weakness and depression give way to a feeling of returning strength and health. It makes no difference whether the ulcerations are in the tissues already named, in the lungs, intestinal tract, or mammæ, or elsewhere, the effect is the same, and the improvement in the local affection generally follows the general constitutional improvement. This condition of weakness seems to attack the general nervous system, affecting the spine, and so we get those cerebro-spinal headaches, or headaches beginning in the nape of the neck and running forward over the head to the eyes, for which *Silicea* is so useful. *Vertigo* also ascends from the nape to head, < looking up. *(Pulsatilla.)*

There seems to be lack of nerve power to resist outward depressing influences. He is cold, or, as Hering puts it, there is *"want of vital warmth, even when taking exercise."* He is sensitive to cold air, takes cold very easily, especially when uncovering the head or feet. On the contrary, he is relieved by *"wrapping up the head" (Magnesia mur.),* or, in other words, by supplying artificially the warmth that he lacks naturally.

I have several times found a *Silicea* child suffering from epileptiform spasms which were always worse at new moon. A few doses of *Silicea* 200th set them all right.

Silicea subjects are often afflicted with offensive foot-sweats *(Sanicula, Psorinum, Graphites)*, which are easily suppressed by getting the feet cold. Such suppression must be remedied, the sweat restored and cured by proper medication or serious results often follow, such as convulsions and other spinal troubles, even locomotor ataxia. *Silicea* is the remedy to restore and cure such sweats by correcting the conditions upon which the sweats depend. *(Baryta carb., Graphites, Psorinum, Sanicula.)*

The *Silicea* patient desires to be magnetized and is relieved thereby. *(Phosphorus.)*

This is one of the remedies of which, like *Sepia, Lachesis, Lycopodium* and others, the old school knows little or nothing, because their chief virtues are only developed in potencies above the 12th.

Silicea is the chronic of *Pulsatilla.*

ACONITUM NAPELLUS.

Fear: of death; of crowds; of going out. Anything, always fearful.

Complaints from exposure to cold, dry cold.

Congestions and inflammations, acute, first stage with great anxiety, heat and restlessness; tosses about in agony; throws off covering. Inflammatory fever.

Pains insuppressable < at night, especially in the evening; neuralgic.

Face very red and flushed, but turns pale on rising up.

Favorite points of attack: Larynx (croup), bronchi (bronchitis), lungs and pleura (pneumonia and pleurisy), joints (rheumatism), heart and circulation (erethism).

Modalities: < in the evening (chest symptoms and

pains); lying on left side; in warm room or warm covering.

> uncovering; kicks the clothes off.

* * * * *

We will now take up what I call the trio of **restless** remedies, viz.: *Aconite, Arsenicum* and *Rhus toxicodendron.*

All are equally restless, yet all are so very different that there is no difficulty in choosing between them. The *Aconite* restlessness is oftenest found in a high grade of synochal or inflammatory fevers. There is no better picture in a few words of the *Aconite* fever than is given by Hering—"Heat, with thirst; hard, full and frequent pulse, anxious impatience, inappeasable, beside himself, tossing about with agony."

The custom of alternating *Aconite* and *Belladonna* in inflammatory affections, which so widely prevails is a senseless one. Both remedies cannot be indicated at a time, and if a good effect follows their administration you may be sure that the *indicated one* cured in spite of the action of the other, which only hindered; or that the patient recovered without help from either. There are many cases of this kind where the doctor is congratulating himself on a cure which was only a recovery, for which he deserves no credit at all. Let us look for a moment at some of the diagnostic differences of these two remedies.

Both have great heat of the skin, but *Aconite* has characteristically *dry, hot skin* and no sweat; *Belladonna* has even greater surface heat, but sweats on *covered parts. Aconite* tosses about in agony with great fear of death; *Belladonna* often has semi-stupor and jerks and twitches.

in sleep. *Aconite* has great distress in heart and chest; *Belladonna* everything seems to centre in the head. *Aconite* fears death without much delirium; *Belladonna* fears imaginary things, with delirium. Thus we might continue to give points of difference. No man who understands the homœopathic art of healing will ever alternate these two remedies.

Aconite is also a great **pain** remedy. If we were to name the three leading remedies in this respect it would be *Aconite, Chamomilla* and *Coffea.* The *Aconite* pains are always attended by the extreme restlessness, anxiety and fearfulness of this remedy. The patient tosses about in agony, "cannot *bear the pain,* nor bear to be touched, nor to be uncovered." Well, you say, all remedies have pain. Not all, and not many so intense pain. *Opium* and *Stramonium* have painlessness oftener than pain. The *Aconite* pains are intolerable and generally worse in the evening or at night. Then we have often alternating with or sometimes even in conjunction with the pains *numbness, tingling,* or *formication.*

In this it resembles *Rhus tox.,* but with *Aconite* the pains predominate, while with *Rhus tox.* the **numbness,** with dull aching and soreness, leads. The pains of *Aconite* are tearing, cutting pains, which drive the patient to desperation. Right here we may as well speak of the leading characteristic of this remedy, for it is almost always present when *Aconite* is clearly indicated. Just one word expresses it: **Fear**—*fear of death* especially, but fear to cross the street, fear to go into society, fear something is going to happen, ever present, undefinable, unreasonable fear. No remedy has it in such a degree as this one. It is the fear as much as the pain that makes the patient so full of that agonized restlessness. The *Arsenic* restlessness goes with extreme prostration and reduced vitality. *Rhus tox.*, on account of the aching pains, which make him want to move for the temporary relief he gets from the movement. *Arsenic* wants to move from place to place, but is *not* relieved. Neither *Aconite* nor *Arsenic* get such relief from movement, nor does *Arsenic* **fear** like *Aconite*, or at least in any such degree. *Aconite*, as a fever remedy, has been greatly abused. Even the old school, astonished at the results of homœopathic treatment, so superior to their so-called anti-phlogistic treatment, and finding *Aconite* so highly recommended and frequently used in inflammatory affections, concluded in accordance with their usual way of reasoning that *Aconite* could be squeezed into their pathological livery and made to do service in all kinds of fever simply because it **was** fever. But they soon found that however useful it might be in some cases of inflammatory fever, it was of no use in typhoids. Thus was generalization from a pathological standpoint again doomed to disappointment, as it always must be. Now many so-called homœopaths have fallen into similar error by concluding that because *Aconite* did quickly cure in some cases having a high grade of fever, that therefore it was always the remedy with which to treat cases having high fever. They even fell into the routine habit of prescribing this remedy for the first stage of all inflammatory affections, and follow it with other remedies more appropriate to the whole case further on. If *Aconite* were the only remedy having inflammatory fever, perhaps we could do no better than to zig-zag the case to a cure this way. Dunham writes: "*Aconite* is never to be given first to subdue the fever and then some other remedy 'to meet the case,' never to be alternated with other drugs for the purpose, as is often alleged, of 'controlling the fever.' If the fever be such as to require *Aconite,* no other drug is needed. If other drugs seem indicated, one should be sought which meets the fever as well, for many drugs besides *Aconite* produce fever, each after its kind."

True words, and as one reads them who has proved their truthfulness and remembers their great author, he feels like exclaiming, "Being dead, yet speaketh." *Aconite* has two very important modalities, viz., fright and dry cold air. We have already noticed the value of the *fear* of *Aconite* as a symptom, connected with acute inflammatory ailments. It is no less a remedy for ailments brought on by fright, either immediate or remote. The patient has received a fright in the dark and is always afraid in the dark afterwards. From fright vertigo comes on, or fainting; trembling; threatened abortion, or suppressed menstruation. Jaundice may be induced by it, and become chronic. There are other remedies for fright, prominent among which are *Opium, Ignatia, Veratrum album,* etc. Now in regard to the *dry, cold air.* No remedy has more prominently acute inflammations arising from dry, cold air. Nineteen out of twenty cases of croup arising from exposure to dry, cold air will be cured by *Aconite.* I live in a locality where croup abounds and have had abundant opportunity to verify this. *Pleurisy, pneumonia* and *rheumatism* also come under this head, and they are, as would be expected, almost invariably accompanied by the high fever, anguish, restlessness and fear so characteristic of this remedy. Any local congestion or inflammation coming from such exposure also comes under the same rule, always providing the other symptoms correspond. The other leading dry air remedies are *Bryonia, Causticum, Hepar sulph.* and *Nux vomica.* Here are some wet weather remedies: *Dulcamara, Nux moschata, Natrum sulphuricum* and *Rhus toxicodendron.* Such things are well to remember, for one positive indication is worth two or three vague ones.

ARSENICUM ALBUM.

Great anguish and restlessness, driving from place to place.

Great and sudden prostration, sinking of vital force.

Intense burning pains.

Intense thirst; drinks often, but little, as cold water disagrees.

Dyspnœa < on motion, especially ascending.

Vomiting and stool simultaneous; < after eating or drinking.

Modalities: < in cold air, from cold things, cold applications; and 1 to 3 A. M. Movement.

> by warm air or room and hot applications; relieved by sweat.

* * * * *

No remedy is more restless than this one. The *Aconite* restlessness comes in the earlier stages of inflammatory diseases, with fever of a high grade. *Arsenicum* in the later stages, after the patient has become greatly reduced in strength, or in low grades of fever like typhoids. The *Aconite* patient tosses to and fro in agony and fear. The *Arsenic* patient is too weak to toss as the anguish and restlessness would incline him to. He cannot move himself around as he desires, but wants to be moved from place to place, or bed to bed, while the least exertion on his own part exhausts terribly. He has fear of death, but not like the *Aconite* fear, but rather an anxiety and a feeling that it is useless to take medicine for he is going to die; he is incurable.

The mental restlessness is as great as the bodily. He has attacks of anxiety that drive him out of bed at night. Even when there is no pain at all he wants to be continually changing place, walking about if strong enough, without any other reason than that he can't keep still. Often the first beneficial effect to be observed in cases calling for this remedy is that the anxiety grows less, the patient lies still, his pain is not so much less, but it does not make him so restless; he can bear it better. This is a good sign and is generally followed by amelioration of all the symptoms. It makes little difference what the disease, if this persistent restlessness and especially if great weakness is also present, don't forget *Arsenic*

Arsenicum leads all the remedies for **burning** sensation, epecially in acute diseases. It is not by any means confined to acute diseases, but is often found in chronic affections, especially of a malignant character or tending to malignancy. I think perhaps *Sulphur* outranks it generally for burnings in chronic affections. There is hardly an organ or tissue in the human system where these burnings of *Arsenic* are not found. This burning, strange as it may seem, is greatly **ameliorated by heat.** Hot applications if they can be gotten in contact with the part, also heat of a warm stove or warm room. This is the exact opposite of *Secale cornutum,* for while the part is objectively cold, it still *burns,* but hot applications are intolerable; they cannot even bear to have it covered; with *Arsenicum,* in throat complaints, in connection with acute catarrh, the burnings in throat and from the excoriating nasal discharge are ameliorated by hot application. The burning in throat is better from eating or drinking hot things. This is the chief modality which enables us to choose between this remedy and *Cepa* and *Mercurius,* for all three have fluent coryza. I once had a case of very severe gastralgia caused by suppression of eczema on the hands. I knew nothing of the suppression, but prescribed *Arsenicum* because the pains came on at midnight, lasting until 3 A. M., during which time the patient had to walk the floor in agony, and there was *great burning* in the stomach. She had but one slight attack after taking *Arsenicum,* but, said she, when I visited her, "Doctor, would that remedy send out salt rheum?" Then I found out about the suppression which had been caused by the application of an ointment, and told her that she could have back the pain in the stomach any time she wanted it, by suppressing the eruption again. She did not want it.

Arsenicum is one of our best remedies for fevers of a typhoid character. So useful is it that Baehr says—"Since *Arsenic* is, more than any other remedy, adapted to the worst forms of infectious diseases it seems wrong to delay its administration until the symptoms indicating it are developed in their most malignant intensity," and further, "our advice, therefore, is that *Arsenic* should be given more frequently than has been customary from the very beginning of the attack, and that we should not wait until the disease has fully developed its pernicious character." I do not think this is sound reasoning or good advice, for I have never found any rule by which I could decide from the beginning that a case would later on develop into a case of the pernicious or malignant character which would ever call for the exhibition of *Arsenic.* While we need not wait for a case to develop to that "most malignant" intensity which calls for *Arsenic,* we would not on the other hand be justified in giving *Arsenic* or any other remedy in anticipation of a condition which might never come. *Arsenicum* is not the only remedy capable of curing these malignant cases, and how do we know after all that it may not be *Muriatic acid* or *Carbo vegetabilis* that will be the remedy after the case is developed. There is no safe or scientific rule but to treat the case with the *indicated* remedy at any and all stages of the disease, without trying to treat expected conditions or future possibilities. It would be out of place here to give all the indications for *Arsenic* in typhoids, as it would take too much space, and they can be found in Raue, Lilienthal or any good work on practice. *Arsenic* is also one of our best remedies in intermittents, especially after the abuse of *Quinine.* Close individualization is necessary here as elsewhere.

Arsenic profoundly affects the alimentary canal from lips to anus. The lips are so dry and parched and cracked that the patient often licks them to moisten them. The tongue is affected in various ways. It may be dry and red, with raised papillæ; or red, with indented edges; or white as chalk or white paint; or lead colored; or dry, brown or black, especially in typhoids. The mouth is dry or aphthous, ulcerated or gangrenous. The throat the same. The thirst is indescribably intense and peculiar, in that notwithstanding its intensity the patient can *take only a little water at a time.* The stomach is so irritable that the least food or drink causes distress and pain, or immediately excites vomiting, or stool, or both together. Cold drinks, ice-water, or ice-cream particularly, disagree and create distress. Vomits all kinds and grades of substances from water or mucus to bile, blood, and coffee ground substances.

The pains in stomach are terrible and aggravated by the least food or drink, especially, if *cold.* The abdominal pains also are intense, causing the patient to turn and twist in all possible shapes and directions. Diarrhœa of all kinds of stools, from simple watery to black, bloody and horribly offensive, and finally the end of the tract is reached and we have hæmorrhoids. Now in every one of these affections, ranging along the whole length of the canal, and from the lightest grade of irritation to the most intense inflammatory and malignant forms of disease, we will be apt to find everywhere present the characteristic *burning* of this remedy, in greater or lesser degree; and the not less characteristic *amelioration from heat,* and also, though not quite so invariably, the *midnight aggravation.*

Arsenicum also has its sphere of usefulness in diseases of the respiratory organs. First, for acute coryza it stands in the front rank, the choice often having to be made between this remedy, *Cepa* and *Mercurius. Arsenicum* has the fluent discharge which corrodes the lips and wings of the nose and more *burning* than the other two remedies. It often follows well after *Mercurius,* if that remedy only partially relieves.

Arsenicum is particularly efficacious in many affections of the lungs, where the breathing is very much oppressed. Respiration is wheezing, with cough and frothy expectoration. Patient cannot lie down; must sit up to breathe, and is unable to move without being greatly put out of breath. The air passages seem constricted. It is especially useful in asthmatic affections caused or aggravated by suppressed eruptions, like pneumonia from retrocedent measles, or even chronic lung troubles from suppressed eczema. I remember a case of asthma of years' standing to which I was called at midnight, because they were afraid the patient would die before morning. Found that her attacks always came on at 1 A. M. Gave *Arsenicum alb.* 30th, and she was completely cured by it.

The symptom by Rollin R. Gregg, "Acute, sharp, fixed or darting pain in apex and through upper third of right lung," is a gem, and has enabled me to cure a number of cases of obstinate lung troubles. In the last stage of pneumonia of old people, with gangrenous expectoration, if the other symptoms correspond, this remedy has often saved life. The burning is often found here as elsewhere. *Arsenicum* is also one of our best remedies in pleuritic effusions.

Arsenicum also affects profoundly the nervous system. To the characteristic restlessness, of which we have said so much, is added **great prostration.** This prostration is present in most diseases, both acute and chronic, where *Arsenic* is indicated. For instance, in typhoids there is no remedy that prostrates more. *Carbo veg.* and *Muriatic acid* equal it, the difference being that the *Arsenic* patient wants to move or be moved constantly, while with the other two remedies there is almost utter absence of any such show of life. Even if not confined to the bed, in acute or chronic diseases the patient is so weak that he is "exhausted from the slightest exertion;" must lie down.

Sometimes this extreme degree of prostration comes on very rapidly.

Here is a picture that shows a condition of things in chronic trouble calling for this remedy. "From climbing mountains, or other muscular exertions, want of breath, prostration, sleeplessness and other ailments." This shows how weak the patient is, and this weakness may be coupled with various forms of disease. You may say it is common for sick people to be weak. True, but the *Arsenicum* patient is weak *out of proportion* to the rest of his trouble, or apparently so; and it is a *general prostration,* not local like the sense of weakness in the chest of *Phosphoric acid, Stannum* and *Sulphur;* or in the abdomen like *Phosphorus;* or in the stomach like *Ignatia, Hydrastis* and *Sepia.* Now I do not see how I can make plainer the value of prostration as an *Arsenic* symptom.

When we come to the tissues we find our remedy almost universally present.

It attacks the *blood,* causing septic changes, exanthemata, ecchymoses, petechiæ, etc.

It attacks the *veins;* varices burn like fire, < at night.

It attacks the serous membranes, causing copious serous effusions.

It attacks the glands, which indurate or suppurate.

It attacks the periosteum.

It attacks the joints; causing pale swellings, burning pains, etc.

It causes inflammatory swellings with burning lancinating pains.

It causes general anasarca; skin pale, waxy or earth colored; great thirst (*Apis* none).

It causes rapid emaciation; atrophy of children.

It causes ulcerations, constantly extending in breadth. The ulcers *burn* like fire, pain even during sleep, discharge may be copious or scanty, the base blue, black or lardaceous.

Anthrax *burning* like fire; cold blue skin dry as parchment, peeling off in large scales.

"Sphacelus," parts look black or *burn* like fire.

"Gangrene," better from heat (worse, *Secale)*.

"Parchment" like dryness, or dry scaly skin.

The skin troubles of this remedy are mostly dry and scaly, and almost always **burning.** It is one of our best remedies for affections caused by retrocedent or suppressed exanthemata, also for suppressed chronic eczemas, etc.

But it is impossible and outside the scope of this work to mention by name all the affections of the tissues in which this remedy is useful.

Notwithstanding this, *Arsenic* is not a panacea. It must, like every other remedy, be indicated by its similar symptoms or failure is the outcome. Its great keynotes are **Restlessness, Burning, Prostration,** and **Midnight Aggravation.**

RHUS TOXICODENDRON.

Dry or coated tongue with a triangular red tip.

Great restlessness, cannot lie long in one position, changes often with temporary relief, tosses about continually.

Lameness and stiffness on beginning to move after rest; on getting up in the A. M. > by continued motion.

Erysipelas or scarlatina with vesicular eruption and characteristic restlessness.

All diseases that put on the typhoid form with the characteristic, triangular red-tip tongue and restlessness.

Stupor and mild, persistent delirium; continually tossing about, with laborious dreams.

Modalities: < when quietly sitting or lying and on beginning to move; wet, cold weather; lifting or straining; getting wet when perspiring. > by continued motion, by warmth, dry air or weather; lying on hard floor (backache).

Muscular rheumatism, sciatica, left side *(Col.);* aching in left arm, with heart disease.

Great sensitiveness to open air; putting the hand from under the bed cover brings on the cough *(Bar., Hep.).*

Back; pain between the shoulders on swallowing.

Cough during chill; dry, teasing, fatiguing, but urticaria over body during heat.

* * * * *

This is the third remedy of our so-called restless trio. This restlessness of *Rhus* is on account of the aching pain and soreness which is temporarily relieved by movement. There is also an internal uneasiness which is purely nervous, which causes the patient to want to be on the move, even when there is no particular pain present; but not nearly to the degree that we find it under *Aconite* and *Arsenicum.*

As in *Bryonia,* so in *Rhus,* the leading characteristic is found in its modality. The aggravation on movement, in the former, is no less marked than the **aggravation** when **quiet** of the latter. The patient tosses and turns from side to side with *Rhus* the same as with *Aconite* and *Arsenicum.* With *Rhus* the change relieves, while with the other two it does not. In *Bryonia,* the more the patient moves the more he suffers, while with *Rhus,* the more and longer he moves the better he feels, until he is exhausted. In acute affections, like scarlatina and typhoid fevers, and even in the hot stage of intermittent fevers, constant movement seems to be the patient's only relief. With chronic diseases like chronic rheumatism the patient must move, suffers on first beginning to move, but as he continues to move, or as he expresses it, "gets limbered up," he feels better. But he cannot long lie comfortably in either the acute or chronic trouble, for the aching comes on and he must move even if it does hurt him at first. The pains causing the restlessness of *Rhus* are not so agonizing as they are under *Aconite* and *Arsenicum,* nor is the prostration so great as under *Arsenicum* nor the excitement so great as under *Aconite.* *Rhus* and *Arsenicum* are often indicated in typhoids, *Aconite* seldom or never, but all three are equally *restless* remedies.

If in genuine typhoid *Arsenicum,* as some think, heads the list, because oftenest indicated, *Rhus* will put in equally strong claims in all other diseases that take on typhoid symptoms. The literal meaning of the term or word typhus is *smoke, stupefaction.* Now in all forms of typhus, known as cerebral, abdominal and pneumotyphus, taking all together, *Rhus* will be as often indicated as any other remedy. Whenever in fevers or even inflammatory diseases the sensorium becomes cloudy (smoky) or stupefaction sets in, with low grade of muttering delirium, dry tongue, etc., we think of *Rhus.* Dry or dark coated tongue, with **triangular red tip,** is especial indication for this remedy. This condition of sensorium and tongue may appear in *dysentery, peritonitis, pneumonia, scarlatina, rheumatism, diphtheria; bilious, remittent,* *typhoid fevers,* etc. It makes no difference what the name or locality of the disease is if the *symptoms* are there. The stupefaction calling for *Rhus* in these diseases is not so profound as that calling for *Hyoscyamus* or *Opium,* but is more on a parallel with such remedies as *Baptisia, Nux moschata, Lachesis* or *Phosphoric acid.* Nor is the delirium so violent as that calling for such remedies as *Belladonna, Hyoscyamus* and *Stramonium.* Both stupefaction and delirium are mild in form, but regular and persistent. Of course the *Rhus restlessness* is present and the patient tosses or turns from side to side, even without knowing of it, or of anything going on around her. She will answer questions and perhaps answer correctly, but afterwards does not know anything that transpired while she was sick, may be for days or weeks.

Rhus, Baptisia and *Arnica* closely resemble each other, and choice is sometimes difficult; but we will try to differentiate them when we come to write upon the two latter.

Cough during chill in intermittents is a characteristic given us by Carrol Dunham, and is very reliable, as I have had occasion to prove.

Rhus acts particularly on fibrous, muscular and cellular tissues. The muscles are stiff and sore. This may be of a rheumatic character, or may have been induced by straining, by heavy lifting or severe muscular exercise of any kind, or it may have been brought on by exposure to cold, especially wet cold.

This strained condition may not be confined to the muscles alone, but may involve the tendons, ligaments and membranes of the joints. Several affections of the muscles of the back and even the spinal membranes (myelitis) may come on from sprain, or by exposure, by sleeping on damp ground, or in bed with damp sheets, or getting wet in a rain storm, especially while perspiring. Indeed *Rhus* is one of our best remedies in lumbago. But it makes no particular difference what muscles are strained or exposed so as to bring on this lameness and soreness the remedy is the same, and if the great characteristic—☞"*Lameness and stiffness and pain on first moving after rest, or on getting up in the morning, relieved by continued motion,*" is present, *Rhus* is the first remedy to think of.

Rhus is also often a remedy for glandular swelling of parotid or submaxillary glands during scarlatina, cellulitis in diphtheria, or orbital cellulitis.

This is also one of our best remedies in skin diseases. No one who has been poisoned by it will doubt that *Rhus* has power to produce skin disease, and of course in accordance with our law of cure we would expect cures by it. We have not been disappointed. The eruption of *Rhus* poisoning is vesicular. *Erysipelas of the vesicular variety,* accompanied by the restlessness and sensorium of this remedy, is quickly cured by it. So, also, is *scarlatina.* If we find the skin red, smooth and shiny, with high grade of fever and delirium *Rhus* would not do any good, but *Belladonna* or some remedy having that kind of skin, etc.

Apis, Cantharis, Lachesis, Ailanthus and others have each their peculiar appearance of the skin in these acute exanthemata. Yet, notwithstanding this, it must be *remembered* that in many cases the leading indication for a remedy will not lie in the skin symptoms, but outside of them.

If in *variola* the eruption turns livid and typhoid symptoms supervene we may rely on *Rhus* for a good effect. Probably no remedy is oftener found useful in *herpes zoster* than this.

Rhus is no less valuable in chronic skin troubles than in acute. *Eczemas* of the vesicular type are often cured by it; there is much itching which is not greatly relieved by scratching. In all such cases of course the constitutional symptoms weigh as much as the local. So far as dose is concerned, I have used it both high and low, and find it useful all along the scale, but I have an M. M. potency made upon my own potentizer which has served me so well, and so many times, that I cannot refrain from speaking of it.

BELLADONNA.

All acute inflammatory diseases present prominent head symptoms, pain, red puffed face, throbbing carotids and delirium, and spasms, or jerks and twitchings.

Eyes staring, red, blood-shot and pupils first contracted, then greatly dilated.

Mouth and throat *very dry, red,* sometimes greatly swollen; all mucous surfaces correspondingly dry and hot.

Pains appear suddenly, and after a while disappear as suddenly as they came.

Skin very red and hot, fairly radiates heat; burns the hand touching it, but sweats on covered parts.

Several inflammations which streak out in radii from a center.

Modalities: < after 3 P. M. or after midnight from uncovering, or draft of air, and lying down; > from covering and head high.

Great liability to take cold; sensitive to draft of air, especially when uncovering the head; from having the hair cut *(Hep.)*; tonsils swell after riding in a cold wind *(Acon.)*.

Imagines he sees ghosts, hideous faces, and various insects *(Stram.)*; black animals, dogs and wolves.

Abdomen tender, distended < by least jar, even the bed; obliged to walk with great care for fear of a jar.

Pain in right ileo-cæcal region, < by slightest touch, even the bed covers.

Pressing downwards, as if the contents of abdomen would issue from the vulva; < standing and sitting erect; worse mornings (compare *Lil., Mur., Sep.)*.

Tongue: Red and dry, with red edges and white coating in the middle; papillæ bright and prominent, like scarlatina *(Acon., Ant. t.)*, offensive, putrid taste in throat when eating or drinking, although food tastes natural.

* * * * *

We now come to consider what I call the trio of delirium remedies—*Belladonna, Hyoscyamus* and *Stramonium*. Many other remedies have delirium, but these three deserve to head the list. *Belladonna* may also be called pre-eminently a head remedy. In most complaints where this remedy is indicated head symptoms preponderate. The *blood* all seems to be rushing to the head. *(Amyl nitrite, Glonoine, Melilotus.)* The head is hot while the extremities are cool. The eyes are red and blood-shot. The face is also red, almost purple red. The carotid arteries throb so as to be plainly visible. There is either great pain, pressure or sense of fullness, or an almost stupid condition. The wild, terrible delirium, if present, may be found with pain, or even with no complaint of pain. In delirium the patient "imagines he sees ghosts, hideous faces and animals and insects." Fears all sorts of imaginary things and wants to run away from them; breaks out into fits of laughter or screams and gnashes his teeth; bites or strikes those around him; in short, performs all sorts of violent acts and is controlled with great difficulty. No remedy has more persistently *violent delirium* than *Belladonna.* One of the characteristic features of *Belladonna* in delirium as compared with the other two remedies is the decided evidence already mentioned of a surcharge of blood in the brain. When the throbbing of the carotids, the heat, redness and congestion of face and conjunctiva go away, the delirium subsides in proportion. *Belladonna* may have delirium with pale face as its alternate, but it is the exception. Even the upper lip is congested and swollen.

In inflammations, which *localize, Belladonna* is in the first stage as often the leading remedy as any other. It does not make much difference **where** they localize, whether in head, throat, mammæ or elsewhere, if they come on suddenly, pursue a rapid course, are red, painful and especially throbbing. It is astonishing how many local inflammations, even a carbuncle or boil, will so disturb the general system and circulation, as to produce the general inflammatory fever, with the characteristic head symptoms calling for *Belladonna,* and no less astonishing how this remedy controls the whole condition, both local and general, when indicated. What! exclaims the believer in local applications, give *Belladonna* internally for a boil on the hand or foot? Yes, indeed, not only *Belladonna,* but *Mercurius, Hepar sulphuris, Tarantula Cuben-*

sis, and many others, and you will not have any need for local medication at all. It is only in the first or congestive or active inflammatory stage that this remedy is in place; but, if properly administered then, it will often abort the whole thing and never leave it to finish all its stages, or if not, so modify as to make it comparatively insignificant.

Belladonna is one of our best remedies in the diseases of children, even vieing with *Chamomilla.* They come *suddenly,* almost without warning. This sudden and intense onset of fever is sometimes duplicated in *Cina* cases, but there is helminthiasis in connection with it. Child is well one minute and sick the next, and one very characteristic symptom in these cases is, the child is very hot, with red face and semi-stupor, but every little while starts or *jumps in sleep as if it might go into spasms.* This condition is often found in children and then *Belladonna* is like "oil upon troubled waters." Remember *Belladonna* inflammations localize more than they do in *Aconite.* I drew the difference between these two remedies in inflammations and inflammatory fevers when writing upon *Aconite.* There is no use of confounding them. Some do so; but, in so doing, only exhibit their ignorance.

There are, in every remedy, symptoms of sensation, circumstance, constitution or modality which are peculiar both to diseases and remedies. These symptoms are not always easily accounted for. The attempt to explain them from a pathological standpoint is not always possible or even necessary were it possible. A simple acceptance of them as facts is often more sensible than to wait long to find the often unfindable. To act as a prescriber upon what we know is better than waiting, because we cannot explain or account for it. For instance, it is not easy to tell why "the pains of *Belladonna appear suddenly and after a time disappear as suddenly as they come,"* while those of *Stannum "gradually increase to a great height and as gradually decline,"* or *Sulphuric acid "begin slowly and decline suddenly,"* or *"gradually increase and suddenly cease,"* but so it is, and the acceptance of these facts enables the homœopathic prescriber to cure his patient, whether hé can explain them or not. Guernsey says—"This medicine is particularly applicable, and in fact takes the lead over all others in cases in which *quickness* or *suddenness* of either *sensation or motion* is predominant." To be sure all these symptoms have their pathological explanation if we could give it; but, acting on our law of *Similia,* we can cure our patients and are not left at sea, without chart or compass, because we cannot explain. We know that these symptoms are the natural outcry of the pathological state, and that the administration of a poison which is capable of setting up a similar outcry cures the patient. What else is necessary? Either this is true, or Homœopathy is a humbug.

The simple fact, abundantly proven, that the remedy having the symptoms corresponding to the symptoms of the patient, cures him, no matter what the pathology, where a cure is at all possible, is one of the greatest discoveries of scientific investigation. Long live the name of Hahnemann, the discoverer.

From our description thus far of this remedy you would expect it to be a good one for *congestive headaches,* and so it is, and not only so, but for neuralgic headaches. Throbbing pains, with the already described evidence of congestion of blood to the head. *Belladonna* headaches, whether congestive or neuralgic, are worse on *stooping forward, bending downward,* or *lying down,* anything that takes the patient out of the perpendicular. *"Worse on lying down,"* in fact, seems to be a very reliable general characteristic. The elder Lippe once told me of a case of suspicious enlargement or swelling and pain of the breast of long standing, which, as he expressed it, seemed likely to prove a case for the surgeon (cancer), which was entirely cured by a few doses of *Belladonna,* to which he was guided by this symptom of the pains being so much worse on lying down. Since then I have observed and verified this symptom in many cases of different kinds. I will not stop to give all the symptoms that might be present in *Belladonna* headaches.

No remedy has greater affinity for the throat. The *burning, dryness (Sabadilla), sense of constriction* (constant desire to swallow to relieve the sense of dryness, *Lyssin),* with or without swelling of the palate and tonsils, is sometimes intense. I once witnessed a case of poisoning in which these symptoms were terribly distressing.

There are two very characteristic symptoms in the abdominal region, viz.: *"Tenderness of the abdomen, aggravated by the least jar, in walking, or stepping, or even the bed or chair, upon which she sits or lies";* and *"pressure downward as if the contents of the abdomen would issue through the vulva, < mornings."* This last symptom is found under other remedies, notably *Lilium tigrinum* and *Sepia.* With *Belladonna* there is often associated with this pressure downward a pain in the back *"as if it would break." "Starting and jumping,"* or "twitching in sleep," or on going to sleep is characteristic.

So also is *"sleepy, but cannot sleep,"* and *"moaning during sleep."*

With *Belladonna* the head likes wrapping up or covering, takes cold when it is uncovered or from cutting the hair *(Silicea)*. *(Glonoine;* can't bear hat on.)

Uniform, smooth, shining, scarlet redness of the skin, so hot that it imparts a burning sensation to the hand of one who feels of it, is very characteristic (H. N. Guernsey).

Convulsions with other symptoms of *Belladonna* are very frequently found under this remedy.

I have here endeavored to give an outline of this great remedy. A volume might be profitably written upon its virtues. No one remedy would be more greatly missed than this, if it were to be expunged from our great Materia Medica, but we must leave it here and proceed to notice

HYOSCYAMUS NIGER.

High-grade delirium, similar to that of *Stramonium* and *Belladonna;* alternating with low-grade delirium, with stupor, equal to that of *Opium*. Face pale.

Grasping at flocks, picking the bed clothes and subsultus tendinum.

Persistent cough, worse lying down, relieved on sitting up, especially in elderly people.

Dementia senilis; fears imaginary things, being poisoned, etc.; sees persons and things that are not present; foolish laughter.

General twitching of all the muscles of the body; in spasms or convulsions.

The mania often takes on the lascivious form. The

patient uncovers and exposes himself, sings and talks amorously.

Fears being poisoned; suspicious and jealous.

Constant staring at surrounding objects, self-forgetful (fevers). Pupils dilated; insensible; small objects seem very large. Sordes on teeth; grating the teeth. Alternates well with *Rhus tox.* (fevers).

* * * * *

Hyoscyamus is as delirious as *Belladonna,* but the high grade of delirium alternates with the low. With *Belladonna* the violent form predominates, while the quiet or stupid form is the exception. With *Hyoscyamus* it is just the other way. The stupid muttering form predominates, with occasional outbreaks of the violent form. The face of the *Belladonna* patient is red, that of *Hyoscyamus* pale and sunken. The *Hyoscyamus* patient is weak and the weakness increases. His violent outbreaks of delirium cannot keep up long on account of weakness. This is not so much so with either *Belladonna* or *Stramonium.* The *Hyoscyamus* patients may begin with the violent form or outbreaks of delirium, but they grow more mild and less frequent, and the low or stupid form increases until there is total unconsciousness; so much so that it sometimes becomes difficult to choose between it and *Opium.*

The case takes on typhoid symptoms fast. The tongue gets dry and unwieldy, the sensorium so cloudy that even if you can arouse the patient to answer questions correctly he immediately lapses right into stupor again. This unconscious condition may continue even with the eyes wide open, staring around the room, but seeing nothing but flocks, at which the patient reaches and grasps; *picks the bed clothes,* indistinctly muttering, or not saying a word for hours. The teeth are covered with sordes; the lower jaw drops; stools and urine pass involuntarily; thus presenting the most complete picture of great prostration of mind and body. This is a picture of *Hyoscyamus* as we find it often in typhoid fever, or typhoid pneumonia (where it is the best remedy I know of), scarlatina and other diseases. It is a wonderful remedy, but not of wide range like *Belladonna.*

Hyoscyamus is not only a great remedy in the acute affections of which we have written, but it is also one of the most useful in chronic manias. If acute delirium passes on into the settled form, called mania, this remedy is still one of our chief reliances. It is much oftener of use here than *Belladonna.* Again, if the mania comes on after an acute disease it is still one of our leading remedies. In these forms of mania there are certain very marked symptoms calling for its use, such as, the patient is very **suspicious;** will not take the medicine because he thinks you are trying to *poison* him, or thinks some plot is being laid against him. He is *jealous* of others, or the first cause of the attack is jealousy. Again, the mania often takes on the *lascivious* form. The patient uncovers and exposes himself, sings and talks amorously. *Hyoscyamus* leads all the remedies for this form of mania.

The patient, like the one in acute delirium of this remedy, is liable to alternate between the mild and violent manifestations; at one time so mild and timorous as to hide away from every one, and again so violent that she will attack, beat, fight, scratch, and try to injure anyone within reach.

The *Hyoscyamus* maniac is generally weak, and so this remedy is found particularly adapted to mania consequent upon the *infirmities of age.* Of course it is useful in all ages if indicated by the symptoms.

The nervous manifestations of this remedy are not confined to the cerebral symptoms; but seem to involve the whole system. As H. N. Guernsey says: *"Every muscle in the body twitches, from the eyes to the toes."* This is one of his chief indications for its use in convulsions, whether epileptic or not. The spasms are generally of the clonic, not the tonic order, as in *Nux vomica* or *Strychnia.* Nor are they so violent as those under *Cicuta virosa;* but the *general twitching* is characteristic in convulsions, as is the *subsultus tendinum* in typhoids.

Hyoscyamus is very useful in a form of dry cough which is aggravated *when lying down* and relieved by sitting up. Here, too, it is particularly useful in old people. I have already referred to its great usefulness in pneumonia. I wish to emphasize it, and believe it to be the leading remedy in the typhoid form of the disease. At least it has performed wonders for me.

It is also very useful in scarlatina of the typhoid form, and is complementary to *Rhus tox.* in those cases. I never alternate the two, but if the depressed sensorium and delirium goes beyond the power of *Rhus* to control I suspend the *Rhus* for a day or two and give *Hyoscyamus,* which will so improve the case that *Rhus* may again come into use and carry it to a successful termination. This is the only alternation I am ever guilty of. It is like that of Hahnemann when he alternated *Bryonia* and *Rhus* in fevers.

STRAMONIUM.

Wildly delirious, with red face and great *loquacity*. **Loquacity**.

Pupils widely dilated; wants light and company; fears to be alone; wants hand held.

One side paralyzed, the other convulsed.

Awakens with a shrinking look; frightened; afraid of the first object seen.

Painlessness with most complaints *(Opium)*. Jerks the head suddenly from pillow in spasms.

* * * * *

The last of the trio is pre-eminently the high-grade delirium remedy, differs from the other two chiefly in the degree of *intensity*.

The raving is something awful. Singing, laughing, grinning; whistling, screaming, praying piteously or swearing hideously, and above all remedies **loquacious.** Again the patient throws himself into all shapes corresponding to his changeable delirium, crosswise, lengthwise, rolled up like a ball, or stiffened out by turns, or, especially, repeatedly *jerks up suddenly his head from the pillow.* Things look crooked or oblique to him.

The whole inner mouth as if raw; the tongue after a while may become stiff or paralyzed. Stools loose, blackish, smelling like carrion, or *no stool or urine.* Later there may be complete loss of sight, hearing, and speech with dilated, immovable pupils and drenching sweat which brings no relief, and death must soon close the scene unless *Stramonium* helps them out.

By way of still further comparison *Stramonium* is the most widely **loquacious.**

Hyoscyamus is the most insensibly **stupid.**

Belladonna in this respect stands half way between.

Stramonium, throws himself about, jerking head from pillow.

Hyoscyamus, twitches, picks and reaches, otherwise lying pretty still.

Belladonna, starts or jumps when falling into or awaking from sleep.

All have times of wanting to escape.

The same state of mind and sensorium is found in chronic and acute manias. I have cured several such cases. One was a lady about thirty years of age, who was overheated in the sun, on an excursion. She was a member in good standing in the Presbyterian church, but imagined herself lost and called me in six mornings in succession to see her die. Lost, lost, lost, eternally lost, was her theme, begging minister, doctor and everybody to pray for, and with her. Talked night and day about it. I had to shut her up in her room alone for she would not sleep a wink or let anyone else.

She imagined her head was as big as a bushel and had me examine her legs, which she insisted were as large as a church. After treating her several weeks with *Glonoine, Lach., Natrum carb.* and other remedies on the **cause** as the basis of the prescription, without the least amelioration of her condition, I gave her *Stramonium,* which covered her *symptoms,* and in twenty-four hours every vestige of that mania was gone. But for the encouragement I gave the husband that I could cure her she would have been sent to the Utica Asylum, where her friends had been advised to send her by the allopaths. I gave her the sixth dilution or potency.

I cured a case just as bad since then with the C. M. potency. I could relate other experiences, just as remarkable, cured with this remedy, but why do so?

Aside from the uses of the remedy, which are the main ones, I will mention now a few symptoms that have been found very reliable guides:

Staggers in the dark or with eyes closed.

Eyes wide open; prominent, brilliant pupils widely dilated.

Desires light and company.

Face hot and red, cheeks circumscribed.

Convulsions, aggravated in bright light.

Mouth and throat dry. *(Bell.)*

Fear of water and aversion to all fluids.

Metrorrhagia, with characteristic mind symptoms.

Great pain in hip disease, or abscesses.

One side paralyzed, the other convulsed. *(Bell.)*

Entire absence of pain. *(Opium.)*

LACHESIS.

Feels very sad and despondent; < after sleeping, or in the morning.

Enemy of all constriction; must loosen everything (neck, chest, throat, abdomen, etc.).

Left-sided affections generally, especially throat, chest, ovaries.

Inflamed parts very tender to touch and of bluish or dark color.

Great weakness and trembling; tongue trembles when protruding it; catches under the teeth (lower).

Blood decomposes, breaks down, hæmorrhages; blood

uncoagulable; ulcers and even slight wounds bleed profusely.

Modalities: < at climacteric; touch, constriction or pressure, sun-heat, after sleeping; > after discharges (suppressed or delayed discharges).

Many complaints connected with the menopause: hot flushes, hot sweats, burning vertex headaches, hæmorrhoids, hæmorrhages.

Great physical and mental exhaustion; trembling in whole body; would constantly sink from weakness.

* * * * *

To Dr. Constantine Hering belongs the honor of introducing and developing the wonderful medicinal properties of this snake poison. If he had never done anything beside this for medicine, the world would owe him an everlasting debt of gratitude. It alone would immortalize him. All this, and more; notwithstanding, Chas. Hempel wrote in his first volume of Materia Medica: "In spite of every effort to the contrary, the conviction has gradually forced itself upon my mind that the pretended pathogenesis of *Lachesis,* which has emanated from Dr. Hering's otherwise meritorius and highly praiseworthy efforts, is a great delusion, and that with the exception of the poisonous effects with which this publication is abundantly mingled the balance of the symptoms are unreliable." Hempel modified his views somewhat, I think, in later editions.

Now, it is interesting to note that in Allen's Encyclopædia of Pure Materia Medica, the verified, and especially the black-typed symptoms, almost all of them, are verifications of provings made with the 30th potency. It is also significant that the provings of Hahnemann's polychrest remedies, mostly made with the potencies, are among the most useful and reliable we have to-day. Some have sought to destroy confidence in the provings of all remedies which are made with the 30th potencies and upwards; not only that, but in their power to cure even when the provings were made with cruder preparations. With us, who know the value of these potencies, all such efforts only excite pity. But many who do not know are misled and prejudiced so as to never dare to test for themselves. To all such we say take no man's ipse dixit, but prove all things, "hold fast that which is true."

Lachesis is a remedy of wide range of action. It has an alternate action on the mind and sensorium, that of excitation and depression. Illustrative of the former are the following symptoms: "Quick comprehension, mental activity with almost prophetic perception, ecstasy, a kind of trance. Exceptional loquacity, with rapid change of subjects; jumps abruptly from one idea to another." This kind of excitation may be found in acute chronic complaints; in the delirium of fevers, or in mania of a settled form. On the side of depression occur: "Weakness of memory; makes mistakes in writing; confusion as to time. Delirium at night; muttering; drowsy; red face; slow, difficult speech and dropped jaw. Feels extremely sad, depressed, unhappy and distressed in mind," and this condition is very apt to be worse on awaking in the morning, or indeed after any sleep, day or night. "Chronic complaints from depressing cause, like long-lasting grief or sorrow." This depressed side of the remedy may also be found in both acute and chronic complaints. Again these opposite conditions may be found alternating in the same person, and a notable fact is that the alternations are extreme. Of course the causes of these conditions of mind and sensorium are varied, but we will often find them in *old topers,* subjects of *broken-down constitution,* and in the troubles incident to the *climacteric age.* Such cases are subject to sudden attacks of giving away of strength, fainting, vertigo from rush of blood to the head causing apoplectic seizure, or opposite symptoms arising from sudden anæmia of the brain. In short, the circulation in *Lachesis* subjects is very uncertain. This is what makes it so valuable in sudden flushes during the climacteric period.

Lachesis has some prominent head symptoms where no other remedy can take its place. It is one of our best remedies for sun headaches; of course it does not compare with *Glonoine* for the immediate effects of sunstroke, but does come in well after the first effects are overcome by that remedy. The patient is troubled with headache every time he is exposed to the sun's heat, and the trouble has become chronic. *(Nat. carb.)*

This is another characteristic symptom, namely weight or *pressure on the vertex. (Cactus, Glonoine, Menyanthes.)* This is found mostly in women suffering at the menopause, and coupled with it in such cases there is sometimes burning on the vertex. *Sulphur* has this symptom, but if it occurred at the menopause the remedy would oftener be found in *Lachesis,* unless, indeed, there were some marked psoric complication. *Lachesis* has a variety of headaches, but I know of only two characteristics that have been of very much value to me in prescribing for them, namely, with the headache *very pale face,* and the patient *sleeps into the headache;* dreads to go to sleep because she awakens with such a distressing headache. These two are very valuable indications, otherwise I would expect to get my indications outside of the headache itself. "Headache extending into the nose, comes mostly in acute catarrh, especially when the discharge has been suppressed or stops after sleep. This kind of headache is often found in hay fever, with frequent and violent paroxysms of sneezing. Now if the hay fever paroxysms of sneezing are decidedly worse after sleeping, even in the daytime, *Lachesis* 2000th may stop the whole business for the season." Being an old hay fever subject myself, I am authority on that statement.

We now come to the action of *Lachesis* on the alimentary tract; first the gums are often swollen and spongy, easily bleeding; when this is found *Lachesis* often follows *Mercury* well. If the gums turn purple the indication is strengthened for *Lachesis*. One of the most characteristic symptoms of *Lachesis* is found in the tongue, especially in diseases of a typhoid type; namely, *puts the tongue out with great difficulty; it is very dry; trembles and catches under lower teeth.* The tongue trembles and is protruded with difficulty under *Gelsemium,* but it is not so dry as in *Lachesis.* This is a sign of great weakness, but in *Gelsemium* it occurs in the very beginning of the fever, while in *Lachesis* it comes later. There is bad odor from the mouth in *Lachesis,* and it may be very dry throughout; or there may be an abundant accumulation of tenacious mucus. Here it again resembles *Mercury.* *Lachesis* is one of our best remedies for sore mouth in the last stage of consumption. This is sometimes a very distressing symptom, and relief for it is often very difficult to find. If *Lachesis* should relieve it, my experience has been that the patients are also greatly relieved in other ways; so much so, indeed, that they think that they are, after all, going to get well. This brings me to notice what I believe I have not spoken of before, that where a cure is no longer possible, and temporary relief is the only thing left, we have the best means of giving it in the homœopathically indicated remedy. Narcotics, counter irritants, so-called tonics, stimulants, etc., do not and cannot compare with the simillimum (if properly administered) in smoothing the pathway to the inevitable termination. *Lachesis* has won its chiefest laurels in affections of the throat.

"Throat and neck sensitive to slightest touch, or external pressure (Sepia); everything about throat distresses, even the weight of the bed covers." This is very characteristic. Another peculiarity is that empty swallowing, or swallowing of saliva or liquids, aggravates a great deal more than swallowing of solids. The pains in the throat run up into the ears. There is much mucus in fauces, with painful hawking. In tonsillitis and diphtheria, swelling of tonsils begins on left side and extends to the right *(Sabadilla).* The pains are aggravated by hot drinks (reverse, *Sabadilla).* All these symptoms are peculiar to *Lachesis,* and are all apt to be very much worse after sleep. In old quinsy subjects, where the trouble always began on the left side, I have often not only aborted the attack, but cured the predisposition thereto.

Sometimes the throat assumes a gangrenous appearance, but if the other indications are present it is an additional indication for its use. *Lachesis* is always one of the first remedies to be thought of in any disease, when it seems inclined to spend its main force in the throat, such as *typhoid fever, pneumonia, scarlatina,* etc.

If the *skin turns purple or bluish,* as if mortification were impending, there is no remedy like it. Not only is *Lachesis* an unusually efficacious remedy for these acute throat troubles, but for those of a chronic form, and the same symptoms are present, even in syphilitic throat troubles. We have placed great stress upon the great sensitiveness of the throat to all touch or pressure; but this does not end it, for, as Lilienthal expresses it, *Lachesis* is the *great enemy of all constriction.* "The pit of stomach sore to the touch, or even to pressure of clothes." "Cannot bear any pressure about the hypochondria." In the abdomen there is "Painful distention, flatulence, which is very annoying, can bear no pressure; the surface nerves are sensitive." "Is obliged to wear clothes, especially about stomach, very loose; they cause uneasiness; even in bed, obliged to loosen and pull up night dress to avoid pressure; dare not lay the arm across the abdomen on account of pressure." "Uterus does not bear contact; has to be relieved of all pressure; frequently lifts the clothes; they cause an uneasiness in the abdomen, even with no tenderness." "Larynx sensitive to least touch, which causes suffocation and feeling of lump in the throat." "During heat, as of an orgasm of blood, he is obliged to loosen clothes about the neck; sensation as though they hindered the circulation of blood, with a kind of suffocative feeling." "Intolerance of tight neck bands." I could no better express the value of this symptom, or great modality of *Lachesis, aggravation from pressure or constrictions,* than by quoting entire from

Guiding Symptoms the above. It does not seem, after such an array of oft-verified symptoms, that more need be said to impress this upon the memory and confidence of any physician. Now, the why of this almost invariable aggravation from pressure of *Lachesis* and almost as invariable amelioration from the same of *Bryonia* I leave for those to explain who pretend to be able to do so. It is, however, another proof of the value of modalities.

Lachesis has some peculiar symptoms of stool and anus. There is an urging, or rather a pressing down, in the rectum, but it is worse when he attempts a stool; hurts so that he must desist. It feels as if the anus were closed. This is somewhat like the constant or rather frequent, though ineffectual, urging to stool of *Nux vomica;* or like the painful constriction of *Lycopodium,* which either prevents stool, or follows after an incomplete and unsatisfactory one. Another marked symptom is that the stools are often *very offensive,* whether formed or not. Then, under *Lachesis,* we have hæmorrhages from the bowels, of decomposed blood, which occur mostly during the course of exhausting, acute diseases, like typhoid. Guernsey gave this: "Flakes of decomposed blood, having form and appearance of perfectly charred wheat straw, in larger or shorter flat pieces; portions more or less ground up." I have met such cases and *Lachesis* was very efficacious, not only in changing the character of the stool, but bringing about general improvement, ultimating in perfect recovery.

This remedy is often of great use in that very common malady, hæmorrhoids; and here you have the constricted feeling, whether the piles are external or blind, and sometimes a beating or throbbing, or as the patient will perhaps express it, a sensation of "little hammers" beating in the rectum. All these symptoms and many more show the affinity of this remedy for the anus and rectum, as they do also its power over disease of the whole alimentary tract.

This is also one of our best remedies in diseases of the female generative organs. In the first place it is eminently an ovarian remedy, and seems to choose by preference the left ovary. It is of use in simple ovarian neuralgia, and from that to actual tumors or even cancer of the left ovary; or the trouble begins in the left and goes to right ovary. (Reverse, *Lycopodium.)* But we may have neuralgia, swelling, induration, suppuration, tumors or cancer of one or both ovaries. Its action in uterine troubles is also very marked. Here is a condition, as expressed in Guiding Symptoms, that I have often verified during climaxis: *"Pains in uterine region increase at times more and more till relieved by flow of blood from vagina; after a few hours or days, the same again, and so on."*

In these cases you almost always have the intolerance of least contact or pressure over the uterine region so characteristic of this drug. The womb prolapses, is at times persistently congested, and obstinate uterine hæmorrhages repeatedly occur. There are hot flashes, hot vertex, pale face and fainting, uterine displacements of various kinds, and deranged capillary circulation, all so common in females at the menopause and especially hæmorrhages. (See also *Crotalus* and *Kreosote.)* Probably there are not three remedies in the whole Materia Medica so often indicated in troubles connected with this period, as *Lachesis.* (*Kreosote,* post-climacteric diseases.) It is often of great use in cancer of either the breasts or uterus. In either case the cancer puts on a bluish or purplish appearance, and if open or fungoid bleeds easily, a dark, decomposed blood. In case of bleeding, the pains and suffering, as in the case of uterine hæmorrhage, are temporarily relieved by it. We would be greatly crippled in the treatment of these various ovarian and uterine troubles without *Lachesis.*

The respiratory organs and chest also come under the influence of this drug. Paralysis of the vocal chords, causing loss of voice; *larynx is sensitive to least touch;* it causes suffocation; it is one of our best remedies in desperate cases of croup, where the child gets worse in sleep; *seems to sleep into it.* Spasm of the glottis; sensation of something running from neck to larynx, stopping the breath. It has great shortness of breath when walking, especially in old topers and in heart affections, when this condition is always the guide to its use. *"The least thing coming near the mouth or nose interferes with breathing; tears off the collar or everything about the neck, throat or chest, because it suffocates."*

Asthma with the same symptoms, has sudden flushes of heat or orgasm of blood; must loosen clothes to prevent suffocation; threatened paralysis of the heart or lungs; dry hacking cough, aggravated by touching throat or larynx, also *cough during sleep,* without awakening or being conscious of it. Here it often cures very obstinate cases of cough after *Chamomilla* has failed, which also has this symptom. For the short dry cough sympathetic with heart troubles, *Lachesis* is often useful. Cough with pain in anus, or stitches in pile tumors. One of our best remedies in *typhoid pneumonia* or *typhoid fever* with lung complications.

Now look out for the *Lachesis* tongue in these cases. *Lachesis* is also one of our most useful remedies in heart troubles, acute or chronic, the peculiar suffocation, cough and aggravation from constrictions being the guiding symptoms.

No remedy more profoundly impresses the nervous system than this. In the first place it causes trembling, not from fright or excitement, but from extreme weakness. In this it resembles *Gelsemium;* both have great trembling of the tongue on trying to protrude it. With both remedies the whole body trembles; but with *Lachesis* she feels faint, as if she must sink right down. This great prostration is both mental and physical, and she does not improve from rest or sleep, but on the contrary *is worse in the morning after sleeping.* With this prostration there are often pain or other troubles with the heart; nausea, pale face and vertigo. Now if this thing goes on the next stage supervenes and paralysis is the end of it. The paralysis is generally left-sided, as are the majority of complaints of *Lachesis,* which is pre-eminently a *left-sided remedy.* This paralysis may come on as a result of apoplexy or cerebral exhaustion; if the latter, there is still great hope of a perfect cure by a judicious use of *Lachesis.* Of course if the lesion is too extensive in apoplexy, and the extravasation of blood too great, there is little hope; but some apparently most desperate cases do recover even then. It is recommended in epilepsy and locomotor ataxia, but I have never seen good effects from it.

There is, however, another place in which I have seen it accomplish much and that is in the languor, weariness and prostration from hot weather. The head not only aches, but the whole body seems prostrated by **sun heat.** *(Antim. crud., Gelsemium, Glonoine, Natrum carb., Natrum m.)*

Worse after sleep, or rather the patient *sleeps into an aggravation,* is a genuine characteristic of this remedy, no matter what the enemies of *Lachesis* say of it. On this line there is one particular symptom to which I wish to call attention, *i. e.,* "As soon as the patient falls asleep, the breathing stops." This is as Hering expresses it. I have oftener found it this way; the patient cannot go clear off into sleep, because just on the verge of it the breath stops and he wakens catching for breath. This is often found in heart troubles, functional or organic, and is very distressing. *Grindelia robusta* has a similar symptom. (Also *Digitalis.)*

I once had a case of very obstinate constipation in an old syphilitic case. He was at last taken with very severe attacks of colic. The pains seemed to extend all through the abdomen, and always came on at night. After trying various remedies until I was discouraged, for he "got no better fast," he let drop this expression, "Doctor, if I could only keep awake all the time, I would never have another attack." I looked askance at him. "I mean," said he, "that I sleep into the attack, and waken in it." I left a dose of *Lachesis* 200. He never had another attack of the pain, and his bowels became perfectly regular from that day and remained so. I could give more cases where this symptom has led me to the cure of ailments of different kinds. It is enough to say that I have no hesitation in adding my testimony to that of others as to the value of this symptom. I think I have said enough about the different symptoms of *Lachesis* to indicate that it is one of the most useful remedies in typhoid fever. I will only add here that it is generally in the second or third week of the disease that it is found indicated. This is one of the differences between it and *Gelsemium*. For the trembling and weakness of *Gelsemium* come early, and if recognized then *Gelsemium* can abort the disease at once. Of course the sensorium, tongue, mouth, throat, abdominal and stool symptoms already spoken of, especially the sleep symptom, help to decide the choice between *Lachesis* and other remedies.

Now upon the tissues. We have swelling on all parts of the body, and one of the most characteristic conditions is the color of them. They are *bluish* verging onto black. (*Tarantula Cub., Anthracinum.*) I never see a swelling of that color but *Lachesis* immediately comes to my mind, and then if I find that they cannot bear to have them *touched*, they are so sensitive, even a poultice is unbearable, because it is so heavy, that settles it. I give *Lachesis* and am seldom disappointed. The blood decomposes, or, as is sometimes said, "breaks down," becomes uncoagulable. This often occurs in typhoid fever, and is of course very serious. The bleeding is easily started, and is very persistent. There seems to be a tendency to hæmorrhagic trouble, so we find *Lachesis* one of our best remedies in purpura hæmorrhagica. Ulcers and wounds bleed profusely; even "small wounds bleed much;" wounds easily become gangrenous. Here *Lachesis* is capable of doing great good. Cancers turned bluish or black, bleed much and often, and burn; blood appears in the urine in many affections, indicating its broken down condition.

We find ourselves drawn out to a greater length on this

truly polychrest remedy than we had anticipated when we began writing. We have also found it a much more useful remedy than we had anticipated from our impressions of it when reading Charles Hempel (for whom we have great respect) in our studenthood. It wears well for those who use it in the 30th potency and upwards. Don't forget that *Lachesis* is pre-eminently a left-sided remedy, as *Lycopodium* is a right-sided one. Left-sided paralysis, ovarian affections, throat troubles, lung troubles, headaches, etc., all make us think of this remedy first because of its positiveness in this respect. Of course, if the other symptoms were present in right-sided affections we would not hesitate to use it. *Lachesis* is often a remedy of great value in skin affections; in scarlatina maligna, black measles, erysipelas, smallpox, malignant boils, furuncles, carbuncles, chronic ulcers, bed sores, fungus hæmatodes, etc. In all these and many other affections appearing upon the surface, the characteristic dark blue color is present, or we need not expect much from this remedy. So far as stages of life and constitution are concerned, I have found it efficacious in all ages and temperaments. But perhaps oftener indicated in thin than in fat people.

Now we bid our old and tried friend an affectionate good-by for a time, and heartily recommend all who have not done so to seek his acquaintance.

NAJA TRIPUDIANS.

Here is a blood relative of *Lachesis,* if serpent poisons may be called relatives, and according to the symptoms arising from the bite of the serpent it ought to be equally valuable as a curative, but it has not yet been found so. Why not? On referring to Allen's *Encyclopædia* we find twenty-nine provers, poisonings and all, for *Lachesis*, and forty-five for *Naja*. Of course, *Lachesis* has been longest in use; but has the difference in time been sufficient to account for the very great difference in utility? Another thing is noticeable; the provings of *Lachesis* were made mostly with potencies as high as the 30th, while those of *Naja* are almost all with the lowest preparation or the crude poison from the bite of the serpent. Does this account for it?

We also notice on referring to the same authority that all the most marked verifications are of symptoms produced by the provings of the 30th of *Lachesis*. Does this indicate that *Naja* must be proven in the potencies to develop its most efficient powers? *Naja* has been found of very decided use in affections of the heart, especially *weak heart (Nux vomica,* tired feeling); diphtheria, where there is impending heart failure or paralysis. Dyspnœa and prostration from weak heart, sympathetic cough in organic diseases with weak heart action. (Dry cough, sympathetic in heart affections, *Spongia.)* Palpitation and bad feeling in heart, < walking. In these troubles, as well as in chronic weakness of heart, there is no doubt of the value of *Naja*. Constantly dwells on suicide like *Aurum*. But further than this I do not know of very many marked successes from its use. Nevertheless, I feel convinced that with further proving and investigation, along the same line as *Lachesis*, it may rival if not outshine it.

CROTALUS HORRIDUS.

Here is another snake poison which, although like *Naja* has been proven only in the low preparations, has a better clinical record. Yet it lacks the clear-cut indications of *Lachesis.* It has shown enough, however, to indicate that it is a remedy of great value. It seems, so far, to have shown its greatest usefulness in diseases which result in a decomposition of the blood of such a character as to cause hæmorrhages from *every outlet of the body (Acetic acid);* even the sweat is bloody. This occurs in the lower fevers of hot climates, such as the bilious remittent fevers, typhoids, and that dread scourge of tropical climates, yellow fever. It is also the chief remedy in diphtheria when the profuse epistaxis occurs which marks many cases of a malignant type. In hæmorrhages of the nose in an old man of broken down constitution, where none of the remedies usually applied did the least good, *Crotalus* acted promptly and no doubt saved the man's life. This was a patient of my own, and, although he had frequent attacks before, he never had another after the *Crotalus.* As would be expected with such a remedy, there is *great prostration* at such bleedings. *Crotalus is right-sided.*

Malignant jaundice is set down as an indication for *Crotalus,* but the yellowness of the skin, so characteristic of *Crotalus,* is after all, I imagine, more of hæmatic than hepatic origin; yet there may be an element of both, as hepatic troubles are so common in hot latitudes where *Crotalus* has gained its greatest laurels.

Crotalus richly deserves proving in the potencies in order to bring out its finer characteristics.

KALI CARBONICUM.

Stitching pains, very characteristic.

Pain in lower right chest through to back.

Anæmia with bloating, especially upper eyelids, which hang down like a bag of water.

Backache, sweat, weakness very great; drops down in chair.

Flatulence great; everything turns to gas.

Heart weak, irregular, intermits.

Modalities: < at 3 to 4 A. M.

After loss of fluids or of vitality, particularly in the anæmic.

Asthma, relieved when sitting up or bending forward, or by rocking *(Ars.)*; worse from 2 to 4 A. M.

Backache, before and during menses.

Complementary to *Carbo vegetabilis.*

* * * * *

This remedy, like some others, finds its leading symptom in the character of its pains. It leads all the remedies for **stitching pains.** *Bryonia* stands next, but there is a very marked difference. The stitching pains of *Bryonia* come on with every movement, and only exceptionally when quiet, while those of *Kali carb.* come on independently of movement. Again, the stitching pains of *Bryonia* are oftenest located in serous membranes, while those of *Kali carb.* are found anywhere and everywhere, and in almost every tissue, *even* to the teeth. One of the favorite localities, however, for this remedy is in the *lower right chest.* This sharp stitching pain is likely to *run right through to the back.* If in pneumonia or pleuro-pneumonia your *Bryonia* has failed when you thought it indicated, and further examination reveals that the stitching pains come on independently of the respiratory movement, *Kali carb.* often helps, and follows well after *Bryonia.* Often the fact is, that *Kali carb.* was all the time the remedy and ought to have been given first. Now, these stitching pains of *Kali carb.* are not by any means confined to the right chest, but we may find them in the left, especially in pleuro-pneumonia, peri- or endocarditis. Remember, also, *Mercurius vivus* in these *lower right-chest pains.* If there should be present at the same time sweat without relief, and the mercurial mouth and tongue, neither *Bryonia* nor *Kali carb.* are "in it."

Another kind of case in which this remedy has achieved signal success, being indicated by the stitching pains, is puerperal fever.

The pains are so sudden and so sharp as to make the patient cry out loudly, and then they are gone. *Kali carb.* has saved some desperate cases of this kind. But it makes no particular difference where the disease is located, if these stitching pains are present, *Kali carb.* should not be forgotten. We cannot too strongly emphasize this.

Kali carbonicum exerts a profound influence over the blood-making processes. The blood lacks red corpuscles. The patient is anæmic, with great debility, skin watery or milky white. This condition is often found with young ladies at the age of puberty. They do not seem to be able to menstruate because of the poor quality of blood and general weakness. They incline to bloat, particularly in face, around eyes and especially upper eyelids, and have much pain and weakness in the lumbar region as well as general weakness. *Kali carb.* is in such cases sometimes successful after *Ferrum* or [illegible] have been wrongly prescribed.

This anæmic condition is also found at the [illegible] and in old age, when the same dropsical tenden[illegible]pear, and the same **characteristic bag-like swellin[illegible]** rather bloating, in the *upper eyelids appears.* In all th[illegible] cases you will generally, or often, at least, find what is called "weak heart." The heart action is irregular or intermittent from very weakness in correspondence with the general muscular weakness. One of the characteristic symptoms which makes us think of *Kali carb.* in these cases is the constant backache of such a nature that the patient feels all the time that the back and legs **must give out.** She drops into a chair or throws herself on the bed completely exhausted. This aching often extends into the hips and down into the gluteal muscles. Patient sweats easily. Farrington says: "This particular sweat, backache and weakness as a combination is not found under any other remedy."

I have already spoken of this remedy somewhat while writing of its stitching pains as an indication for its use in diseases of the chest, but I did not there do it full justice. It is not only a great remedy for pneumonia, pleurisy and heart troubles, as there spoken of, but goes much further and becomes very useful in incipient and even with advanced cases of phthisis pulmonalis. I have seen a case pronounced incurable by several old experienced and skillful physicians, Dr. T. L. Brown among them, get well under a dose once in eight days of *Kali carb.* The disease was located mainly in the lower right lung, with profuse expectoration of matter of pus-like appearance, pulse 120, greatly emaciated, no appetite, and quite a large

13he lung. This man is still alive (twenty-five c-er), hale and hearty. Such service from any y makes a man fall in love with it. There is a *time* acteristic for this remedy which is very valuable in est affections, viz., *aggravation at* 3 A. M. It may be found in cough, consumption, hydrothorax, asthma, and ropsies attending heart disease. The father-in-law of Dr. T. L. Brown, an anæmic old man, was apparently near his end with hydrothorax and general dropsy. Dr. Brown was a skillful prescriber, but in this case had utterly failed to even relieve. In consultation with Dr. Sloan, after carefully reviewing the case, the fact appeared, through the daughter of the patient, who had been his nurse all the time, that all his symptoms were aggravated at 3 A. M. Now *Kali carb.* 200 was given, and with such miraculous results that in an incredibly short time the old man was well and never had a return of that trouble. He lived for several years after, and, finally, did not die of dropsy at all. The day of miracles is not past yet. Hahnemannian Homœopathy performs them still.

I cannot persuade myself to leave this remedy yet, although I have given its chief uses.

I must call attention still further, even at the risk of repeating somewhat, to some very important symptoms. In regard to the nervous system I have already spoken of the *great debility* which I have called *muscular debility,* but there is a weakened condition of the nerves which renders them very sensitive which is well described in the symptoms found in the Materia Medica. "Very easily frightened, shrieks about imaginary appearances; *cannot bear to be touched;* starts when touched ever so lightly, especially on the feet." These are valuable indications for *Kali carb.* *Then don't forget the "bag-like œdematous swelling in the upper eyelids."* It goes with many affections and is invaluable as a guiding symptom. "Sticking pain in the throat (pharynx), as if a fishbone were sticking in it" (see *Hepar sulphur., Dolichos, Nitric acid* and *Argentum nitricum).*

"Great sensitiveness of epigastric region, externally." "Stomach distended, sensitive, feels as if it would burst." "Excessive flatulency, everything he eats or drinks appears to be converted into gas." "Fullness, heat and great distention in abdomen immediately after eating a little." "Abdomen distended with wind after eating." All these stomach and abdomen symptoms indicate the value of this remedy in dyspeptic conditions. They make us think of *Carbo vegetabilis, China officinalis* and *Lycopodium clavatum,* but remember *Kali carb.* and that it is especially adapted to *broken down, aged people who are anæmic. "Sitting up, leaning forward,* relieves in chest affections." The patient is also aggravated by lying on the affected side. Don't forget this, for it may enable you to choose between it and *Bryonia,* which has the reverse.

Now in what I have written I do not pretend to have told all, and if I thought that any young physician would be led to rely alone upon this work of mine or be led away from thorough study of the Materia Medica instead of to it I would stop writing.

KALI BICHROMICUM.

Affections of the mucous membranes with discharge of tough, stringy, adherent mucus, which can be drawn out into long strings.

Formation of jelly-like mucus on mucous membranes.

Round deep ulcers, as if cut out with a punch.

Diphtheritic membranes on mucous surfaces.

Migratory pains, which appear and disappear suddenly.

Pains appear in small spots, which can be covered by a silver dollar or the point of the finger, especially in the sick headache, which is preceded by blindness.

Yellow coating at base of the tongue; or dry, smooth, glazed, cracked tongue.

Rheumatism alternating with dysentery or diarrhœa.

Gastric complaints; bad effects of beer; loss of appetite; weight in pit of stomach; flatulence.

Nose; pressing pain in root of nose; discharge of "clinkers," plugs.

* * * * *

"Affections of any mucous membrane with discharges of tough, stringy, adherent mucus, which can be drawn out into long strings." No remedy has this more prominently than this one. *Hydrastis* comes near to it, and *Lyssin* may approach it when from the mouth or throat; also *Iris versicolor.*

But *Kali bich.* produces and cures this kind of discharge from nose, mouth, fauces, pharynx, larynx, trachea, bronchi, vagina and uterus.

And the action of the drug does not stop here but goes on to the formation of tough membrane, on the same surfaces. Again it causes and cures ulcerations of the mucous membranes. These ulcers are peculiar, *"deep as if cut with a punch, edges regular."* I remember one case of years ago in which such ulcers appeared in the throat of a woman. One had eaten up through the soft palate into the posterior nares, and the whole palate looked as though it would be destroyed by the ulcerative process if not speedily checked. The case had a syphilitic look to me and had been under the treatment of two old school physicians for a long time. I gave *Kali bich.* 30th, and to say that I was astonished at the effect (for it was in my early practice) is putting it mildly, for the ulcers healed so rapidly, and her general condition, which was very bad, correspondingly improved, that in three weeks from that time she was well to all appearance and never had any return of the trouble afterwards, or for years, at least as long as I knew her. I forgot to state that she also had the stringy discharge, though not so profuse as I have often seen in other cases.

I once cured a dog that had a sore mouth and throat, from which the saliva hung in strings, and dragged on the ground as he staggered along. People who saw him said he was mad, but I think not, as he did not snap or bite or have suffocating spasms.

Kali bichromicum is one of our sheet anchors in the treatment of disease of the mucous membrane of the nose. Not only in inflammations of an acute character, which are attended with stringy discharges, but also of a chronic kind known as "chronic catarrh." In these cases the patient often complains of much pressure at the root of the nose *(Sticta pulm.)*, and especially if an habitual discharge becomes suddenly suppressed. *Slugs and clinkers* form in the nose, which form again and again after removal. Sometimes there discharge tough green masses or hard plugs. This process of chronic inflammation may go on from bad to worse, until ulceration sets in to such an extent that the whole septum may ulcerate away. I have known a case in which the apparently "punched

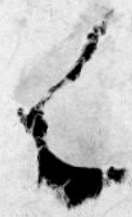

out" ulcers ate a hole right through the septum. This may be syphilitic or not. If in syphilitic cases the destructive process should attack the bones *Kali bich.* may still be of use, though I should expect to be obliged to resort to *Aurum met.* or some more deeply acting remedy.

I have likewise found in those troublesome cases of chronic post-nasal catarrh, where the dropping back into the throat is stringy, or those crusty or pluggy formations occur, this to be a good remedy, and it has gained me some fast friends.

In its formation of membranes in the throat it is as positive as any other remedy, and when the membrane extends downward into the larynx, causing membranous croup, I believe no remedy excels it. I have with it cured many cases of diphtheritic croup, and of late years never give it below the 30th potency, because abundant experience has convinced me that it does better than the low triturations.

Kali bichromicum has been of use in the treatment of stomach troubles. The vomiting is often of the ropy character, and here also, as in nose, mouth and throat, we may have formed "round ulcers." But short of actual ulceration we have a form of dyspepsia, in which this remedy is very useful. It is often found in drunkards, especially *beer drunkards.* There is great weight in the stomach, fullness, a distress *immediately after eating* (like *Nux moschata),* but not like *Nux vomica,* which comes on two or three hours after, nor like *Anacardium,* which also comes on two or three hours after eating, and then the pain continues until he *eats again, which relieves.*

There are two appearances of the tongue which may be present in conjunction with these stomach troubles; one

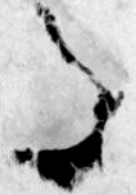

is a yellow coating at the base *(Mercurius prot.* and *Natrum phos.)*, the other a dry smooth glazed or red cracked tongue. This latter tongue is found more often in connection with dysentery in which *Kali bich.* has sometimes done good service.

There is one kind of discharge which comes from mucous membranes of which I have not yet written, "jelly-like mucus." *(Aloe socotrina.)* It may come from nose, posterior nares, vagina or anus. This is especially found in dysentery where the stools have by some other remedy changed from an appearance "like scrapings" to the jelly-like form. Of course leucorrhœas of both the ropy and jelly-like variety come under this remedy and many fine cures have resulted from its use. It is no less so in affections of the respiratory organs, in coughs, croup, bronchitis, asthma, and even in consumption. The chromic acid element in this combination of *Kali* seems responsible for the ropy mucus, as no other *Kali* has it in any such degree.

There are a few more points about this remedy that ought not to be omitted. The pains are peculiar. They appear in **small spots,** which can be covered with the point of a finger. This is markedly so with the pains in the head. In sick headache often so. Farrington says: "There are quite a number of remedies having blind headache, but *Kali bichromicum* is the best of them." The blindness comes on before the headache; then, as the headache begins, the blindness disappears. (See *Iris versicolor* and *Natrum mur.)* Then the pain settles in **a small spot** and is very intense. Again, the pains of *Kali bichromicum* appear and disappear suddenly. This is like *Belladonna.* Then, again, they fly from one place to another like *Pulsatilla.* There are five remedies having markedly wandering or erratic pains, viz.: *Kali bichromicum, Kali sulphuricum, Pulsatilla, Lac caninum* and *Manganum aceticum.* *Kali bichromicum* does not stay as long in a place as *Pulsatilla* does, nor is there so much disposition to swell. *Kali sulphuricum* is most like *Pulsatilla* in all its symptoms (see Boericke & Dewey's *Twelve Tissue Remedies).* The *Manganum* pains shift crosswise from joint to joint, while *Lac caninum* alternates sides, being worse on one side one day and on the other the next, etc. Then, again, *Kali bichromicum* alternates *symptoms;* for instance, rheumatic and dysenteric symptoms alternate. (Also, *Abrotanum.*) *Platina* alternates back symptoms, with general mind and bodily symptoms.

Kali bichromicum is particularly adapted to fat, light-haired persons, or children disposed to catarrhal, croupy, scrofulous or syphilitic affections. Dr. Drysdale deserves much credit for what he has done for the profession by introducing this truly great remedy.

KALI HYDROIODICUM.

Cough with profuse, thick, green, salty expectoration, from deep down, as if from mid-sternum, with pain through to back; great weakness and night sweats.

Stitches through the lungs; in middle of sternum; through sternum to back or deep in chest; < walking.

Irresistible desire for open air; walking in open air does not fatigue; periosteal rheumatism.

Intolerable bone pain, especially at night; syphilitics.

Syphilitic affections, especially after the abuse of *Mercury.*

Glandular swellings; interstitial infiltration.

Hepar sulphur. antidotes its over-use.

* * * * *

This is one of the drugs so greatly abused by the old school that I confess to not having prescribed it much; in the first place, from my prejudice against it, and, in the second, because it never had so thorough a proving as did *Kali carb.* by Hahnemann.

There is one condition of the respiratory organs in which I have found it of great value. When after a hard cold a long-continued cough is the consequence, or it may be after an attack of pneumonia. The patient seems as if running into consumption. There is profuse expectoration from low down, deep in the chest, as if it came from mid-sternum, with pain through to between the shoulders *(Kali bichrom.) (Kali carb.,* lower right chest through to back), and there are exhausting night-sweats and great general weakness. I have repeatedly cured such cases where consumption seemed inevitable.

In the beginning of my practice I used to dissolve two to four grains of the crude salt in a four-ounce vial of water and direct to take a teaspoonful of this preparation three times a day, until it is half used, and then fill up with water and continue taking the same way until cured; filling up the vial every time it was half used. But several years ago, having a marked case of this description and feeling sure of my remedy, I gave it in the 200th potency as an experiment. This case also made fully as speedy a recovery as the others treated with the crude drug, so since then I often prescribe it in the potencies. There are two other remedies that may dispute the place with *Kali hyd.* in such cases, viz., *Sanguinaria* and *Stan-*

num. In all the expectoration is profuse and thick, but in *Stannum* the matter tastes *sweet,* in *Sanguinaria* the breath and sputa are very *fœtid,* even to the patient (also *Sepia* and *Psorinum),* while in *Kali hyd.* it is *salty* to the taste *(Sepia).* With *Kali hyd.* and *Stannum* the expectoration is often thick, green; not so much so with *Sanguinaria.* Sometimes with the *Kali hyd.* there is a frothy or soap-suds-like appearance of the sputa, but the heavy, green, salty expectoration seems to me to be more characteristic. The frothy expectoration is found in œdema of the lungs and may occur in Bright's disease. I have more than once gotten the reputation of curing consumption in such cases as I have been describing, and I don't know but I deserved it, at least I was never known to deny it.

Kali hydroiodicum as used by the old school is given either as a sort of specific against syphilis, or more often syphilis complicated by their abuse of mercury, or again as an **alterative** in scrofulous affections, without much reason. Now, what is an alterative? Here is the definition: "A medicine which gradually induces a **change** in the habit or constitution, and restores healthy functions without sensible evacuation." Isn't that rather sweeping? How is that for a school of medicine that claims to be the custodian of all medical science? Isn't that about what we would like to do in every case—*restore healthy function,* without sensible evacuation? How would *Kali hydroiodicum* do then for a panacea? There are, however, many so-called alteratives according to this definition; which shall we give? It is just here that we homœopaths believe that such vague general terms as alterative, tonic, narcotic, etc., are too unmeaning for purposes of close prescribing, and therefore misleading. They allow the doctor to prescribe too loosely a *class* of remedies, instead of the particular remedy of that class best adapted to the individual case.

We claim, therefore, great superiority for our system of prescribing, which is based upon a system of close drug proving, which brings out the closest, finest shades of difference between remedies belonging to a class of remedies. There must be no substitution of one for the other, if we would do the finest prescribing possible.

It requires but little comparison between the Materia Medicas of the two schools to show the wide difference in this respect.

There is said to be a place for the use of this remedy in pneumonia. I have not had experience with it here, but on account of its reputation I give it, and may use it if occasion requires.

I give you Farrington's words for it: "Pneumonia, in which disease it is an excellent remedy when hepatization has commenced, when the disease localizes itself, and infiltration begins. In such cases, in the absence of other symptoms calling distinctively for *Bryonia, Phosphorus* or *Sulphur,* I would advise you to select *Iodine* or *Iodide of Potassa.* It is also called for when the hepatization is so extensive that we have cerebral congestion, or even an effusion into the brain as a result of this congestion. The symptoms are as follows in these cases:

"First they begin with a very red face, the pupils are more or less dilated, and the patient is drowsy; in fact, showing a picture very much like that of *Belladonna.* You will probably give that remedy, but it does no good. The patient becomes worse, breathes more heavy, and the pupils more inactive to the light, and you know then that you have serous effusion into the brain, which must be checked or the patient dies." So far good. But now even Farrington *dulls*—all great men sometimes do. He says, "why did not *Belladonna* cure?" "He who prescribes by the *symptoms* alone in this case would fail, because he has not taken the totality of the case." What does Farrington mean? Does he mean that in his picture of *Belladonna* he had the totality of the case without the hepatization, or does he mean that the hepatization was the totality without the other symptoms? Here are the two horns of his dilemma—which would he take? I contend that all the other symptoms of the case, without the hepatization, was not the totality of the case. The hepatization was one, and only one, of the totality of symptoms. Now he says—"Put your ear to the patient's chest, and you will find one or both lungs consolidated." Well, I should call that a very important *objective* symptom, and one that could not be left out of the *totality* of the case. Remember that both subjective and objective symptoms must enter into every case in order to make the totality complete.

So after all, in true Hahnemannian fashion, I claim that he who prescribes, being guided by *all the symptoms,* will not and cannot fail where a cure is at all possible. These are and must be our infallible guide, or *Similia Similibus Curantur* is not true. (See Kafka's case, Hom. Clinic, page 73, 1870.)

Guiding Symptoms, Vol. VI, page 441, records this—"Distends all the tissues by interstitial infiltration; œdema, enlarged glands, tophis exostoses; swelling of the bones." Then of course it cures such distentions of the tissues.

Great mistakes and abuses of the remedy, and irreparable injury to the patient, often follow the use of remedies on such vague or single indications, that is of course if we prescribe on them alone. That would be like trying to prescribe for pneumonia from the single indication *hepatization*. This is only one symptom, and that one may occur under *any remedies*. If we say, or could say, interstitial distention of the tissues with certain other symptoms peculiar to that remedy, then could we differentiate between it and other remedies. But to use a remedy simply as an absorbent because it has secured absorption in some other case, is simply to fall back into the indiscriminate generalization and routinism of the old school. *Kali iodatum* is called an anti-syphilitic. So is mercury. *Sulphur* is called anti-psoric, and *Thuja* anti-sycotic. That is well to begin with, but the "end is not yet." There is a large class of remedies for each of these miasms and *the one* (indicated by all the symptoms or the characteristic symptoms) *out of the class* is the one to select for the cure of each individual patient.

The very fact that *Kali iodatum* has been too generally and indiscriminately used is the reason why it is a great question as to whether humanity has been most blessed or cursed by it. We homœopaths have much to do in combating the evils produced by the abuse of both these drugs, and *Hepar sulphur.* is *one* of the best antidotes. Most of the reported cures with this remedy *Kali iod.* are made with the low or crude preparations of the drug. I think it can be used lower than most drugs without injury, and yet I believe we do not know half its remedial power as developed by our process of potentiation.

KALI MURIATICUM

Is one of the so-called "Bio-chemic" remedies, or one of the twelve tissue remedies, claimed by Schuessler to be able to cure all the ills that flesh is heir to. It has not been proven enough to know half its real value. Clinical use in the potencies, ranging from the 3d to the 30th, has proven that it is a remedy of undoubted great value. It is of use in the second stage of inflammations or the stage of interstitial exudation in any part of the body, and here it is not, so far as yet known, attended with the danger of *Kali hydroiodicum.* If it had been used in the massive doses of the latter remedy, we might have had more deleterious results than we now know of. I have seen enlarged joints after acute rheumatism rapidly reduced to normal size under its action, sometimes after they had resisted other remedies a long time; but I do not know of any characteristic symptoms for its use in preference to other remedies. It is also a remedy for tonsillitis after the acute inflammatory symptoms have been checked by *Aconite, Belladonna,* or *Ferrum phos.* I have found it very efficacious in deafness from inflammation and closure of the Eustachian tube. I began using it in the 3d or 6th, but have better success with the 24th potency. A great many cases of chronic incurable deafness might have been cured by this remedy if used early. *Mercurius dulcis* may be mentioned in this connection, as it was not when we wrote of the *Mercuries,* as another remedy for these Eustachian troubles. Of course you would be apt to have some other mercurial symptoms which would perhaps enable you to choose between the two remedies. *Kali mur.* is likely to come into use more from a clinical introduction than from provings. That is what Hering used to call a remedy born by breech presentation. It is possible, but not right or natural.

APIS MELLIFICA.

Burning, stinging pains (like bee stings); eyelids; throat; panaritium or felon, hæmorrhoids, ovaries (especially right one), breasts (mastitis), skin (erysipelas, urticaria, carbuncles).

Great œdema; general or local (face, ears, eyelids, especially lower); throat (diphtheria); genitals (especially scrotum); skin (erysipelas and urticaria); everywhere; general anasarca, abdomen. These œdemas are accompanied with the characteristic pains, or no pain at all.

Stupor, with sharp, sudden, shrill cries in brain disease *(crie encephalique).*

Thirstlessness, especially in dropsies and during heat of intermittents.

Skin alternately dry and perspiring.

Suffocative; feels as if every breath would be his last, especially in dropsical conditions or hot stage of intermittents.

Modalities: < after sleep, on touch (very sensitive), from heat and warm room; > cold room or air and cold applications.

Bad effects from suppressed or retrocedent exanthemata; measles, scarlatina, urticaria.

Involuntary diarrhœa, with sensation as if anus were wide open.

* * * * *

It seems to me that in this remedy also the leading characteristic is to be found in its sensation—*burning,* **sting-**

ing *pains*. They are sharp and quick, like the sting of the bee. These pains are as characteristic of this remedy as are the *itching-like chillblains of Agaricus,* or the burnings of *Arsenicum* and *Sulphur;* but the burnings of *Apis* are relieved by cold, while those of *Arsenic* are relieved by heat. The stinging appears in many diseases, and kinds of tissue. In the serous membranes or the brain coverings, when we get those "shrill, sudden piercing screams"—"*cri cerebrale,*" which attend such dangerous affections as hydrocephalus, cerebro-spinal meningitis and typhus cerebralis, *Apis* is the remedy. Again we get these pains in the mucous membranes, as in the throat and hæmorrhoids, and the burning is almost always more or less present at the same time. It is also found very prominent in the ovaries. It has proved a very valuable remedy in cancers, even open ones, when this stinging, burning pain was present; also in panaritium. I have seen rapid cures follow its exhibition in felon. Hering puts it—"*redness and swelling with stinging and burning pain in the eyes, eyelids, ears, face, lips, tongue, throat, anus, testicles.*" (> by cold applications ought to be added.)

So we see how generally the system comes under the action of this remedy. In skin affections, especially the acute exanthems, this is the grand leading symptom, and is especially indicated in affections of the brain and meninges caused by a sudden suppression of skin diseases.

The next general condition for which this remedy seems to be as near specific as any remedy can be is an infiltrated cellular tissue; an œdematous or dropsical condition. This condition obtains almost from the beginning of inflammatory affections and extends to the stage of exudation, and even to chronic dropsical states. In those intensely violent and rapid cases of diphtheria in which the whole throat fills right up with œdematous swelling, the vulva hanging down like a transparent sac filled with water *(Kali bichromicum, Rhus toxicod.)*, and the patient is in imminent danger of death by suffocation from actual closure of the throat and larynx, there is no remedy like *Apis.* The stinging, burning pains may be present in these cases; or what is **more** dangerous still, because there is no complaint until the case is far advanced, is an *absolutely painless* condition. *Baptisia* has painlessness in throat affections, but the swelling is not so rapid as *Apis,* and there is no œdema. A number of years ago I was called to Watkins Glen, N. Y., in consultation in a very bad case of diphtheria. One had already died in the family and four lay dead in the place that day. Over forty cases had died in the place and there was an exodus going on for fair. Her attending physician, a noble, white-haired old man, and withal a good and able man, said, when I looked up to him and remarked I was rather young to counsel him: "Doctor, I am on my knees to anybody, for every case has died that has been attacked." The patient was two rooms away from us, but I could hear her difficult breathing even then. *Apis* was comparatively a new remedy then for that disease, but as I looked into her throat I saw *Apis* in a moment, and a few questions confirmed it. I told the doctor what I thought and asked him if he had tried it. He said, no he had not thought of it, but it was a *powerful blood poison;* try it. It cured the case, and not one case that took this remedy from the beginning, and persistently, died. It was the remedy for the *genus epidemicus.* See my report of this in Vol. XII., *Hahnemannian Monthly.*

This œdematous condition of *Apis* may be found in almost any part of the body, but is especially prominent in mouth and throat, eyelids and face, *around* the eyes (*Phosphorus,* whole face); lower lids hang down like bags of water. (*Kali carb.,* upper lids.) In erysipelas the swelling of the skin is of this œdematous appearance, and generally with stinging pains. Sometimes the œdema increases until it forms large blister-like bags of water.

The dropsical effusion may be general or local. It is found in the thoracic cavity, in ovaries, in abdominal cavity, scrotum, and genitals of females. One peculiar symptom which helps to choose between it and other remedies in dropsy is the almost absolute *absence of thirst* (with thirst, *Acetic acid, Arsenic* and *Apocynum*).

I will now, in addition to what I have written, call attention to some particular affections and symptoms in which *Apis* should be remembered. A very important symptom not yet mentioned is *tenderness or sensitiveness to touch,* as if bruised. This is particularly true in the abdominal, uterine, and ovarian regions, but is not by any means confined there, for we may find the whole surface of the body exceedingly sensitive to touch; even the hair seems sore (*China officinalis*). This condition is often found in cerebro-spinal meningitis and is a strong indication for *Apis.* In erysipelas this tenderness is often present, and is found under *Hepar sulphur.* as well as *Apis.*

The sleep of *Apis* is either very restless, or in brain diseases there is *deep stupor,* interrupted occasionally by *piercing screams.* Never forget *Apis* then. In all inflammatory affections and in intermittent fevers, if you find the patient *alternately dry and hot, or perspiring,* think again of *Apis.*

No remedy has this alternation so strong as *Apis*. *Sensation as if every breath would be his last* is very characteristic, and occurs not only in dropsical troubles of the chest, but seems also to be a nervous symptom. In scarlatina *Apis* is especially indicated if the eruption is retarded or retrocedent and serious brain troubles result, and it is no less efficacious in post-scarlatinal dropsies if the symptoms do not indicate some other remedies.

CANTHARIS VESICATORIA.

Frequent urging to urinate, with straining and cutting, burning pains.

Small unsatisfactory quantity passed at a time, or bloody urine.

Excessive *burning* pains (eyes, mouth, throat, stomach, intestinal tract; all the mucous surfaces and skin).

Stringy and tenacious discharges from the mucous membranes.

Nearly all complaints accompanied with the characteristic urinary symptoms.

Erysipelas, with blebs or large blisters filled with water and burning pain; useful for surface burns (locally).

Uncontrollable anguish, furious rage, frenzied delirium; strong sexual desire, both sexes.

Disgust for everything; drink, food, tobacco.

Dysenteric stools, bloody and shreddy, like scrapings from intestines, with tenesmus in rectum and bladder.

* * * * *

If I were to select the one remedy with which to prove the truth of the formula similia, etc., I think this would be the one. There is no remedy that so surely, and so violently, irritates and inflames the urinary organs, and no remedy so promptly cures such irritation when it puts on the *Cantharis* type or form, which it often does.

H. N. Guernsey wrote: "It is a singular fact, though known to most practitioners, that if there be frequent micturition attended with burning, cutting pain, or if not so frequent and the cutting, burning pain attends the flow, *Cantharis* is almost always the remedy for whatever other suffering there may be, even in inflammation of the brain or lungs." He might have added in the throat, and mucous membranes all through the intestinal tract, even to the rectum and anus, and in the pleura or on the skin.

He also wrote: "*Cantharis* should always be remembered and studied in treating affections of the air passages when the mucus is tenacious." *(Hyrastis, Kali bichrom., Coccus cacti,* etc.) I had the pleasure of verifying the truth of this in the case of a lady who had suffered a long time with bronchitis. The mucus was so profuse, and tenacious, and ropy, that I thought of *Kali bichromicum,* and thought it must be the remedy; but it did not even ameliorate, and she got worse all the time, until one day she mentioned that she had great cutting and burning on urinating, which she must do very frequently.

On the strength of the urinary symptom, for I knew nothing of its curative powers on the respiratory organs at that time, I gave her *Cantharis.* The effect was magical.

It is needless to describe the mutual delight of both physician and patient in such a case, for it was astonishing the rapidity with which the perfect and permanent cure of the case was accomplished.

Let us notice still further the effects of this remedy

upon the urinary organs by calling attention to a few symptoms that have been both produced in proving and cured *ab usu in morbis.* I have learned to place the *highest estimate* upon such symptoms. To be sure there are many symptoms in our great Materia Medica that have come to us through clinical sources only, and very valuable ones, too. But they cannot be received with such implicit confidence on short acquaintance as those that are both pathogenetic and clinical. They should always be separated when possible, as they were in "Hull's Jahr" of old. Here are a few of them. *"Violent pains in bladder, with frequent urging to urinate, with intolerable tenesmus." "Violent burning cutting pains in the neck of the bladder." "Before, during, and after urinating fearful cutting pains in the urethra." "Constant urging to urinate; urine passed drop by drop with extreme pain." "Urine scalds him; it is passed drop by drop."*

No homœopathist meeting these symptoms in a case would fail to think of *Cantharis* at once, no matter what else ailed the patient, as it has cured the most diverse and varied diseases when occurring in conjunction with these urinary symptoms. How any physician of any school can deny the truth of *similia similibus curantur* in the light of such testimony or proof can only be accounted for on the principle of "none so blind as those who will not see."

Cantharis has also very decided action upon the skin. In erysipelas it is sometimes the best remedy, and choice has to be made between it and *Apis,* which also sometimes has *great urinary irritation* in such cases. In the *Apis* cases there is apt to be more *œdema;* in *Cantharis* more *blistering.* In *Cantharis* the *burning* is more intense than under the *Apis,* while in the latter there is more *stinging.* The urinary symptoms, if present, are very much more intense under *Cantharis.* Again, the mind symptoms of the two remedies are quite different. In the *Apis* cases, aside from the stinging pains which make the patient cry out sharply at times, especially if the eruption inclines to "go in" and attack the membranes of the brain, the patient may not be so very restless and complaining; but in the *Cantharis* case the patient is uneasy, restless, dissatisfied, distressed, sometimes moaning or violently crying; wants to be moved about constantly. The mind symptoms actually make one think of *Arsenicum album,* and when we take into account the intense burning it is doubly so. So that it would be very easy to get confused between these two remedies, as well as *Cantharis* and *Apis.* If great thirst is also present it would make us think of *Arsenic.* And now we are upon the skin, *Cantharis* is a great remedy for burns, both locally as an application and internally for the more chronic conditions and sequelæ. In all skin troubles where blebs or watery vesicles form, which burn and itch, or when touched burn and smart, we do well to remember *Cantharis,* and look further to find more symptoms, if present, to corroborate it. Hering used to challenge skeptics to burn their fingers, and then cure them by dipping the fingers into water medicated with *Cantharis.* So great was his faith in it.

I will call attention to a sensational symptom of *Cantharis* which I believe is underestimated in practice. It is the sensation of **Burning.** If any remedy deserves to be placed alongside *Arsenicum* for burning, it is this one. I will quote so as to bring all together, in a way to impress upon our memory the burnings of *Cantharis.* "Inflammation of the eyes particularly, when caused by a *burn.*" "*Burning* in mouth, throat, and stomach." "Great thirst, with *burning* pain in throat and stomach." "Violent *burning* pain in stomach in region of pylorus." "Violent *burning* pain and heat through whole intestinal tract." "Passage of white or pale-red tough mucus with the stool like scrapings from intestines, with streaks of blood; after stool colic relieved, *burning,* biting, and stinging in the anus." "Great *burning* pain in the ovarian regions." "Peritonitis with *burning* pain, abdomen sensitive and tenesmus of the bladder." "*Burning* and stinging of the larynx, especially when attempting to hawk up tough mucus." "*Burning* in the chest."

We have already spoken of the *burnings* connected with affections of the urinary organs, and also of the *burnings* of the skin in erysipelas and other eruptions upon the surface.

This seems to me to be sufficient to impress upon the reader the value of this symptom belonging to this remedy. I will close by calling attention to its effect upon the membranes to *increase their secretion.* This action is positive and is a valuable indication for its use.

TARANTULA HISPANIA.

This spider poison has like other spider poisons very positive nervous symptoms. It acts upon the uterus and ovaries, and upon the female sexual organs generally. "In case of hyperæsthesia or congestion of these organs, which set up a general hysterical condition, states simulating spinal neurasthenia, sensitive and painful back, excessive restlessness, and impressibility to excitements, music, especially, where there is constant inclination to keep the hands busy *(Kali bromatum)*, and again especially if accompanied by sexual desire or pruritus of the genitals, *Tarantula* is able to accomplish much." Choreaic conditions, which are often the outcome of an advanced stage of the above described nervous condition, are peculiarly amenable to this remedy. Twitching or jerking of the muscles in conjunction with other troubles should always call to mind this remedy, with which such jerkings are so characteristic. It has a restlessness in women similar to the restlessness in men of *Phosphorus*, viz., cannot keep quiet in any position; must keep in motion, though walking < all the symptoms. This remedy is not yet as thoroughly understood as it should be. Another spider ought to be mentioned in this connection, viz., the

TARANTULA CUBENSIS

Or the hairy spider. It is one of the most efficacious remedies for boils, abscesses, felons, or swellings of any kind, where the tissues put on a *bluish color*, and there are *intense burning pains*. We used to think we had two great remedies in *Arsenicum* and *Anthracinum* for these swellings; but *Tarantula Cubensis* is simply wonderful. I have seen felons which had kept patients awake night after night walking the floor in agony from the terrible pains so relieved in a very short time that they could sleep in perfect comfort until the swellings spontaneously discharged, and progressed to a rapid cure. This remedy should receive a thorough proving. It is a gem.

MYGALE LASIODORA

Is also a spider poison, and has cured cases of chorea. The cases seem to have been of a very violent nature, and the *twitching in the facial* muscles is predominant. This remedy also ought to be fully proven.

ARANEA DIADEMA.

Another spider which Grauvogl classed with his so-called hydrogenoid remedies, *i. e.*, the patient always suffered, with whatever she had, *most in wet weather.* It is well to remember such positive modalities, for it may narrow down the case to a few remedies from which our curative must be chosen; for instance—*Aranea, Natrum sulphuricum, Dulcamara, Nux moschata, Rhus toxicodendron, Rhododendron*—all have these wet weather aggravations, and we will be apt to find our remedy there if the patient is characteristically worse in wet weather.

THERIDION CURASSAVICUM.

Vertigo, with nausea, on closing the eyes, or the least noise.

Over-sensitiveness of nerves; scratching on linen or silk, or crackling of paper is unbearable.

Pain running through upper left chest to shoulder.

* * * * *

Theridion curassavicum is another spider poison proven by Hering. There is one peculiar and characteristic symptom under this remedy, which has been verified by myself and others—*"Vertigo with nausea especially on closing the eyes."* Allen puts it—vertigo **on closing the eyes** *(Lach., Thuja),* on opening them, *Tabacum;*

on looking upward *(Puls., Sil.)*; **from any even least noise;** aural or labyrinthine (Meniere's disease).

Again **"every sound seems to penetrate through the whole body, causing nausea and vertigo."** *Asarum* has a somewhat similar symptom which is worth remembering. *"Over-sensitiveness of nerves,* **scratching of linen or silk,** crackling of paper is unbearable." *(Ferr., Tarax.)*

The vertigo occurs in different affections of the head or stomach, and cures the whole trouble when it is present. It seems like a small thing to "go by," but no smaller than "vertigo, worse on lying down, and turning the head" *(Conium),* or "vertigo on looking upward" *(Silicea, Pulsatilla)* and many other symptoms of other remedies which have been verified many times. Another symptom which seems to be very valuable in chest affections is, *"pains run through upper left chest to shoulder." (Phthisis florida* has been cured on this symptom for a guide, if given early.) This is like *Myrtus communis,* with which I have helped many cases having that peculiar local symptom. *(Sulphur, Pix liquida* and *Anisum stellatum* also have it.)

Dr. Baruch says: "In rachitis, caries and necrosis it apparently goes to the root of the evil and destroys the cause."

COCCUS CACTI.

We now leave the spider family, but as we are dealing with small fry of the insect order we will notice the *Coccus cacti,* a small bug or insect which infests the plants of the cactus species of Mexico and Central America. It has made its best record in curing affections of the respiratory organs. Whooping cough with expectoration of much tough, ropy white mucus. This mucus comes in large quantities and is often accompanied with gagging and vomiting, which seems to expel the mucus from the stomach. Sometimes a bronchial catarrh remains after whooping cough, which has this kind of expectoration. Here this remedy will sometimes clear up the whole case. This is all I know of its virtues *ab usu in morbis*. Now we come to a little pest of womankind all over.

CIMEX LECTULARIUS.

It has one characteristic symptom which has been verified. "Sensation as if the tendons were too short." There is sometimes actual contraction as if the legs cannot be stretched out. This has been verified in intermittent fevers, and only the other day (a short time ago) Dr. Brewster, of Syracuse, told of a case in which he was guided by this symptom.

A man was driving a fractious horse that started to run away with him. Thinking to give him enough of it he let the horse run, and when tired of running whipped him into running more until he had run him up a hill several miles long. The road over which he passed was very rough, and the man was so bruised and sprained about the buttocks and legs that he was confined to the house for a long time in consequence. It finally settled into what seemed likely to be a permanent contraction of the tendons of the lower limbs. No remedy relieved, until the good doctor bethought him of a case of intermittent fever which he had cured twenty years before, being guided by this symptom. He gave the patient a dose of Jenichen's 600th potency of *Cimex*, with immediate result, and cure of the case. "Honor to whom honor is due," even if it be a bed-bug.

CHAMOMILLA MATRICARIA.

Very irritable mood; snaps and snarls; will not speak or answer civilly; *mad.*

Exceedingly sensitive to pain, which makes her mad; numbness alternates with, or attends, the pains; sweats with the pains.

Excessive uneasiness; anxiety; agonized, tossing about; will only be quieted by carrying the child about.

High fever with sweating, especially on the head; thirsty; one cheek red and hot, the other pale and cold.

Dentition diarrhœa; green stools, foul odor like rotten eggs, much colicky pain, abdomen bloated.

Cough dry < at night, *when asleep,* from tiekling in throat pit; < cold weather and every winter.

Especially adapted to children and nervous, hysterical women.

Violent rheumatic pains drive him out of bed at night; compel him to walk about.

Burning of soles at night; puts feet out of bed.

Numbness with the pains.

* * * * *

Charles J. Hempel called this "the catnip of Homœopathy," because it was particularly adapted to nervous affections, especially of children. This is one of the remedies that finds its leading characteristic symptoms in the *mind* of the patient. To "boil down" all the different ways in which the *Chamomilla* mind can be and is expressed: *"The patient is cross, ugly, spiteful, snappish.* She knows it, admits it, and so does every one else. She will return mean, uncivil, spiteful answers to her best friends, and then confess her fault, to repeat it again and again, and stoutly affirms she cannot help it, she feels so." This state of mind is always present in the marked *Chamomilla* case, whether it be adult or child.

Of course the young child cannot give vent to its feelings by talking, so it comes as near to it as it can by whining and crying, sometimes it seems without cause, and also when it shows by fever, diarrhœa, teething and many other complaints that it is actually sick and suffering. It wants this or that thing, puts out its little hand for it, and when it is offered pushes it away and points to something else, to reject it in turn. Now the child does not know what it wants, but the homœopathic physician does. It wants a dose of *Chamomilla.* This peevish disposition in which nothing pleases, takes possession of the child, mother, father or any and all grades and classes of subjects when *Chamomilla* is the remedy, and it is found in connection with all kinds of diseases. It is also especially adapted to ailments *brought on* by fits of anger. In short, it is the leading *anger remedy* of the Materia Medica.

The other leading anger remedies, or, for ailments brought on by anger, are *Aconite, Bryonia, Colocynth, Ignatia, Lycopodium, Nux vomica, Staphisagria.*

It is also one of the leading remedies for **pain,** and there is this peculiarity about it, the pain is not always in proportion to the gravity of the case, and we often see, for instance, in labor, a great deal harder pains of which the patient does not complain half so loudly. But in the *Chamomilla* case the patient is exceedingly *sensitive* to the pain and exclaims continually, "Oh; I cannot bear the pain." Many times have I met this condition in labor cases, and in the majority of them the cross, peevish snappish, condition of mind accompanying, and seen it changed in a short time to a mild, uncomplaining, patient state, by a single dose of *Chamomilla* 200th.

This sensitiveness to pain is not confined to labor cases, but I have often observed it in neuralgias, toothache, rheumatism, etc., and the same happy results follow its use.

This condition of sensitiveness is often found in coffee drinkers, or in those who have been addicted to narcotics. *Chamomilla* is very useful here. There is another sensation which is often found in conjunction with, or sometimes alternating with, this pain or sensitiveness, and that is **numbness.**

It is found in rheumatism or paralytic states and is very characteristic. The pains of *Chamomilla* are oftener aggravated by heat than otherwise, but are not on the other hand, like *Pulsatilla,* ameliorated by cold. In fact, the patient is often very sensitive to cold, and cold air brings on troubles for which this remedy is specific. I now call to mind a very painful case of rheumatism of the left shoulder in a middle-aged man. It was in my earlier practice, when I was prescribing for names more than I do now, and of course he got *Aconite, Bryonia* and *Rhus toxicodendron,* etc., but no relief. A wiser man was called in consultation and the patient was quickly cured by *Chamomilla.* When I asked the counsel what led him to prescribe this remedy he answered *numbness with the pains.*

Another condition which is met by this remedy is *restlessness* and *sleeplessness.* You will remember that we gave as the great trio of restless remedies *Aconite, Arseni-*

cum and *Rhus tox.* That was right, but we did not say that those were all the restless remedies. Here we have another in *Chamomilla.* Let me quote: *"Violent rheumatic pains drive him out of bed at night, and compel him to walk about."* (*Rhus tox., Ferrum met., Verat. alb.*) *"Excessive uneasiness, anxiety, agonized tossing about, with tearing pains in the abdomen." "The child can only be quieted by carrying it on the arms will not be quiet unless carried."* (Opposite *Bryonia.*) These symptoms represent in a few words the restlessness of this remedy. But some will ask, isn't this similar to your *trio* of restless remedies? It is; but there are shades of difference and concomitant symptoms that decide between them all. And the true Hahnemannian is the man to recognize them. There is no particular overwhelming fear, fear of death, etc., under *Chamomilla* as there is under *Aconite.* The patient is maddened; driven to desperation under *Chamomilla;* does not care whether she dies or not; had *rather* die than *suffer so,* and so we might draw lines of differentiation between this and other restless remedies, but it would take too long. Each physician must get a habit of doing this for himself. In his ability to do this lies the superior skillfulness of the homœopathic practitioner. Without this he can only hope for indifferent success at most, and will be driven to all sorts of experiments, adjuvants, surgical measures and so forth which might be avoided, much to his own credit, and the advantage of his patient. The sleeplessness of the *Chamomilla* patient is owing to the pain and excessive nerve sensibility and this remedy procures sleep by overcoming these troubles, which make the patient sleepless. Now there are a few symptoms, when occurring in conjunction with the peculiar mind and nervous symptoms of this remedy, that confirm the choice of it, such as

"Warm sweat on the head wetting the hair."

"Pressing earache in spells; tearing pain extorting cries."

"Ears particularly sensitive to cold air."

"One cheek red and hot, the other pale and cold."

"Face sweats after eating or drinking."

"Toothache if anything warm is taken into the mouth." (*Pulsatilla.*)

"Toothache recommences when entering a warm room."

"Teeth feel too long."

"Dentition with diarrhœa of green stools smelling like rotten eggs."

"Hot and thirsty with the pains; also fainting." *(Hep. sul.)*

"Gastralgia in coffee drinkers; constrictive pain, or as if a stone were in the stomach." *(Nux vom.)*

"Wind colic; abdomen distended like a drum; wind passes in small quantities without relief."

"Stools green, watery, corroding *(Sulph.)*, like stirred eggs."

"Stools hot, smelling like rotten eggs."

"Metrorrhagia dark coagulated blood, flowing in paroxysms."

"Menstrual colic, also following anger."

"Labor pains press upward, or begin in back, and pass off down inner side of thighs."

"Rigidity of os, pains unendurable."

"After-pains also unendurable."

"Children have spasms, from fit of anger in the nurse."

"Cough from tickling in throat pit."

"Cough dry, worse at night, especially *while asleep,* does not waken when coughing." *(Calcarea ost., Psorinum.)*

"Chronic cough, worse in winter or cold weather."

"Body chilly and cold; face and breath hot."

"Heat and chill intermingled." *(Ars. alb.)*

"Skin moist and burning hot." *(Bell.)*

This does not by any means cover all the symptoms which indicate *Chamomilla,* but when they do occur it is strongly indicated and shows something of the range and usefulness of this remedy when given according to homœopathic rules.

COFFEA CRUDA.

All senses more acute; reads fine print easier; smell, taste and touch acute; unusual activity of mind and body; full of ideas, quick to act, no sleep on this account, etc.

Affections from sudden surprises, especially joyful surprises; very emotional.

Pains insupportable, drive to despair; exasperation, tears, tossing about in agony; great sleeplessness.

Headache, from over-mental exertion, thinking, talking; one-sided, as from a nail driven into the brain *(Ign., Nux);* as if the brain were torn or dashed to pieces; < in open air.

Jerking toothache; relieved by holding ice water in the mouth; returns when water becomes warm.

* * * * *

Coffea cruda, like *Chamomilla,* acts strongly upon the nervous system. Indeed in nervous troubles, where the patient has not been addicted to the coffee habit, it often takes precedence. If on the other hand he is a coffee drinker, *Chamomilla* is the remedy. Doctor Teste, of Paris, used to say that coffee was responsible for a large proportion of the neuralgias of France. The *Coffea* patient is a subject of very great general exalted sensibility. See Hering's characteristic cards. *"All the senses more acute, reads fine print easier, smell, taste, and touch acute, particularly also in increased perception of slight passive motions." "Unusual activity of mind and body." "Full of ideas, quick to act, no sleep on this account." "Lively fancies, full of plans for the future."*

These symptoms portray, as plainly as words can, the nervous conditions calling for this remedy.

It makes one think of *Chamomilla,* but the **mind** of *Chamomilla is not there.* On the other hand, it makes one think of *Aconite,* but the fear of death **is** not there. Hering used to recommend *Aconite* and *Coffea* in alternation in painful inflammatory affections, where the fever symptoms of the former and also the nervous sensibility of the latter were present, and I know of no two remedies that alternate better, though I never do it, since I learned to closely individualize. *Coffea* is especially adapted to mental shocks, such as *sudden surprises, especially joyful surprises, excessive laughter and playing, disappointed love, noises, strong smells,* etc. It is also adapted to *variable* moods; *first crying then laughing, then crying again.*

Coffea also vies with *Chamomilla* and *Aconite* as a *pain* remedy. *"Pains insupportable, drive to despair." "Exasperation, tears, tossing about in great anguish."* Here again we would not give *Coffea* in an habitual coffee drinker, but *Chamomilla* rather.

The particular localities where these pains mostly occur are in the head, where the pain is generally one-sided, feeling *"as though a nail were driven into the head." Ignatia* has a similar headache, and it generally occurs in hysterical subjects. Then the choice may have to be made between these two remedies.

Prosopalgia, which is often traceable to bad teeth, and *Coffea* has a very peculiar toothache, in the fact that the tooth is easy as long as he *holds cold water upon it.* Remember *Chamomilla* toothache is often caused by taking *warm* things into the mouth, but is not relieved by taking cold things like *Coffea.*

Dysmenorrhœa, with excessively painful colic. If there are large *black clots* and *Coffea* does not relieve, follow with *Chamomilla.* Pains threatening abortion, or after-pains, or very severe unbearable labor pains are often relieved by this remedy. In short, for pains anywhere, which seem intolerable, and there are no other especially leading symptoms, *Coffea* is to be remembered.

The same over-excitability, so characteristic of this drug, causes great *sleeplessness,* and *Coffea* has won to itself great credit as a *sleep* remedy. In my experience and observation, it works best here in the 200th potency. And there is no more beautiful verification of the truth of *Similia* than just here, for it *causes great sleeplessness* in many people when taken in large quantities. Cough and sleeplessness after measles (a very common occurrence) is wonderfully relieved by it, and it is sleep, not narcosis, and never injures or sickens the patient like the *stupor* of the opium preparations.

IGNATIA.

Remedy of paradoxicalities. Head better lying on painful side, moody, goneness not > by eating, sore throat < by swallowing, thirst during chill, face red during chill, etc.

Sad, sighing, changeable, moody disposition.

Twitching or spasms, or convulsions from exciting or depressing emotions, fright, etc.

All-gone, weak, empty sensation in stomach not > by eating.

Anal troubles (piles, prolapsus, soreness and pain after stool, pains shooting up into abdomen).

Adapted to emotional, hysterical subjects.

Modalities: < slight touch, smoking, coffee; > lying on painful side; hard pressure; profuse watery urination.

Cough; dry, spasmodic; not relieved by coughing; the longer he coughs the more the irritation to cough increases.

Pain; in small circumscribed spots; over-sensitive *(Cof., Hep.).*

In most cases *Ignatia* should be given in the morning.

Ignatia bears the same relation to the diseases of women that *Nux* does to bilious men.

* * * * *

Ignatia is another one of the long list of our nervous remedies. Its peculiar mental symptoms, like those of *Aconite, Chamomilla, Nux vomica* and many others, are most characteristic. Like these remedies, it seems to exalt the impressionability of all the senses; but unlike the others, it has in it a marked element of sadness, and disposition to *silent grieving.* Anyone suffering from suppressed, deep grief, with long drawn sighs, much sobbing, etc., and especially if inclined to smother or hide that grief from others, is just the subject for this remedy. She desires to be alone with her grief. *Sighs much* and seems so sad and weak. The weakness is complained of right in the pit of the stomach. She feels weak, faint, and *"all gone"* there. Another equally characteristic state of mind is a **changeable mood.** No remedy can equal *Ignatia* for this. *Aconite, Coffea, Nux moschata* and a few others have it, but *Ignatia* in the greatest degree. And so this remedy becomes one of our best in the treatment of hysterical affections. The patient is at one time full of glee and merriment, to be followed suddenly with the other extreme, of melancholy sadness and tears, and so these states of mind rapidly alternate. Again, we have in *Ignatia* an impatient, *quarrelsome, angry mood* (but not to the degree of *Chamomilla)* at times. Again the *Ignatia* patient is, because of her excessive impressibility, easily frightened. Here it becomes one of our best remedies for the effects of fright, vying with *Aconite, Opium* and *Veratrum album.* In short, *Ignatia* may justly be termed pre-eminently the remedy of **moods.**

Aside from its mental symptoms, it is a great nervous remedy. It acts upon the spine as decidedly as *Nux vomica,* affecting both motor and sensory nerves. It is one of our best remedies for spasms or convulsions, and is especially adapted to spasmodic affections originating in mental causes, as after *fright, punishment of children* or other strong emotions. In one case of puerperal convulsions, other remedies having failed to do any good, the consulting physician while observing the patient during one of the spasms noticed that she came out of it with a succession of long drawn sighs. He inquired if the patient had had any recent mental trouble, and learned that she had lost her mother, of whom she was exceedingly fond, and whom she had mourned for greatly, a few weeks before. *Ignatia* 30th quickly cured her. Again, short of actual convulsions, *Ignatia* has, in a most marked degree, **twitchings** all over the body, hence it becomes one of our best remedies for chorea, especially if caused by fright or grief on the mental side, or teething or worms on the reflex irritation side. There is only one remedy that comes near it for these twitchings and that is *Zincum metallicum.* Of course, *Agaricus, Hyoscyamus, Cuprum met.*, etc., come close, and some might think are equal. *Veratrum viride,* when better known, may lay claim to high rank here. *Ignatia* is sometimes recommended for paralysis, but will be found, I think, exceptionally useful, and that mainly in hysterical cases, which are not of a very dangerous character. Like *Aconite, Chamomilla* and *Coffea, Ignatia* is *over-sensitive* to *pain.*

Ignatia, like its male partner, *Nux vomica,* is a great remedy for headaches of nervous, especially hysterically nervous, subjects. That would be about the same as saying, that while *Nux vomica* is adapted to nervous men *Ignatia* is the same for women, which is quite true. You will remember that hysterical, nervous headaches are often one-sided. Hence *Ignatia* is such an efficient remedy for headaches as expressed in these words: *"Headache as if a nail were driven out through the side of the head relieved by lying on it."* These headaches come on in highly nervous and sensitive subjects, or in those whose nervous systems have suffered from over-anxiety, grief or mental work. The *ever-changeable and contradictory* symptoms so characteristic of the drug show here as elsewhere. Not only does the pain in head change locality, but at one time the pain will come on gradually and abate suddenly (like *Sulphuric acid),* or, like *Belladonna,* it will come on suddenly and abate as suddenly as it came. Like *Aconite, Gelsemium, Silicea,* and *Veratrum album,* the headache often terminates with a *profuse flow of urine.* That is often the case in headaches of nervous hysterical women. *(Lac defloratum,* profuse flow *during* headache.)

Finally the headaches are aggravated by coffee, smoking, the abuse of snuff, inhaling tobacco smoke, alcohol, close attention, from pressing at stool, and, while it is sometimes relieved while eating, is aggravated soon after. The *Ignatia* headache is sometimes accompanied by hunger like that of *Psorinum.* It is also < by cold winds, turning head suddenly, stooping, change of position, running, looking up long, moving the eyes, noise and light.

It is ameliorated by *warmth, lying on it, soft pressure, external heat and profuse flow of limpid urine. Ignatia* has some strong throat symptoms. In the first place it has the so commonly observed symptom called *"globus hystericus,"* or as if a lump came up from the stomach into the throat as if she would choke. She swallows it down but it comes right back and is very distressing. It is especially apt to come if she gets *grieved* and wants to cry. These are of course purely nervous sensations, but *Ignatia* goes further, and also cures real serious affections of the throat like tonsillitis and diphtheria. In these cases the real characteristic symptom is, that the pain and suffering in the throat is *relieved by swallowing* or is worse between the acts of deglutition. *(Capsicum.)* A very peculiar symptom for such troubles, for such cases are generally *aggravated* by swallowing, hence we would not expect to frequently find a case in which this would be the remedy; but such cases do arise occasionally and baffle us if we haven't the remedy. Here is where Homœopathy, as we say in base ball, "scores some of its best runs," and the satisfaction of curing such a case with an *unusual* remedy is, to say the least, very gratifying to him who performs the cure. With *Ignatia* cases, in addition to the aggravation when not swallowing, there is sometimes aggravation when swallowing liquids and relief from swallowing solids. This is like *Lachesis,* you remember, but is the reverse of *Baptisia,* which can swallow liquids only; the least solid food gags. It is necessary to keep these correspondences and opposites in mind, for it often enables us to make what are called "snap shot" prescriptions and save much time, study and suffering.

Some of the particularly valuable "guiding symptoms" of *Ignatia,* in addition to those already noticed, are *"extreme aversion to tobacco smoke."* This is a general aversion and aggravates many, many complaints. *"Weak, empty, gone feeling at the pit of the stomach."* In the case of *Ignatia* this symptom is apt to be accompanied by a disposition to *sigh* or take a long breath. Two other remedies have this symptom of goneness in the stomach as prominently as *Ignatia.* They are *Hydrastis* and *Sepia.* The other symptoms must decide between them. This weak feeling in the stomach in *Ignatia* is sometimes described as a feeling of flabbiness, as though the stomach *hung down relaxed. Ipecacuanha* has a similar feeling. Sometimes we come across very severe cases of gastralgia in women of hysterical tendencies. Here this remedy is the first to be thought of.

Ignatia has as positive action upon the anus and rectum as does *Nux vomica. Prolapsus of the rectum* is marked.

(Ruta graveolens.) Like *Nux vomica* it has frequent desire for stool, but in place of stool, or with it, comes the prolapsed rectum. The patient is afraid to strain at stool, to stoop down or lift, for fear of the prolapsus. A contractive sore pain follows after a stool and lasts for an hour or two. This is like *Nitric acid,* which has the same symptom only after a loose stool. There is also some pain in anus without reference to stool. Dunham, that prince of observers, gave us the characteristic: *"Sharp pains shooting upward into the rectum." (Sepia* has similar pains in uterus.) It is a gem, and has often been verified. So we see that *Ignatia* is one of our important anal and rectal remedies.

This remedy is also very unique in its fever symptoms. There is no disease in which we are better able to show the power of the potentized remedy to cure, than intermittent fever. Chronic cases that have resisted the Quinine treatment for years are often quickly and permanently cured by the 200th and upwards. The following symptoms indicate *Ignatia:* 1st. *Thirst during chill* and in no other stage. 2d. Chill relieved by *external heat.* 3d. Heat aggravated by *external covering.* 4th. *Red face during the chill.* Here are four legs to the stool, and we may sit upon it in perfect confidence. No other remedy has thirst during chill and in no other stage. In *Nux vomica,* you will remember, the chill is not relieved by the heat of the stove, or the bed, and during the heat *Nux vomica* must be covered, as the least uncovering brings back the chill. So we see that notwithstanding the alkaloid of both drugs is strychnia they differ widely when we come to apply them to the cure of the sick. The red face during chill led me to the cure of an obstinate case, and after I noticed the red face I also noticed that the boy was behind the stove in the warmest place he could find. The 200th promptly cured. Two other cases in the same family, at the same time, and from the same malarious district, were cured, one by *Capsicum,* 200th, the other by *Eupatorium perfoliatum,* same potency. The former had chill beginning between shoulders, in the latter the chill in the A. M., great pain in bones before, and vomiting of bile at the end of chill. I do not know but I have mentioned these three cases before; but it will bear repeating, for it illustrates the *efficacy of potencies* in obedience to our great law of cure. Can any reasonable man doubt such evidence?

COCCULUS INDICUS.

Weakness of cervical muscles, can hardly hold the head up.

Weakness in small of back as if paralyzed; gives out when walking; can hardly stand, walk or talk.

Hands and feet get numb; asleep.

Headache with nausea and vomiting; gets faint and sick on rising up or riding in carriage or boat.

General sensation of weakness; or weak, hollow, gone feeling in head, stomach, abdomen, etc.; < by loss of sleep or night watching.

Great distention with flatulent colic, wind or menstrual colic; crampy pains, inclined to hernia.

Modalities: < sitting up, moving, riding in carriage or boat, smoking, talking, eating, drinking, night watching; > when lying quiet.

* * * * *

Farrington says: "*Cocculus* acts on the cerebro-spinal

system, producing great debility of these organs. * * * It causes a paralytic weakness of the spine, and especially of its motor nerves; thus we find it a certain and frequent remedy in paralysis originating in disease of the spinal cord. * * * It is especially indicated in the beginning of the trouble, when the lumbar region of the spine is affected; there is weakness in the *small of the back* as if paralyzed; the small of the back gives out when walking. There is weakness of the legs, and by the legs I mean the entire lower extremities; the knees give out when walking, the soles of the feet feel as if they were asleep, the thighs ache as if they were pounded; first one hand goes to sleep, then the other; sometimes the whole arm goes to sleep and the hand feels as if swollen. These symptoms lie at the foundation of the symptomatology of the whole drug; they all seem to depend upon spinal weakness." Dunham says: "Its sphere of action is preeminently the system of animal life; the voluntary muscular system first, and then the sensorium are the primary seats of action. Nausea extending to the point of vomiting and accompanied by faintness and by severe vertigo when lifting the head is a characteristic symptom." Hughes says: "It influences the voluntary muscles rather than the intellectual powers; with this Hahnemann's provings entirely agree." Pareira says: "It acts rather on the voluntary muscles than the intellectual powers." We have given these quotations from different authors in order to find whether they afforded us much help from a practical standpoint. Dr. Hughes says the provings of Hahnemann corroborate these generalizations. We quote from the provings:

"Weakness of the cervical muscles with heaviness of

the *head, muscles seem unable to support the head.*" *(Calc. phos., Verat. alb.)* "Paralytic pain in the small of the back, with spasmodic drawing across the hips, which prevents walking." "His knees sink down from weakness, he totters while walking and threatens to fall to one side."

"At one time his feet are asleep, at another the hands." "The hand trembles while eating, and the more the higher it is raised." "Now one hand, now the other, seems insensible and asleep." "The soles of the feet go to sleep, while sitting." "General attacks of paralytic weakness, with pain in the back."

All these are verified symptoms from Allen's *Encyclopædia of Pure Materia Medica.* They are in the simplest terms, and while they do agree with the statements of the above quoted learned men, acting upon the spine and motor muscles, could be applied to the cure of the sick according to the directions of Hahnemann by any layman of ordinary intelligence. Thus is the practice of curative medicine simplified, being delivered from speculative theorizings of dreamers, and if it will cure the sick in the case of a *Cocculus* patient, it will by the same unerring law of "symptom covering" do it in every curable case.

We might sum up the whole action of this remedy upon the nervous system in one word, viz., *prostration,* but what does that amount to for purposes of prescribing. Many remedies prostrate fearfully, but each one has its *peculiar kind* of prostration, and when men, like I heard a celebrated surgeon in a homœopathic college do, make their boast that they prescribed on physiological ground, without any regard to symptomatology, I can but feel that such know little or nothing of the art of homœopathic prescribing, no matter what their other attainments. According to Hahnemann's teachings symptomatology leads in scientific prescribing, no matter what the pathological condition.

Aside from the symptoms which attend the general prostration and spinal trouble, or coupled with them, we have the following which are characteristic. "Confusion or stupefaction of the head, increased by eating and drinking." "Vertigo, as if intoxicated and confusion of the mind." "Whirling vertigo on rising up in bed; which compelled him to lie down again." "Sick headache with nausea and inclination to vomit." "All these symptoms are made particularly worse by riding in carriage or boat." Sea-sickness. (Sea-sickness > on deck in fresh cold air.) (*Tabac.*) The headaches and vertigo of *Cocculus* are different from *Bryonia,* notwithstanding the fact that both are made worse by rising up in bed. In *Bryonia* and some other remedies the sickness at the stomach precedes the headache which in *Cocculus* is exactly the reverse. Painful sensation of weakness or *emptiness* in the head is found under *Cocculus* and is in keeping with the general weakness. This sensation of *emptiness,* which is another name for *weakness,* is a general characteristic of *Cocculus,* and is found in head, abdomen, bowels, chest, heart, stomach; in short, in all internal parts. The nausea of *Cocculus,* which is so constant a symptom of the headaches, is something like that which is so characteristic of *Colchicum,* viz.: "Extreme aversion to food, caused even by the smell of food, although with hunger." With *Colchicum* there is more pronounced nausea, as well as aversion. The patient is nauseated *even to faintness.* There is with *Cocculus* a metallic taste in the mouth.

The sensorium comes under the same profound depression that invades the general nervous system. The patient is sad, absorbed within himself, brooding, moody, silent, sits in a corner buried in sad thoughts, etc. This is particularly the case in nervous fevers. *Depression, depression, depression.* *Cocculus* has some very important symptoms in the abdominal and uterine regions.

One is *great distention of the abdomen.* This is found in both flatulent colic and dysmenorrhœa. In flatulent colic, for which it is so valuable a remedy, the patient complains of a sensation as if the abdomen were full of sharp sticks or stones. The attacks are often at midnight. The flatus seems here and there, and passage of it does not seem to relieve much, for new forms again take its place.

Then again there seems to be great pressure in the inguinal region as if *hernia* would occur. In dysmenorrhœa, in addition to the distention, there are *griping, cramping* pains, which are very severe, and also a remarkable degree of *weakness. She is so weak that she can hardly stand, walk or talk.* This is very characteristic and, so far as weakness goes, resembles *Carbo animalis,* but in *Cocculus* it is in line with the general prostration of the remedy, while in *Carbo animalis* the **flow** weakens her. In *Cocculus* the flow may not be at all excessive, but on the contrary may grow less and less and a leucorrhœa appear in its stead, or even between the menses also. This is the way we have to differentiate between remedies if we are successful in practice.

Now, if I were to give the four great characteristic symptoms of this remedy they would be these:

1. Weakness of cervical muscles, with heaviness of head.

2. Affections caused or < by riding in cars, carriage or boat.

3. Sensation of weakness, or hollowness in various organs.

4. Ill effects from loss of sleep, night-watching or over-work. *(Causticum, Cuprum met., Ignatia, Nitric acid.)*

What would you add, my brother?

CONIUM MACULATUM.

Vertigo, especially < on turning the head, or looking around sidewise, or turning in bed.

Swelling and induration of glands, after contusions or bruises.

Cancerous and scrofulous persons with enlarged glands.

Urine flows, stops and flows again intermittently, prostatic or uterine affections.

Breasts sore, hard and painful during menstrual period.

* * * * *

This is another of the so-called spinal remedies. I will not, as I did under *Cocculus,* quote what authorities say from a pathological standpoint. All seem to agree that it paralyzes from below upwards, and the poisoning of Socrates with it is adduced in illustration. It ought to be a remedy for locomotor ataxia. The strongest characteristic I know, from a homœopathic standpoint, is its peculiar vertigo, which is much aggravated by *turning the head sidewise.* *(Coloc.,* turning head to left.) Turning over in bed is the same. Some say *lying down in bed and turning over.* I have found that it is not so much the *lying down* as it is the turning of the *head sidewise*, whether in an upright or horizontal posture.

I once treated a case of what seemed to be locomotor ataxia with this remedy.

The patient had been slowly losing the use of his legs; could not stand in the dark; and when he walked along the street would make his wife walk either ahead of him, or behind him, for the act of looking sidewise at her or in the least turning head or eyes that way would cause him to stagger or fall.

Conium cured him. It would always aggravate at first, but he would greatly improve after stopping the remedy. The aggravation was just as invariable after taking a dose of Fincke's c. m. potency as from anything lower, but the improvement lasted longer after it.

Taking an occasional dose from a week to four weeks apart completely cured him in about a year. It was a bad case, of years' standing, before I took him.

I have often verified this symptom in the vertigo of old people, where it is most frequently found; but it also often accompanies various affections in all ages, and especially is found in ovarian and uterine affections. I know of no remedy that has this symptom so strongly.

There is a form of ophthalmia in strumous subjects which calls for *Conium* in preference to any other remedy, and the peculiar, prominent and uncommon (as Hahnemann says, Organon, paragraph 153) symptom is, *photophobia, intense, out of all proportion to the objective signs* of inflammation in the eye. The pains are worse at night and terribly aggravated by the least ray of light, relieved in dark room and by pressure.

There may or may not be ulcers on the cornea. *Conium*

is also one of our best remedies for falling of the eyelids, as are three other remedies, viz.: *Gelsemium, Causticum* and *Sepia.* "Swelling and induration of glands, with tingling and stitches after *contusions or bruises.*" Many cases of lumps or swellings in the breasts (for which *Conium* seems to have a particular affinity) have disappeared under the action of this remedy. Even cancerous affections of breasts *(Asterias rubens),* uterus and stomach have been helped or cured, especially if the trouble seems to have originated in a *blow or injury* to the part. It is perhaps the first remedy to be thought of in all cases of tumors, scirrhous or otherwise, coming on after contusions, especially if they are of stony hardness and heavy feeling. *Conium* and *Silicea* both have hardness of mammæ, *Conium* right, *Silicea* left nodules *(Carbo animalis, Conium, Silicea);* acute lancinating pains. *(Asterias.)* Again it is to be especially considered if at every menstrual period the breasts become *large, sore and painful,* aggravated by the *least jar or walking.*

In all the scirrhous affections of the breast, womb or other parts the pains of *Conium* are burning, stinging, or darting, and may make one think of *Apis mellifica.* The other symptoms must then decide between them.

Conium has marked action upon the sexual organs. In the male there is great weakness of the organs. He has intense desire and amorous thoughts, but is unable to perform. He has emissions at the very thought or presence of a woman. The erections are insufficient, last only a short time, or "go back" on him in the act of embrace, and he suffers with weakness and chagrin afterwards. This affects the mind and hypochondriasis of the bluest blue takes possession of him. This condition of mind may obtain in both sexes; as a result of too free, and also especially too **infrequent** indulgence; or, excessive abstemiousness. Hence *Conium* becomes a good remedy for old bachelors and old maids. If the vertigo is also present in such cases *Conium* is sure to be of great benefit.

Intermittent flow of urine is very characteristic. (Clematis.) One might think that this was owing to a paralytic condition of the bladder. I don't know; but I do know that the symptom often occurs in the hypertrophy of the prostate gland incident to old age and *Conium* helps. "Sweats day or night; *as soon as one sleeps or even when closing the eyes,*" is a characteristic found under no other remedy that I know of. (Reverse *Sambucus.)*

Dr. Adolph Lippe once made a splendid cure of a complete one-sided paralysis in a man 80 years of age with this remedy, and was guided to it by this symptom. I think it would be rather a difficult task to give a correct pathological explanation of such a symptom; but there is a reason, and whether we can give it or not we can cure it if we have a corresponding one appearing under a remedy; where a cure is at all possible.

It is interesting to follow out the connections of symptoms. Take for instance the single prominent symptom of *Conium,* **vertigo.**

Vertigo on *turning* the head, Con., Calc. ost., Kali c.
" " *moving* the head, Bry., Calc. ost., Con.
" " looking up, Puls., Silic.
" " looking down, Phos., Spig., Sulph.
" from odor of flowers, Nux v., Phos.

Vertigo on *watching,* or loss of sleep, Cocc., Nux vom.
" " the *least noise,* Therid.
" while *walking,* Nat. m., Nux v., Phos., Puls.
" " studying, Nat. m.
" " or after eating, Grat., Nux v., Puls.
" as if whirling, Bry., Con., Cyclam., Puls.
" " the bed turned, Con.
" with fainting, Nux vom.
" " staggering, Arg. nit., Gels., Nux v., Phos.
" " eyes closed, or in dark, Arg. n., Stram., Therid.
" " dimness of sight, Cyclam., Gels., Nux v.
" when rising from seat, Bry., Phos.
" " " " stooping, Bellad.
" " " " bed, Bry., Chel., Cocc.
" " stooping, Bell., Nux, Puls., Sulph.
" " ascending, Calc. ost.
" " descending, Borax, Ferrum.
" " lying, Con.
" must lie down, Bry., Cocc., Phos., Puls.
" occipital, Gels., Sil., Petrol.
" after sleep, Lach.
" " suppressed menses, Cyclam., Puls.

A good understanding of such connection often starts the prescriber on the "short cut" route to the remedy in a case.

ÆSCULUS HIPPOCASTANUM.

Sense of *fullness* and pulsation in various organs and veins (especially plethoric), as if too full of blood.

Constant dull backache across sacrum and hips;

< walking or on stooping (piles, leucorrhœa, displacements, etc.).

Sense of fullness, and as of sticks in the rectum (hæmorrhoids).

Mucous membranes of mouth, throat, rectum are swollen, burn, dry and raw.

Coryza; thin, watery, burning; rawness and sensitive to inhaled cold air.

Frequent inclination to swallow, with burning, pricking, stinging and dry constricted fauces *(Apis, Bell.)*.

* * * * *

This is one of the remedies that is not so remarkable for its wide range of action as it is for positiveness within its range. Almost all its usefulness, so far as known, centers in its action in the lower back and pelvic region and ever prominent is this characteristic: *Constant dull backache, affecting sacrum and hips, much aggravated by walking or stooping.* It is one of our leading remedies for hæmorrhoids, and in addition to this backache there is a feeling of *fullness, dryness,* and sticking as if the rectum was *full of sticks.* There is not the tendency to protrusion or prolapsus that there is in *Ignatia, Aloe, Podophyllum* and some other remedies, and the backache is often greatly out of proportion to any external evidence of piles. This feeling of *fullness* seems to be a sort of general characteristic of *Æsculus,* but is especially prominent in the pelvic cavity.

These symptoms are often found in conjunction with other affections besides hæmorrhoids, such as uterine displacements, and inflammations; and some very bad forms of *leucorrhœa* have been promptly cured by this remedy. There is another quite valuable symptom in these pelvic troubles, viz.: *throbbing* or *beating* sensations, that calls for *Æsculus*. I have seen equally good results from the use of this remedy in the 3d, and the potencies.

I have used *Æsculus* with very good results in coryza and sore throat. The coryza is very much like the *Arsenic* coryza, thin, watery, and burning, but what characterizes *Æsculus* here is sensation of rawness; *sensitive to inhaled cold air.* In the throat it has the same sensation of rawness, both in the acute form, and also in chronic follicular pharyngitis, for which it is often a good remedy. It may be that age and use will develop more uses for this remedy.

ZINCUM METALLICUM.

Inability to develop or hold out the rash in eruptive diseases, can't expectorate or menstruate, is > if can.

Cannot take stimulants, as they aggravate in general.

Fidgety feet, *must move* them constantly.

Twitching of single muscles all over the body.

Violent trembling all over, so as to shake the bed; lost nerve control.

Weakness and weariness in nape of the neck; < holding head long in one position; backache < sitting.

Modalities: < from wine; > by restoration or development of eruptions, during menses, restored expectoration, seminal emission, discharges generally.

Defective vitality, brain and nerve power wanting; to comprehend, to memorize.

Child cries out during sleep; rolls the head from side to side; face alternately pale and red.

* * * * *

This metal seems to act principally upon the nervous system. I think it is Burt who says: "What *Iron* is to the blood, *Zinc* is to the nerves." If we examine the provings and clinical records of *Zinc,* we find that it seems to have the power to arouse or strengthen the nervous system in its inability to supply force to carry on functions necessary to health or the elimination of disease products from the system. This is speculation. What are the facts? 1st. If scarlatina or other eruptive diseases do not properly develop the eruption, on account of too great weakness of the patient, as evidenced by general depression of pulse, temperature, etc., *Zinc* is very useful.

Other remedies have such or similar trouble, *Cuprum,* for instance; but in *Cuprum* the eruption has been suppressed by some outward cause. *Zinc,* it has never come to the surface, or it has been out, and has receded from lack of vitality or strength to hold it there. *Sulphur* may be the remedy, but the cause is then more often apt to be traceable to psora.

This weakness shows in other ways, as, for instance, in asthma. The patient *can't expectorate,* but as soon as he can he is relieved; or again she *cannot menstruate,* and is relieved of her suffering while menstruating. *(Lachesis.)*

There is another peculiarity connected with this characteristic. The nervous weakness of the *Zincum* patient is that he can take no wine or stimulants. You would think that a little wine would at least temporarily relieve; on the contrary, it aggravates all the sufferings, even though taken in small quantities. Of course other remedies have this aggravation from wines or stimulants, like *Glonoine, Ledum, Fluoric acid, Antimonium crudum,* etc., but I think *Zinc* stands first.

The nervous debility of *Zinc* shows in other ways also. There is sometimes *aching and weariness in the nape of the neck,* as if it had been held in one position too long, < by writing or other long continued labor. The backaches are worse while *sitting* and better when moving about. This would call to mind *Rhus toxicodendron,* but with *Zincum* you would not get the *general* aching relieved by continued motion, as in the case with *Rhus. Pulsatilla* has it also, but generally in connection with menstrual irregularities. The remedy most resembling *Zinc* in this particular is *Cobaltum.* Both these remedies have this symptom in consequence of sexual excesses or weaknesses, but in *Zinc* an emission temporarily relieves the pain and in *Cobalt* it does not. The most characteristic of all the symptoms of *Zinc* in connection with its general nervous weakness, is: *"An incessant, violent fidgety feeling in the feet or lower limbs; must move them constantly."* This is present in many, if not almost all, of the affections for which *Zinc* is *par excellence* the remedy.

There is also sometimes present "burning along the whole length of the spine." This burning is purely subjective, for there is no actual local increase of temperature. Another characteristic of this remedy is, *"twitching and jerking of various muscles."* I spoke of this symptom when writing upon *Ignatia.* I would place *Zincum, Ignatia* and *Agaricus* in the van of all remedies for causing and curing these general twitchings.

Another symptom for which this is one of our best remedies is, *general trembling.* This is also from prostration.

The patient loses control over his motions, although he is not yet paralyzed. Paralysis may come later if this condition is not remedied.

A word or two about the importance of this remedy in

brain troubles. It makes little difference whether the affection of the brain arises from suppressed eruptive diseases, dentition, typhus fever or disease of any other name or nature, if the symptoms indicating the remedy are present. Allow me to relate a case from my own practice illustrating its curative value in typhoid.

A young lady about 20 years of age complained, a week before I was called, of weakness, or feeling of general prostration; headache, and loss of appetite, but the greatest complaint was of prostration. She was a student and her mother, who was an excellent nurse, attributed all her sickness to overwork at school, and tried to rest and "nurse her up." But she continued to grow worse. I prescribed for her *Gelsemium* and followed it with *Bryonia* according to indications, and she ran through a mild course of two weeks longer, and seemed convalescing quite satisfactorily.

Being left in a room alone, while sleeping and perspiring, she threw off her clothes, caught cold and relapsed. Of course the "last state of that patient was worse than the first." The bowels became enormously distended, profuse hæmorrhage occurred, which was finally controlled by *Alumen,* a low form of delirium came on, the prostration became extreme notwithstanding the hæmorrhage was checked, until the following picture obtained—staring eyes rolled upward into the head, head retracted; complete unconsciousness, lying on back and sliding down in bed, twitching, or rather intense, *violent trembling all over, so that* she shook the bed. I had nurses hold her hands night and day, she shook and trembled so; hippocratic face, extremities deathly cold to knees and elbows, pulse so weak and quick I could not count it, and intermittent; in short, all signs of impending paralysis of the brain. The case seemed hopeless, but I put ten drops of *Zincum metallicum* in two drams of cold water, and worked one-half of it between her set teeth, a little at a time, and an hour after the other half. In about one hour after the last dose she turned her eyes down and faintly said, *milk*. Through a bent tube she swallowed a half glass of milk, the first nourishment she had received in 24 hours. She got no more medicine for four days, and improved steadily all the time. She afterward received a dose of *Nux vomica* and progressed rapidly to a perfect recovery. So *Zincum* 200th can, like other metals, perform miracles when *indicated*.

STANNUM METALLICUM.

Sinking, empty, all-gone sensation in stomach *(Chel., Phos., Sep.)*.

Sad, despondent, feels like crying all the time, but crying makes her worse; faint and weak, especially when going downstairs; can go up well enough.

Colic > by hard pressure, or by laying abdomen across knee or on shoulder *(Col.)*; lumbrici; passes worms.

Leucorrhœa; great debility; weakness seems to proceed from chest.

Prolapsus, worse during stool, so weak she drops into a chair instead of sitting down. While dressing in the morning has to sit down several times to rest.

Great weakness in chest, can hardly talk, with general debility, which centers in the chest.

Loose cough; with heavy, green, sweet expectoration.

Pains gradually increase to a great height, and as gradually subside.

* * * * *

Another metallic remedy. The leading characteristic is *great weakness in the chest (Argentum met.)*; so weak cannot talk. No remedy has this symptom so strongly as tin. It is present, not only in the laryngeal and lung troubles for which *Stannum* is such a great remedy, but in *great debility. So weak she drops into a chair*, < going down stairs (*Borax; Calc. ost.* up stairs). It is found in connection with uterine displacements and leucorrhœas of thin, debilitated subjects and has made brilliant cures in such cases. Of course in the lung, bronchial, and laryngeal affections, this symptom is *very* prominent. In these troubles there is generally very profuse expectoration with the cough, and the matter raised tastes *very sweet,* or it may be exceptionally salty. For the salty expectoration I would sooner think of *Kali iod.* or *Sepia.* In all three of these remedies the expectoration may be thick, heavy, and green or yellow in color. Both *Stannum* and *Kali iod.* have profuse night sweats, but the *Stannum* has greater sense of weakness in the chest (cannot talk) than any of the others. Another very characteristic symptom of *Stannum* is that the *pains gradually increase to a great degree of intensity and then as gradually decrease.* (See *Platinum.*) This pain is of course neuralgic, may be located anywhere in the tract of a nerve, but has been often verified in prosopalgia, gastralgia and abdominal colic.

These pains are ameliorated by pressure, like *Colocynth* and *Bryonia;* so if *Colocynth* fails, which is generally first thought of in abdominal pains relieved by pressure, *Stannum* may relieve, and especially if the attacks have been of long standing or the patient seems to have a chronic tendency thereto. If in children, the patient is relieved by carrying it over the point of the shoulder, the shoulder pressing into the abdomen. The *Stannum* patient is generally very sad and despondent, feels like crying all the time. *(Nat. m., Puls., Sepia.)* I have often verified the above symptoms and have seen equally good effects from the 12th, 30th, 200th and 500th (Boericke & Tafel) potencies.

PLATINA.

Pride and over-estimation of one's self; looking down on others; things look small to her.

Genitals exceedingly sensitive, but excessive sexual desire; nymphomania, with ovarian troubles; prolapsus or profuse menses.

Pains increase gradually and as gradually decrease *(Stann.)*; sometimes attended with numbness *(Cham.)*.

* * * * *

This remedy may be studied in three relations: in its relation to the mental, nervous and sexual systems. It has curious mental symptoms. Here are three of them: "Pride and over-estimation of one's self; looking down with haughtiness on others." "Illusion of fancy, on entering the house after walking an hour, as if everything about her were very small, and all persons mentally and physically inferior, but she herself physically and mentally superior." "Changing moods, gay and sad alternately." This last symptom is like *Ignatia, Crocus, Nux moschata* and *Aconite,* and *Platina* has another symptom like *Aconite*—"fear of death." Now the first two symptoms above mentioned might appear to some as of no practical value in the treatment of the sick. There is no pathological explanation for them beyond the fact of a generally disordered mind, which might take any other form of hallucination. But this is a valuable indication and found under no other remedy. I was led by it to prescribe the remedy in a very obstinate case of insanity which had resisted the skill of several allopathic physicians of note, and they had finally decided that the case must be sent to the insane asylum. The parents, however, who were quite wealthy, could not consent to that, and were induced to try Homœopathy. I gave her *Platina* on the strength of this mental indication, which was very prominent, coupled with another prominent symptom, which also appears under this remedy, viz., "physical symptoms disappear and mental symptoms appear," and *vice versa.* The physical symptom was a pain the whole length of the spine. This was the symptom alternating with the mental one. It was one of the most brilliant cures I ever saw. Improvement began the first day and never flagged, and she remained well now 15 years, with never a sign of return.

The nervous symptoms outside the brain symptoms calling for *Platina* are: 1st. "The pains *increase gradually* and as *gradually decrease.*" 2d. "The pains are attended with numbness of the parts." This first symptom you will remember is like *Stannum,* but the *Platinum* patient is not characteristically so weak as the *Stannum* one. The second one is like *Chamomilla,* but the *Platina* patient is not so unvaryingly ugly as the *Chamomilla* one. Both are great mental remedies, however, and if any question arises (as there may) a close study of them in their entirety may be necessary.

In regard to the gradual outset of the pains of *Platina* and *Stannum, Belladonna* has exactly the opposite; but

Belladonna more resembles the *Platina* in its brain symptoms.

Sexual organs. "Nymphomania aggravated in the lying-in; tingling or tittilation up into the abdomen." "Excessive sexual desire, especially in virgins; premature or excessive development of sexual instinct." "Genitals excessively sensitive; cannot bear to be touched; will almost go into a spasm from an examination, and almost faint during intercourse." "Metrorrhagia or profuse menses; blood black and clotted."

Ovarian trouble and prolapsus with the profuse menses and excessive sensitiveness of the genitals to touch or coition. All these are very strong indications for this remedy. All these symptoms, mental, nervous, spasmodic, sexual, etc., would indicate that *Platina* ought to be a good remedy for that protean malady, hysteria, and so abundant experience has proven it to be. Here again I have, as in the case of *Zincum* and *Stannum,* found the higher preparation of the drug most potent for good, though in a case of insanity I used the 6th, not having it high at that time.

Platina has a form of constipation similar to *Alumina, i. e., the stools adhere to the anus like soft clay.*

SELENIUM.

Here is another metal that, like *Stannum,* has for its most characteristic condition, excessive weakness. But the weakness of *Selenium* does not, like *Stannum,* seem to centre in any particular locality. It is more general. He is so weak that he is easily exhausted from any kind of labor, either mental or physical. This debility may follow any exhaustive disease like typhoid fever, or may come from seminal emissions. The weakness of *Selenium* shows itself as much in the male sexual organs, as it does generally. Erections are slow and weak, emissions of semen too rapid in coition and he is cross and weak afterwards. Sexual desire strong, but he is *physically impotent.* Has seminal emissions two or three times a week, and gets up with weak, lame back after them. Prostatic fluid oozes while sitting, during sleep, when walking, or at stool. If this weakness has been of long standing, he begins to emaciate, especially in the *face, hands* and *thighs. (Acetic acid.)* This is a picture of the *Selenium* prostration. Aside from or connected with it are a few other characteristic symptoms, such as constipation, the stool being of such immense size that it cannot be discharged without mechanical aid. *(Sanicula.)* It must be picked away with the fingers. Involuntary dribbling of urine while walking, or after urinating or stool. *(Sarsaparilla* dribbles while sitting.)

Bad effects from drinking too much tea; all complaints are aggravated by it. Irresistible longing for spirituous liquors. Hoarseness, must often clear the throat of mucus especially at the beginning of singing. Irresistible desire for stimulants, wants to get drunk but feels worse after it. Very forgetful in business, but during sleep dreams of what he had forgotten. I have never used this metal below the 200th potency.

PHOSPHORUS.

Tall, slender, narrow-chested, phthisical patients, delicate eyelashes, soft hair, or nervous, weak persons who like to be magnetized. Waxy, half anæmic, jaundiced persons.

Anxious, universal restlessness, can't stand or sit still. < in dark or when left alone, before a thunder storm.

Burnings prominent in every place, as in mouth, stomach, small intestines, anus, between scapulæ, intense, running up spine, palms of hands, heat begins in hands, spreads to face.

Craving for cold things, ice cream, which agrees, or cold water, which is thrown up as it gets warm in the stomach. Must eat often or he faints. Must get up at night to eat.

Sinking, faint, empty feeling in head, chest, stomach and whole abdominal cavity.

Cough, < twilight till midnight, < lying on left side, > on right side. Right lower lobe most affected.

Diarrhœa, profuse, pouring out as from a hydrant; watery with sagolike particles or dysenteric, with wide open anus.

Apathetic, unwilling to talk, answers slowly, moves sluggishly.

Constipation: fæces slender, long, dry, tough and hard like a dog's; voided with difficulty.

Hæmorrhagic diathesis; slight wounds bleed profusely, hæmoptysis; metrorrhagia worse; vicarious, from nose, stomach, anus, urethra in amenorrhœa.

Cannot talk, the larynx is so painful; cough, going from warm to cold air, laughing, talking, reading, eating, lying on left side (*Dros., Stan.*).

* * * * *

As a general characteristic, **Burning** is almost as strong under this remedy as under *Arsenicum* and *Sulphur.* There is no organ or tissue in which it may not be found, from the outer skin to the innermost surface of every tract or parenchyma. It may be subjective only without actual rise of temperature, or it may attend organic changes in malignant diseases, with great rise of temperature. The sensation of *burning* in an intense degree should always place *Phosphorus* in the front rank for consideration. Again, there is perhaps no remedy having stronger action on **The Nervous System.** It attacks it in its very citadel of strength, the brain and spinal cord, producing softening or atrophy with all its attendant symptoms in their order, as prostration, trembling, numbness, and complete paralysis. It does this in both acute and chronic form of disease.

It will be found in acute typhoids as well as in that slowly progressive disease, locomotor ataxia. Its causes may be sudden, like pneumonia, typhus, exanthematic diseases, croup, bronchitis, when vitality reaches its lowest ebb, or may arise in a condition undermined by grief, care, or excessive mental exertion; excess in venery or onanism.

Its action at the first may be characterized by a burning heat in various parts, and especially in the skin, with restless moving and anxiety, especially at twilight. Over-sensitiveness of all senses, such as external impressions, light, odors, noises, touch, etc., and later when organic changes have taken place the other extreme, of loss of motion, sensation, and sensitiveness obtains.

In the former state there is one very characteristic symptom, *the patient moves continually, can't sit or stand still a moment.* Instead of fidgety feet, like *Zincum,* he is *fidgety all over.* *Phosphorus* affects every tissue. The blood becomes broken down or impoverished. Chlorosis and pernicious anæmia obtain. *Apis* and *Kali carb.* also each have anæmia or a pale waxy or what is called bloodless appearance of the patient. They all have œdema or bloating, and there is one peculiar difference in the face between them. In *Kali carb.* the upper lids bloat and hang down like a bag of water. In *Apis* it is more in the lower lids, while in *Phosphorus* they bloat all around the eyes; and the whole face bloats. Under *Phosphorus* the blood becomes so broken down that it will not clot any more, and we have purpura hæmorrhagica. Even in apparently healthy tissues we have this strong characteristic discovered by Hahnemann, viz.: *"Slight wounds bleed much."* This is what is called the hæmorrhagic diathesis, and much to be feared, as many persons having it may bleed to death from any slight abrasion; and this same tendency to bleed extends to fungoid growths like fibroids, fungoids, cancers, etc., and are very dangerous and troublesome.

Then again *Phosphorus* attacks the bones in the form of necrosis. It is so especially of the lower jaw, but is also true of other parts, as the vertebræ; and I once cured a very extensive and long standing case of caries of the tibia with it.

Fatty degeneration of heart, liver and kidneys, with the characteristic anæmic condition, should call attention to this remedy. General emaciation, rapid or slowly progressing like atrophy in children, also comes under its tissue destroying power.

And so we find it to be a remedy of wide range and great power. But it is never enough for the homœopathist to know simply the action in general upon any organ or set of organs. He must know how it acts differently from other remedies when acting upon the same tissue or

13

organs. Now while *Phosphorus* acts upon the mind, to cause "great anxiety and restlessness" as in other remedies, *Aconite, Arsenicum,* etc., it must be remembered that it is the anxiety and restlessness that precedes another state.

It belongs to a stage of irritation in the brain and nervous system which if not checked will go on to organic changes, which will be attended with a very different set of symptoms, such as come for instance from actual brain softening in which appears *apathy, sluggishness; talks slowly, is indifferent or won't talk at all.* There is one particular symptom worthy of note: *the patient fears to be left alone;* is afraid; afraid of the dark, in a thunder storm, etc. This is more during the irritable stage of which we have spoken. *Phosphorus* is a great remedy in typhoids, especially with lung complications, and here we often get stupor and low muttering delirium like *Lachesis,* but while *Lachesis* is worse after sleep, *Phosphorus* is generally better, if he can get to sleep. In the late stage of brain or nervous troubles, calling for this remedy, we find the patient losing all ambition to do anything; either mental or physical labor is shunned. There is great indifference. He cannot think with his usual clearness; cannot apply himself to study or mental operations, ideas come slowly or not at all. Again the patient is sometimes amative, or like *Hyoscyamus* shamelessly exposes himself.

There is no remedy that covers a greater variety of mind symptoms arising from brain trouble than *Phosphorus.* No remedy produces greater vertigo, with a longer list of various connections. I have found it one of the best and oftenest indicated for *vertigo of the aged.*

Chronic congestion to the head is characteristic, and the sense of burning in the brain is prominent; the heat and congestion seems to *come up from the spine.*

Heat running up the back is more characteristic of this than any other remedy. Deafness is prominent, and is peculiar, in that it is especially *deafness to the human voice,* a common symptom in the aged. The most frequent use I have made of the remedy in nose affections is in a chronic catarrh, in which the patient frequently blows *small quantities of blood from the nose;* the handkerchief is *always* bloody.

As I said when writing upon the tissues, the face of *Phosphorus* is characteristically pale and bloated around the eyes, but in pneumonia we often find circumscribed redness of the cheek upon the side of the lung inflamed. This is also true with *Sanguinaria.* About the mouth and tongue I do not know anything particularly characteristic. It has a peculiar symptom of the throat. *The food swallowed comes up immediately as if it had never reached the stomach.* This is supposed to be due to spasmodic stricture of the œsophagus.

Under appetite and thirst we have some very valuable indications for this remedy.

Hunger is one, must eat often or he faints; right after or soon after a meal, is hungry; hungry in the night; must eat. He is relieved by eating, but is soon hungry again. This calls to mind *Iodine, Chelidonium, Petroleum, Anacardium,* etc.

The thirst is also peculiar. He wants *cold things,* like *Pulsatilla,* but *as soon as they get warm in the stomach they are vomited.*

Some people have an abnormal craving tor salt, or salt

food, and eat too much of it. *Phosphorus* is a good remedy to counteract the bad effects. *(Nat. mur.)*

We have many kinds of vomiting under *Phosphorus,* but nothing characteristic except the one already mentioned.

We have already spoken of the hungry, faint feeling in the stomach. Sometimes this is described as an empty, gone feeling, and here again we think of such remedies as *Ignatia, Hydrastis, Sepia* and others; but *Phosphorus* does not stop here with this sensation, but extends through the *whole abdomen.* No remedy has this feeling in the abdomen so strong as *Phosphorus.* Under stool and rectum occur some very characteristic symptoms also, for instance: Stools profuse, watery, *pouring away as from a hydrant,* with lumps of white mucus, like *grains of tallow.* Stools bloody, with small white particles like opaque frog-spawn. Stools involuntarily oozing from a *constantly open anus,* or dysenteric stools with wide-open anus and *great tenesmus.* Constipation; fæces slender, *long, dry, tough like dog stools.* No remedy has a richer array of stool symptoms, and as we see by the above few select ones, some of them are very unique and have often been verified. It will repay any physician to carefully and frequently look them over.

This remedy powerfully excites the sexual appetite in both sexes. It is almost irresistible, and leads the patient into a mania in which he will expose himself. This is succeeded by the opposite extreme of impotence, though the desire remains after the ability to perform is gone. Of course, these sexual symptoms are accompanied with concomitant symptoms of the drug.

Upon the female sexual organs *Phosphorus* is true to

its general hæmorrhagic tendencies; if the menses do not appear, there is often *vicarious bleeding* from the nose or lungs instead. *Phosphorus* is *bound to bleed.* It is so with cancer of the womb or breasts also. They bleed easily. Upon the *respiratory organs* also this is one of our greatest remedies. Beginning with the voice and larynx, it causes and cures *great* hoarseness. Patient can hardly make a loud noise, and is apt to be worse in the evening or fore-part of the night. There is *pain in the larynx,* worse by talking, or can't talk at all on account of it. In croup, it sometimes comes in after *Aconitum* and *Spongia* have failed. The disease has progressed downward until it involves the bronchi and parenchyma of the lungs. It is of indispensable value here, and, also when, after the violence of the affection seems to have abated, the patient hoarses up every evening and seems to be *inclined to relapse.*

In bronchitis the cough is tight, worse from evening to midnight, also from *speaking, laughing, reading aloud (Argentum met.), cold, and lying on left side.* The patient suppresses the cough with a moan just as long as he can, because it hurts him so. The whole body *trembles* with the cough.

It has great oppression of breathing in both acute and chronic affections of the lungs. There is *heaviness, as of a weight on the chest.* In pneumonia, for which *Phosphorus* is one of our best remedies, it attacks by preference the *lower half of the right lung.* It is apt to be indicated by the symptoms, either at the beginning of the stage of hepatization, when it puts a stop to the further progress of the disease, but its more frequent application comes in where the stage of hepatization is past and we want to break it up and promote absorption or resolution. Here it has no equal, as I am fully convinced by abundant experience.

Now, do not misunderstand and give the remedy blindly on a pathological indication only. If you do you will sometimes fail, and ought to. But I repeat, this remedy will oftener be found the indicated one here than any other. After the hepatization begins to break up, other remedies like *Tartar emetic, Sulphur* and *Lycopodium* will come in.

In pleuritis you will find stitches in the *left* side increased by lying upon the left side. Remember in both affections *Phosphorus* is characteristically increased by lying upon the left side.

In tuberculosis, it is oftenest indicated in the incipient stage with the symptom of cough, oppression and general weakness already mentioned; but I have often found it indicated in the later stages, and if given very high and in the single dose and not repeated have seen it greatly benefit even incurable cases. If given too low and repeated it will fearfully aggravate.

One of the most characteristic symptoms of this remedy is, *"feeling of intense heat running up the back."* Again the burning may be in spots along the spine. Also it has intense heat and burning between the scapulæ. (See also *Lycopodium.)*

These, like the rest of the burnings of *Phosphorus,* often occur in diseases of the spine and nervous system, but not necessarily so. Like *Zinc,* these burnings may be purely subjective, but are none the less valuable as therapeutic indications.

Another very characteristic symptom of *Phosphorus* is

burning of the hands. It is as strong as the burning feet of *Sulphur,* and is found both in acute and chronic diseases; cannot bear to have the hands covered. The flashes of heat all over (which *Phosphorus* has) *begin* in the hands and spread from there even to the face. It now remains to call attention to the **Constitution of Phosphorus.**

1. "Tall, slender persons of sanguine temperament, fair skin, blonde or red hair; quick, lively perception and sensitive nature."

2. "Tall, slender phthisical patients, delicate eyelashes, soft hair."

3. "Tall, slender women disposed to stoop."

4. "Young people who grow too rapidly and are inclined to stoop."

5. "Nervous, weak persons who like to be magnetized."

Now, in number four there is not the tendency to grow fat, like *Calcarea carbonica,* but tall, and you will notice that the *Phosphorus* element in *Calcarea phosphorica* takes away the fat producing property of the *Calcarea* element.

Now, in closing, we desire to say we have only touched upon the wonderful virtues of this drug, which must be studied in its entirety. Enough, however, we trust to convince of its great value.

SEPIA.

Bearing down pains, must sit close and cross her legs to keep something from coming down out of the vagina.

Sense of fullness in the pelvic organs, and pressure down into the anus, as if a ball or weight; oozing of moisture.

Flushes of heat and perspiration at the climacteric.

Painful sense of emptiness or goneness at the pit of the stomach.

General relaxation, weak, faints while kneeling at church; falling womb and pelvic organs; drooping eyelids, weak back < on walking.

Cachectic, yellow face, with yellow saddle across face and nose; moth patches; ringworms.

Modalities: < standing, mental labor, sexual excess, jar, after sleep, laundry work; milk (diarrhœa), climacteric, kneeling at church, > sitting with legs crossed, loosening clothes, open air.

Sensation of a ball in inner parts; during menses, pregnancy, lactation, great sadness and weeping. Dread of being alone; of meeting friends, indifferent, even to one's family, to one's occupation; to those whom she loves.

Headache: in terrific shocks; pressing, bursting < motion, stooping, mental labor, > by pressure, continued fast motion.

Urine: deposits a reddish clay sediment, which adheres to the vessel; fœtid, offensive, must be removed from room.

Enuresis: bed wet almost as soon as the child goes to sleep; during first sleep, violent stitches upward in the vagina.

Dyspnœa; < sitting, after sleep, in room, > dancing or walking rapidly.

* * * * *

This is another of our wonderful remedies of which the dominant school knows nothing, except they have learned it from us. Its chief sphere of action seems to be in the abdomen and pelvis, especially in women. No remedy produces stronger symptoms here. We quote from different but equally good observers.

"Sensation of bearing down in the pelvic region, with dragging pains from the sacrum; or feeling of bearing down of all the pelvic organs." (Hahnemann.)

"Labor-like pains accompanied with a feeling as though she must cross her legs and 'sit close' to keep something from coming out through the vagina." (Guernsey.)

"Pain in uterus, bearing down, comes from back to abdomen, causing oppression of breathing; crosses limbs to prevent protrusion of parts." (Hering.)

"Prolapsus of the uterus, of the vagina, with pressure as if everything would protrude." (Lippe.)

"Experience has shown its value in cases of ulceration and congestion of the os and cervix uteri. Its use supercedes all local applications." (Dunham.)

No higher authority than the united testimony of these five of our best observers could be brought to show the action ot *Sepia* upon the pelvic organs.

Now when we come to examine the provings in Allen's *Encyclopædia,* we find that these symptoms were mainly produced by Hahnemann and his provers, and Hahnemann advocated proving remedies in the 30th, and some of them were produced by the 200th, especially those most strongly verified by black-faced type.

We confess that we cannot understand how so many question the value of potencies for proving or curing, and most of all do we wonder at Dr. T. F. Allen himself "going back" on potencies above the 12th. Such a course looks very much to us like "kicking against the pricks" or, in other words, trying to fight the truth. But we must be charitable.

Sepia, like *Sulphur,* affects the general circulation in a very marked manner. *Flashes of heat* with *perspiration* and *faintness* is almost as characteristic of this remedy as of *Sulphur.* But there are, with *Sepia,* more apt to be associated with them the pelvic symptoms already given, and they are also more apt to occur in connection with the *climacteric.* Indeed, these flashes often seem with *Sepia* to start in the pelvic organs and from thence to spread over the body.

But this irregularity of circulation extends as far as that of *Sulphur.* The hands and feet are hot alternately, that is, if the feet are hot, the hands are cold, and *vice versa.* There is not so much *sensation* of burning with *Sepia* as with *Sulphur,* but there is actual heat, and the venous congestion, which seems to be the real state of the organs where the pressive bearing down et cetera is felt, is also accompanied with much throbbing and beating.

This local congestion to the pelvic organs is not simply sensational. There are actual displacements in consequence of it, and the long continued congestion results in inflammations, ulcerations, leucorrhœas and even malignant or cancerous disorganizations. Induration with a painful *sense* of stiffness in the uterine region is characteristic.

This pelvic congestion also affects the rectum in a marked degree. The rectum prolapses, there is a sensation of fullness, or of a foreign substance as of a *ball or weight,* and oozing of moisture from the rectum. Indeed, the rectal and anal symptoms are almost as strong as the uterine and vaginal. It is impossible to enumerate all the symptoms connected with the circulatory disturbances of *Sepia* in such a work as this, only a general study of the Materia Medica can do it.

The urinary organs come in for their share of symptoms. The same pressure and fullness consequent upon the portal congestion reaches here. We will now proceed to give what we have found to be particularly valuable symptoms under the various organs in this region. "Pressure on bladder and frequent micturition with tension in lower abdomen." "Sediment in the urine like clay; as if clay was burnt on the bottom of the vessel; urine *very offensive (Indium),* can't endure to have it in the room, it is reddish or may be bloody." This is found mostly with women. With children there is one peculiar symptom which has often been verified. "The child always wets the bed during its *first sleep.*"

Upon the male organs I have found it particularly useful in chronic gleet. There is not much discharge, but a few drops, perhaps, which glue up the orifice of the urethra in the morning; but it is so persistent and the usual remedies will not "dry it up." In my early practice I used to use a weak injection of *Sulphate of Zinc,* but it used to annoy me that I could not do it without resorting to local measures. *Sepia* does it in the majority of cases and *Kali iodatum* will do it in the rest. I have, where there was a thick discharge of long standing and the smarting and burning on urinating continued, several times finished the case with *Capsicum.*

As a rule, this long continued slight, passive gleety discharge is a result of weakness of the male genitals, as is shown by a flaccidity of the organs and frequent seminal emissions. The emissions are thin and watery. *Sepia* covers all of this and often sets all to rights in a short time.

The mind symptoms of *Sepia* are like *Pulsatilla,* in that she is sad and cries frequently without knowing the reason why. So if in a tearful mind with uterine disturbances *Pulsatilla* should fail you, the next remedy to be studied is *Sepia.* But there is another condition of mind not found under *Pulsatilla* or any other remedy in the same degree, and that is, that, notwithstanding there is no sign of dementia from actual brain lesion, the patient, contrary to her usual habit, *becomes indifferent to her occupation,* her house work, her family or their comfort, *even to those whom she loves the best.* This is a very peculiar symptom and a genuine keynote for the exhibition of *Sepia.*

Upon the head *Sepia* is one of our best remedies in hemicrania of women of the *Sepia* temperament, and who are suffering from uterine trouble which we have already described. Another peculiar headache is, that the pain comes in *terrific shocks,* so as to *jerk* the *head* in spite of the patient.

There are three remedies that have prominently drooping eyelids *(Causticum, Gelsemium* and *Sepia).* Of course, the other symptoms must decide which is the one indicated in the case at hand. So far as the *nose* is concerned *Sepia* is often of use in chronic catarrh. I had a case in which the discharge was thick, bland and in large quantities. *Pulsatilla* would relieve the catarrhal trouble but would, at the same time, increase the menstrual flow too much, but *Sepia* cured both. The choice will sometimes have to be made between *Kali bichromicum* and *Sepia* in these chronic catarrhs, but it is generally easy, although the local symptoms are much alike.

"Yellow saddle across upper part of cheeks and nose,

and *yellow spots on the face,"* is a characteristic of great value, but the yellowness and yellow spots do not always stop here. You may find them in abundance on the abdomen. The whole surface of the body may be yellow like jaundice. The face of the *Sepia* patient is the most "tell tale" face I know, and if you find it upon a woman you may always find her leading symptoms in connection with her menstrual and uterine functions.

There is one symptom of *Sepia* upon the stomach that is also very characteristic, viz., a "painful sensation of emptiness, *goneness* or faintness." The patient will call it an "all gone" feeling. Of course you remember that *Ignatia* and *Hydrastis Canadensis* have this symptom very strongly. Other remedies also have it in more or less marked degree but none so strongly in connection with uterine symptoms as *Sepia,* unless perhaps it be *Murex purpurea,* and you will not often have much difficulty in choosing between these last two if you carefully examine all the symptoms. I have often thought that this symptom, so persistent and severe, might be due to the actual emptying of the upper abdomen by the prolapsed womb, dragging everything after itself into the pelvic cavity. It is so in *Stannum* and *Lilium tigrinum,* and the weakness of the natural supports (ligaments) of the uterus being *remedied* (not supplanted by the pessaries and artificial supports of various kinds) the distressing symptoms disappear. *Vomiting in pregnancy* with this "all gone" feeling is often cured by *Sepia;* also the *thought or smell (Colch.)* of food sickens her. I mentioned the "sense of weight or a ball in the rectum" when writing of the pelvic congestion of *Sepia.* This sensation is not relieved by stool. *Sepia* is a remedy for constipation, and that of a very obstinate character. Like *Selenium* it has great straining; but manual aid is necessary to accomplish the stool. This is mostly in children.

I once cured a very obstinate case of entero-colitis (so-called cholera infantum), after the complete failure of two eminent allopaths, with *Sepia,* the leading symptom being, *"always worse after taking milk."* Oozing of moisture from the anus finds its remedy here sometimes, but oftener in *Antimonium crudum.* The *Sepia* patient is very weak. "A short walk fatigues her very much." She *faints easily* from extremes of cold or heat, after getting wet, from riding in a carriage, while kneeling at church, and on other trifling occasions. This fainting, or sense of sinking faintness, may be found in pregnancy, child bed, or during lactation; or, again, it may come on after hard work, such as "laundry work;" so it has come to be called the "washer woman's" remedy. *Phosphorus* has washer woman's toothache.

SKIN. "Itching often changes to burning when scratching." *(Sulph.)* "Soreness of skin; humid places in bend of knees." "Brown spots in face, chest, abdomen; chloasma." Herpes circinatus. "Large suppurating pustules constantly renewing themselves." "Acarus itch, pruritus; tettery eruptions, etc." *Sepia,* like *Sulphur,* has many forms of eruption on the skin, and indeed there is great general resemblance between these two antipsorics. They follow each other well. Of course that is always providing they are indicated by the symptoms, which is often the case. I do not believe in the so-called incompatibles as some do. I should give *Causticum* after *Phosphorus, Silicea* after *Mercury,* or *Rhus tox.* after *Apis mel.* if I found them *indicated.*

MUREX PURPUREA

Is a remedy which, though not extensively proven, bids fair to become exceedingly useful. So far as we know, it comes nearer to *Sepia* than any other remedy and the characteristic difference between them is, that with *Murex* there is great, *almost uncontrollable sexual desire,* while with *Sepia* there is a lack of or aversion to the same, especially with prolapsus.

Both remedies have *"sinking, all gone"* sensation in the stomach; also "bearing down" sensation, as if *internal organs would be pushed out, must sit and cross limbs to ameliorate the pressure,* but the sexual irritation and desire of *Murex* is excited by the least contact of the parts. *(Orig., Zinc.)*

Again, *Murex* has a *sore pain in uterus,* something like *Helonias,* which is expressed as "conscious of a womb," feels it more when she moves, **it is so sore and tender.** *(Lyssin.)*

Two other remedies must be remembered in nymphomania, viz., *Lilium* and *Platina.*

LILIUM TIGRINUM.

Great bearing down, as if pelvic contents would press out through the vagina; > by pressing up with the hand or sitting down *(Sepia* crosses the legs).

Sensation of constriction in heart with uterine troubles.

Frequent desire for stool and urine with uterine displacements, tenesmus.

Tormented about her salvation.

Listless, yet does not want to sit still; restless, yet does not want to walk; hurried manner, desire to do something, yet no ambition; imperative duties, inability to perform them.

Depression of spirits: disposition to weep; aversion to food; indifferent about anything being done for her.

* * * * *

Lilium tigrinum is one of the remedies that closely resembles *Sepia* in its action on the uterine organs. This symptom, for instance, *"weight, with feeling as if the pelvic contents would pass out through the vagina if not prevented by pressure with the hand* (pressing up against the vulva, *Lilium tig.),* or by sitting down." There is no remedy that is more efficacious for uterine displacement than *Lilium.* The persistent bearing-down feeling in the uterine region of *Lilium* is attended with a feeling as if the pelvic viscera, indeed the whole abdominal contents, were being dragged downward, even from the chest and shoulders, towards the vagina.

The choice between *Lilium* and *Sepia* might not always be easy. The *Sepia* case is more likely to be a chronic one. On the other hand, the *Lilium* case is more intense, painful and distressing. The *Sepia* cachexia, of course, would decide easily in its favor, if it is markedly present There is more urinary irritation, or frequent desire to urinate, with *Lilium;* indeed this is sometimes so severe as to make one think of *Cantharis.* Again, rectal irritation and distress is often found in conjunction with the urinary, in this respect reminding one of *Merc. cor., Capsicum* or *Nux vomica.*

With the uterine we often have quite an array of very severe heart symptoms. There are sharp quick pains, and much fluttering of the heart. This remedy also has in a marked degree the great characteristic symptom of *Cactus grandiflorus, "sensation as if the heart were constricted or held by an iron band."* This symptom, associated with the many other heart symptoms, has sometimes led to a prescription of *Cactus*, when *Lilium* was the remedy and *vice versa*. The uterine symptoms are sometimes masked so as to be over-looked for the time by the violence of the heart symptoms. All these heart, urinary, and rectal symptoms seem to be mainly reflex, while the real trouble is centered in the uterus and its appendages.

The mind is also very markedly affected under *Lilium*. Here it may resemble *Pulsatilla* for tearfulness; doubts her salvation, like *Veratrum album*, *Sulphur* and *Lycopodium* and a constant *hurried* feeling, as of *imperative* duties with utter inability to perform them. (See *Argentum nitricum.*)

VIBURNUM OPULUS

Is a remedy of undoubted value in painful womb troubles. It has been used for painful dysmenorrhœa in different potencies to the 30th, and in tincture. It seems to be particularly efficacious in the neuralgic form of the disease. I have found that the symptom, *pain beginning in the back and going around to loins and to uterus, ending in cramps there,* is the most remarkable indication. With this symptom present, I have seemingly checked an impending abortion, and in one case even after a slight flow of blood was present.

Actæa racemosa, Chamomilla, Caulophyllum, Magnesia phos. and *Viburnum* are all excellent remedies in neuralgic dysmenorrhœa. In *Actæa*, the pains are in back, through hips and down the thighs. In *Chamomilla*, they make the patient mad and she says she cannot bear them.

With *Caulophyllum* the pains are very intermittent and spasmodic, screams with the pains.

With *Magnesia phos.* hot applications to the hypogastrium ameliorate more or less.

Of course we have many other remedies for this painful affection, among which are *Pulsatilla, Cocculus, Cuprum, Cactus, Belladonna, Platina,* etc.

For particular indications, we must refer to our Materia Medica.

SECALE CORNUTUM.

Passive hæmorrhage, everything open and loose, no action, *in thin, scrawny, cachectic women.*

Great coldness (objective) of the surface, yet the patient cannot bear to be covered.

Numbness, crawling and paralysis; formication as of mice creeping there, all parts of body.

* * * * *

Secale cornutum is a remedy capable of great good, but is, perhaps, as much misused as Quinine. Its power to contract the uterus is undoubted, and for this reason it is often given when other remedies would do better. It has power to control hæmorrhages that few other remedies, if any, can surpass. It is said to do this by contracting the capillaries. But we must remember that other remedies control hæmorrhages, and whether they do it by contracting the capillaries, by their action upon the blood itself, or other specific action, makes no difference, so long as they *control it.* Some physicians are always giving *Ergot* in post-partum hæmorrhages on this **contracted** theory, without ever thinking of anything else. They always give it in material doses to get, as they term it, the *physiological* effect. I have never, in a practice of thirty-five years, used it in this way, but have always been able to control such hæmorrhages. *Secale* is not often indicated in active post-partum hæmorrhages. If there is a tendency to passive hæmorrhage, everything open and loose, no action, *in thin, scrawny, cachectic women* (muscles flabby), there is no remedy like it, and the potencies are much better than the tincture or wine of *Ergot* in massive doses. This is also true in menorrhagias and metrorrhagias unconnected with pregnancy. The blood is dark, liquid and flowing worse on the slightest motion.

The constitution, temperament and age of the patient are of great importance, for it is particularly adapted to *feeble, thin, scrawny, cachectic women of lax muscular fibre, subject to passive hæmorrhages* from all outlets of the body; also old, decrepid persons.

This remedy *(Secale)* is often abused on account of its power to produce muscular contractions of the womb. Now in regard to this as with hæmorrhages, it is capable of doing all that it ought to be called upon to do, in the potencies.

I fully agree with Cowperthwaite, who says: "To give it in parturition to hasten delivery, as is the practice of the old school, is simply inexcusable." On the other hand, I agree with Dr. H. N. Guernsey, "that it is useful when labor pains are weak, suppressed or distressing, in weak, cachectic women, in the 200th dilution," and have verified it beyond question.

The practice of giving the fluid extract in such cases, as is done by some physicians calling themselves homœopathic, ought to be sufficient cause for expelling them from a homœopathic society. It seems to me to be confession of either inexcusable laziness or ignorance.

We have a long list of remedies of undoubted value for weak labor pains with specific indications for their use, and when so indicated they are more efficacious and less dangerous than *Secale* in massive doses of fluid extract with no other indications than uncontracted uterus or weak pains. The men who prate learnedly of getting the *physiological* effects of *Secale* in massive doses had better ask themselves if the same result gotten with the potentized remedy homœopathically applied, is not just as much in accordance with the physiological law, and much more scientific from a homœopathic standpoint. Weak pains remedied by the indicated homœopathic drug bring on *natural* labor, while large doses for the same purpose of an unindicated one do not and never can produce *natural labor.* It is nothing more or less than drug poisoning.

Here is one symptom of *Secale* that is of inestimable value: "*Great coldness* (objective) *of the surface* yet the patient cannot bear to be covered." This is oftenest found in cholera and cholera infantum; but it is also found in senile gangrene. The feet and toes may be objectively as cold as an iron wedge, but the patient is distressed beyond endurance by having them covered. I saw one marked case of this kind. All the toes were attacked with dry gangrene. A few doses of *Secale* (high) afforded great relief, and checked the progress of the disease for a long time.

Camphora has the same symptom in a marked degree in choleraic disease. *Camphora* seems to be most efficacious for the first stage or early collapse in the course of the disease, before the discharges have become offensive, putrid or dark colored. *Secale* has burning in the feet *(Sulphur)* and cramps in the calves *(Sulphur)*.

If, however, we should prescribe on this alone it would make no difference which we prescribed, but they are very unlike in their entirety. *Sulphur* does not have the degree of collapse of *Secale,* nor the icy coldness of surface with subjective burning. So we see the folly of one symptom prescribing after all.

We must have the keynote symptom, of course, but it must harmonize with the rest of the case. *Secale* has "burning of all parts of the body, as if sparks were falling on them." It also has *numbness,* crawling and paralysis of the extremities. This is due to its action on the spinal chord. In addition to the coldness of the skin already noticed, we must state that the skin looks *dry,* wrinkled and is insensible often, or there may be much *formication* under, as if mice were creeping there.

CAULOPHYLLUM THALICTROIDES

Is another very valuable "woman remedy," because of its specific action upon the uterus. It deserves a thorough reproving. I cannot better show its virtues than by reporting a case.

A married lady, aged 40, with wry neck of long standing, was seven months' pregnant. She was attacked with *severe pains and swelling of all the finger joints.* The only way she could get relief from the intense pain so that she could rest or sleep at all was by enveloping her fingers in mustard. I prescribed *Caulophyllum* 3d, which relieved the finger pains, but brought on such severe labor pains that I was obliged to discontinue it for fear of premature labor. Then the bearing-down pains ceased, and the finger pains returned and continued in full force until she was delivered of her child, when they also ceased for two or three days. Then the lochia, instead of decreasing, gradually or normally, increased until it amounted to a metrorrhagia. *The flow was of a passive nature, dark and liquid.* There was great sense of weakness and *internal trembling* (not visible externally) and now, to crown her suffering, the terrible finger pains returned again. I was afraid of the *Caulophyllum,* although it seemed indicated, because it brought on the bearing-down pains when I gave it before. But after giving *Arnica, Sabina, Secale* and *Sulphur,* without the least improvement, I concluded to try *Caulophyllum high.* I did so in the 200th potency and cured the whole case promptly and permanently. Now this was a perfect *Caulophyllum* case, and if I had given it properly in the first place I have no doubt I would have saved that woman all unnecessary suffering.

I have given this remedy in long-continued passive hæmorrhage from the uterus after miscarriage when I had the characteristic weakness and sense of *internal trembling* present. It has often regulated irregular spasmodic labor pains, and has also often relieved pains of the same character in dysmenorrhœa. I repeat, this remedy deserves a careful reproving.

ACTÆA RACEMOSA.

Nervous symptoms, twitchings, spasms, convulsions, neuralgias; chills without shaking < at menstrual period.

Muscular rheumatism; stiff neck, drawing head back;

can't turn the head; rheumatism of the belly of muscles, by preference.

Headaches *pressing outward;* or upward, as if top of head would fly off, or into eyes (ciliary neuralgia), or down nape into spine.

Gloomy, sad, *sleepless;* thinks she will go insane.

Menorrhagia; pains run through hips into thighs, passing down.

Climacteric; infra-mammary pains left side, persistent.

Modalities: < menstrual period and during climacteric.

* * * * *

Actæa racemosa is another remedy which exerts a strong influence upon the female organism. The nervous system manifests its action in a multitude of symptoms, many of them being what is known as hysterical in character. There are twitchings, spasms, convulsions, neuralgias and mental symptoms in abundance. She shivers (nervous chill without coldness), faints, talks incessantly, frequently changing subjects; is grieved and troubled, with sighing, or is *very gloomy with sleeplessness;* thinks she is going insane, etc.

In the head there are severe pains, *pressing outward,* as if the top of the head would fly off, or *running into the eyes,* which ache fearfully; or the pains settle in the *occiput and shoot down the neck.* There are very few, if any, remedies that have worse ciliary neuralgia than *Actæa racemosa.*

In the female sexual organs it cures "pains in the uterine region, darting from side to side." The menstrual function is performed irregularly. Sometimes the flow is scanty, but more generally profuse, and we have the mental and nervous symptoms above enumerated in abundance, with these irregularities. It is one of our best remedies in menorrhagia, when there is *"severe pain in the back, down the thighs and through the hips, with heavy pressing down,"* as I have often proven. It is also excellent in *infra-mammary pains in the left side* during the climacteric, as I have also proven.

Also in backache and spinal irritation sympathetic with uterine troubles. It cures sharp lancinating pains in various parts, either nervous or muscular, if they are connected with uterine disturbances. In rheumatism the affection attacks the *belly of the muscle* by preference. *Actæa* is a many-sided remedy and adapted to nervous troubles of many forms.

SABINA

Is one of our best remedies for profuse flowing from the female genital organs, as in menorrhagia, metrorrhagia, abortions, or after labor.

These hæmorrhages are apt to occur in paroxysms, worse from motion *(Secale)*, blood dark *(Kali nit.* and *Cyclamen)*, and clotted *(Crocus)*, or partly clotted and partly fluid and watery *(Ferrum)*, the clots being black; from loss of tone in the uterus; *(Caulophyl.)* after abortion or parturition, with *pain from back to pubes.* This pain from back to pubes is its grand keynote, and may be found, not only in flooding, but in threatened abortion and menstrual troubles generally. There is sometimes present the general characteristic of *Pulsatilla,* "aggravation from warm air and in a warm room, and amelioration in open, cool, fresh air," and in cases of too profuse menstruation; but you cannot give *Pulsatilla* because it increases the already too profuse flow. Here is where

Sabina comes in, for it has the same aggravation and amelioration *with* the profuse flow. This is an important diagnostic difference between the two remedies and is reliable.

Sabina is indicated in threatened abortion at the third month, especially if the characteristic pain from back to pubes is present. If the pains begin in the back and go around from there and end with cramps in the uterus, *Viburnum opulus* is the remedy. This kind of pain seems as characteristic for *Viburnum* as is the other for *Sabina.*

Sabina has arthritic swelling of the wrist joint; also of the toe joints. This, if occurring in conjunction with its profuse flow from the genitals, may make the choice of remedy lie between it and *Caulophyllum* in some cases. The ovaries sympathize very much with the uterine troubles of *Sabina,* especially after abortion, or suppressed gonorrhœa, or leucorrhœas.

HELONIAS DIOICA.

Anæmic women, with prolapsus; worn out with hard work, mental or physical.

Heaviness in pelvic region, languor, pain or burning in back, with *continual consciousness of a womb, sore and tender.*

Better when mind is off herself.

* * * * *

I have found this remedy of use in a generally debilitated condition of women, with many and various complaints or symptoms in the region of the uterus, for instance: *Prolapsus from atony,* enervated by indolence and luxury; *worn out with hard work, mental or physical;* muscles burn and ache; so tired cannot sleep (Dr. H. C. Allen).

There is almost always associated with it a more or less anæmic condition. This anæmia may seem to be consequent upon too profuse menstruation or flooding, or it may exist entirely independent of any such cause. In these cases I have often found albumen present in the urine, sometimes in large quantities, especially in pregnant women, and seen rapid improvement and disappearance of the albumen under the action of this remedy.

The fact that these anæmic and debilitated states are found, both under profuse and scanty discharges of the uterine organs, seems to indicate that the local symptoms are secondary, or a consequence of general debility and impoverished blood. Again, the fact that *Helonias* cures both conditions equally well seems to corroborate it.

What are the symptoms? The *leading* symptoms are anæmia, great general weakness and languor, and great lowness of spirits or profound melancholy. This condition of mind is temporarily relieved by diversion. She is always better if she can get her mind off herself; dragging weakness in sacral region; various displacements of womb, but more especially prolapsus; pain in the back, with lameness, stiffness and weight, and heat or burning in lumbar region; back feels tired and weak; continual *consciousness of a womb,* it is so *sore and tender (Pyrogen*—distinct consciousness of a heart). Now this condition and these symptoms are often found at the age of puberty, during pregnancy and after labor, and here *Helonias* is indeed a blessing. I have found it efficacious in the 2d and the 30th, according to susceptibility of the patient. *Helonias* deserves a thorough proving in the potencies. Compare with *Aletris.*

ERIGERON, TRILLIUM, MILLEFOLIUM

Are three remedies having a reputation for their power to control hæmorrhages. *Erigeron* has cured epistaxis, with congestion to the head, red face *(Melilotus)* and febrile action. Hæmatemesis, with violent retching and burning in the stomach. Bleeding from hæmorrhoids, with burning. Hæmoptysis and blood spitting. Hæmaturia, with stone in the bladder and uterine hæmorrhage. The only marked symptom in addition to the hæmorrhage that should lead to its selection over other remedies of this class, especially in its hæmorrhages from the pelvic organs, is the marked violent *irritation of the rectum* and bladder. Here we must remember also *Cantharis, Lilium tig.* and *Nux vomica.*

Trillium, from clinical use, seems to be a genuine hæmorrhage remedy. The blood is bright red, whether of the active or passive kind of hæmorrhage. It is especially useful in **menses every two weeks,** *lasting a week and very profuse.* Here a choice may have to be made between it and *Calcarea ost.* and *Nux vomica.*

It resembles *China in flooding, with fainting, dim sight,* and *noises in the ears.* Of course, *China* would be the best for the after effects of such a hæmorrhage.

There is sometimes with such flooding a relaxed sensation as if the hips, sacro-synchrondroses and small of back would *all fall apart;* wants to be *bound together.* This should doubly indicate it in post-partum hæmorrhage.

It is also especially useful at the climacteric with the

above symptoms. It has cured hæmorrhages from other organs, but I have no experience with it there.

Millefolium is the only one of the three that has seemed to have *produced* hæmorrhages in its pathogenesis. Hahnemann says of it: "*It causes nose-bleed.* It causes hæmaturia." Clinical use has verified it.

The blood from the different organs is generally bright red, like that of *Aconite,* but the anxiety of that remedy is not there. In fact, no great fear is present in the cases where I have used it. Sometimes the blood in the urine forms in the bottom of the vessel a *bloody cake.* When a young man I was troubled for a long time with frequent attacks of profuse epistaxis. Dr. T. L. Brown prescribed for me several times, but without success. I became weak from loss of blood. Finally my old grandmother told me to chew yarrow root, and showed me the plant growing in my father's yard. I did so and was quickly cured. While on my vacation at Blue Mountain Lake, in the Adirondacks, I met a man there in the last stage of consumption. He had his medicine from his doctor in New York with him. He was spitting daily large quantities of blood, with severe cough, and his *Secale* was not able to control it in the least. He finally said to me: "Doctor, can you do anything to stop this bleeding?" I stooped down (I did not want that patient on my hands) and pulled up a little root of yarrow growing at our feet, handed it to him and told him to chew it. He looked surprised, but did so, liked the taste of it and kept on chewing. It stopped his bleeding and soothed his cough so much that he dug up a basket of yarrow and took it home with him. That controlled the bleeding. He went to Florida for the winter, but died the next spring. It is especially recommended for hæmorrhages after a fall or other injuries. If *Arnica* failed in such a case I would think of *Millefolium.*

DIGITALIS PURPUREA.

Extremely slow, intermittent pulse; weak heart; or rapid, very irregular pulse.

Respiration; irregular, difficult, slow, deep or performed by frequent deep sighs; sometimes stops on dropping off into sleep.

Excessive jaundice, with slow, weak heart, and ashy-white stools.

Faintness or sinking at the stomach; feels as if he would die if he moved.

Blueness of skin, eyelids; lips, tongue; cyanosis. Distended veins on lids, ears, lips and tongue.

* * * * *

Very much has been said and written upon this as a heart remedy. It is called a cardiac tonic, but Homœopathy knows no such thing as a tonic in medicines. The only tonic, in the sense of something to impart strength or tone to the human organism, is nourishing food. If *Digitalis* is capable of correcting a diseased condition, it does so by opposing its own power to cure to the power that is making the patient *sick,* which is called disease.

The leading characteristic of *Digitalis* is *a very slow pulse.* This may alternate with a very quick pulse, and between the two *we may* sometimes get a very irregular or intermittent pulse.

One day I saw an old but very strong man staggering across the road toward my office. I thought he was drunk, but on closer observation I noticed that his face looked purple, his lips bluish, and I stepped out and helped him in. He sat down and could not for a few minutes speak a word, but sat and struggled for breath. His pulse was very irregular and intermittent. When he could speak, he told me that for a number of weeks past he had been having these spells, had fallen several times and been obliged to go into the stores and sit, before he could go along the streets. Auscultation revealed hard, blowing sound with first beat of the heart. He had had inflammatory rheumatism in his younger days. He had been obliged to give up all manual labor and dared not go away from home on his business, that of bridge builder. Said he expected to die with this heart disease. I gave him *Digitalis* 2, a few drops in water. In a few days I saw him shoveling snow from the walk in front of his dwelling. "Hello," he said, "I have no heart disease;" and I saw him often after that and he told me that that medicine cured him of "those spells."

A young man of good habits was taken with nausea and vomiting. He was drowsy, and after a couple of days he began to grow very jaundiced all over. The sclerotica were as yellow as gold, as was, indeed, the skin all over the body, even to the nails. The stools were natural as to consistence, *but perfectly colorless,* while the urine was as *brown as lager beer,* or even more so. Where you could see through it, on the edge of the receptacle, it was yellow as fresh bile. The pulse was only *thirty beats per minute,* and often dropped out a beat.

This was a perfect *Digitalis* case of jaundice, and this remedy cured him perfectly in a few days, improvement in his feelings taking place very shortly after beginning it; the stools, urine and skin gradually taking on their natural color. The characteristic slow pulse was the leading symptom to the prescription, for all the rest of the symptoms may be found in almost any well-developed case of severe jaundice.

In dropsies, consequent on heart disease, *Digitalis* is often the remedy, and in these cases the skin is more apt to be bluish, as from venous stagnation, than in those cases dependent on renal disease.

Among the troubles consequent upon weak heart action with slow pulse that are particularly amenable to *Digitalis* are vertigo (this is often found in the aged); dropsy of brain, chest, abdomen or scrotum; passive congestion of the lungs.

Among the more characteristic symptoms, aside from the slow pulse, are:

"Blueness of skin, especially eyelids, lips, tongue, and nails; cyanosis."

"Faintness or sinking at stomach; feels as if he were dying."

"Sensation as if the heart would stop beating if she moved." (*Gelsemium,* if she did *not* keep moving. *Lobelia,* as if it would cease any way.)

"Respiration irregular, difficult, performed by frequent deep sighs."

"Great weakness and general sudden sinking of strength."

When going to sleep the breath fades away and seems to be gone; then wakes up with a gasp to catch it, cannot get to sleep on this account. (*Grindelia* and *Lachesis.)*

CACTUS GRANDIFLORUS.

Constriction of the *heart,* as if an iron band prevented its normal movement; < lying on left side.

Constriction, general; of heart, chest, bladder, rectum, uterus, vagina, etc.

Hæmorrhages in connection with heart troubles; nose, lungs, stomach, rectum, bladder.

Palpitation; day or night; worse when walking and lying on left side; approach of menses.

Fear of death; believes the disease incurable.

* * * * *

Cactus grandiflorus is another great heart remedy, and its grand characteristic is not at all like *Digitalis.* It is a "sensation of constriction of the heart, *as if an iron band prevented its normal movement."* (*Iodine* has a sensation as if heart was *squeezed together. Lilium tigrin.,* as if *grasped and released alternately. Lachesis, constriction on awaking,* throws off covering; *Arsenicum alb.,* constriction or oppression *on walking.)* This sensation of *constriction* is not confined to the heart, but is found in the chest, bladder, rectum, uterus, vagina; in short, it seems to be a general characteristic for this remedy, as does that of *fullness* for *Æsculus hippocastanum.*

The heart troubles of *Cactus* are quite apt to be caused by inflammatory rheumatism, where it is one of our best remedies. Among the symptoms found, more or less connected with heart troubles, for which *Cactus* is indicated, are:

Heavy pain on vertex like a weight (*Glonoine; Lachesis* at climacteric), a frequent symptom in persons suffering with heart troubles, cerebral congestion, profuse epistaxis, hæmatemesis, hæmorrhages from anus, hæmaturia or hæmoptysis. *In any hæmorrhages, seeming to be in sympathy with heart trouble,* think of *Cactus.*

Now, besides the leading characteristic of *Cactus* on the heart, we have other chest and heart symptoms which are very valuable. Oppression of chest or difficult breathing, as if the chest could not be expanded, with this sense of band-like constriction.

"Periodical attacks of suffocation, with fainting, cold perspiration on face and loss of pulse."

"Fluttering and palpitation of heart, increased when walking or *lying on left side.*"

"Great irregularity of heart's action, intermittent pulse, valvular murmurs in organic diseases of heart."

"Palpitation < lying on left side *(Nat. mur.).*

"Œdema of left hand, foot and leg."

"Rheumatism of all joints, *beginning in upper extremities." (Ledum* in lower.)

"Numbness of the left arm" (*Aconite;* aching, *Rhus toxicod.*).

"Cactus is a remedy of not very wide range; but of paramount importance in its sphere."

SPIGELIA ANTHELMINTICA.

Violent beating of the heart, shakes the chest; sometimes audible several inches away.

Left-sided neuralgias of head, face and eyes; pains increase and decrease with the rising and setting sun; watering of the eye, on affected side.

Modalities: < from motion, noise, inspiration, moving eyes, cold, damp, rainy weather; rising sun; > quiet; dry air, setting sun.

* * * * *

In this we have another valuable heart remedy. The pains in the heart in this remedy are as severe as those under *Cactus* and the action is more violent than under either *Cactus* or *Digitalis*. It is so violent as often to be *visible to the eye through the clothes, shaking the whole chest, and the sounds are often audible several inches away*. It is not only a very valuable remedy in acute attacks of the heart but in chronic valvular affections following the acute attack, where we have the loud blowing sounds and *attacks of violent palpitation*. I have seen the violent attacks of palpitation quickly relieved, and not only that, but the valvular troubles gradually and perfectly cured, under the action of this remedy. In these troubles the patient can often only lie on *the right side (Phos., Nat. mur.), or with the head very high;* least motion < *(Naja)*. It is one of our best remedies for neuralgic affections of the head, face, and eyes.

The headaches are generally one-sided, beginning in the occiput and extending forward, and settling over the left eye (right, *Sang.* and *Silicea)*. They are aggravated by the least noise or jar. They *increase with the rising of the sun and decrease with its going down (Natrum mur., Tabacum)*, and the eye on the affected side often runs clear water. *(Chelidon. maj.*, right side with water gushing out.)

Spigelia is very useful in ciliary neuralgia, the pain being of the same character as the headaches. The pains are also stabbing, running through into the back of the head, or like *Actæa,* they press outward, as if the eyeballs were too large for the sockets *(Comocladia)*.

In any or all of the above-named affections, for which *Spigelia* is so efficacious, the patient is made worse from motion, noise, inspiration or moving the eyes, and especially in *cold, damp, rainy weather.* It makes us think of *Bryonia, Kalmia* and *Natrum mur.*, and *Actæa* (motion), *Belladonna* (noise), and *China* (touch, especially light touch). It is certainly a very valuable remedy, though not one, so far as known, of very wide range of action.

KALMIA LATIFOLIA

Ought to be noticed just here, because it seems, at first sight, so much like *Spigelia,* and Hering says it follows *Spigelia* well in heart disease.

Both remedies have severe neuralgia of the face, but *Kalmia* is oftenest right-sided, *Spigelia* left. Both have pains in eyes, worse on turning them, but *Kalmia* has a sense of stiffness *(Rhus tox.* and *Natrum mur.). Spigelia* eyes hurt as if too large for the orbit. Both affect strongly the heart, and are useful in heart troubles of rheumatic origin. Both have violent, visible, tumultuous action of heart; *Spigelia* is invariably so, while *Kalmia* has at times remarkable *slowness* of the pulse (like *Digitalis).* The *Kalmia* form of rheumatism, like *Cactus,* goes from above downward *(Ledum* from below upward), and the pains in *Kalmia* shift suddenly. If we were called to a case of migratory rheumatism, and the heart seemed to be suffering, we would think of *Kalmia* before *Pulsatilla,* of course all the *other* symptoms taken into consideration. The pain of *Kalmia* often extends down to left hand *(Rhus).*

So far as the neuralgic symptoms of *Kalmia* are concerned, they are not much like *Spigelia,* except that they locate in the face, and are very violent. The sides and time of aggravation are different, and *Kalmia* is not often found involving the whole head, like *Spigelia.* Hering mentions that with *Kalmia* "weakness is the only *general* symptom with neuralgia." The neuralgic pains of *Kalmia* are sometimes attended with, or followed by, **numbness** of the parts affected, in this resembling *Aconite, Chamomilla, Gnaphalium* and *Platina.* It is to study up the points of resemblance of remedies having a particular affinity for the same region or organ, and to note also more particularly the *differences,* that perfects the true homœopathic prescriber. No kind of labor will bring better returns.

IPECACUANHA.

Persistent nausea, *which nothing* relieves, in many complaints.

Headache as if bruised, all through the bones of the head, down into root of tongue, *with nausea.*

Stools as if *fermented,* or as *green as grass,* with colic and *nausea.*

Hæmorrhages from uterus; profuse, bright blood and heavy breathing, *with nausea.*

Spasmodic, or asthmatic cough; great depression and wheezing breathing; child becomes rigid and turns blue.

Backache, short chill, long fever, heat usually with thirst; raging headache, *nausea;* and sweat last; *nausea* during pyrexia.

Better than Quinine, in intermittents, or after its abuse, the symptoms agreeing.

* * * * *

Ipecacuanha leads all the remedies for *nausea.* Any

not being at all relieved by vomiting, just as sick after as before—this is what we mean by *persistent* nausea. This should at once call attention to this remedy. It is often found in connection with gastric troubles from dietetic errors, and the choice will sometimes be between *Ipecacuanha* and *Pulsatilla,* because both are useful in gastric disturbances caused by indulgence in mixed diet—pastry, ice-cream, pork, fatty food, etc. *Pulsatilla* may be considered the better, while the food is *in* the stomach. *Ipecacuanha* after it is *out,* but the nausea persists notwithstanding.

Again, with *Pulsatilla* the tongue is often coated, like *Antimonium crudum,* while with *Ipecacuanha* there may be a slight coating, or the tongue may be perfectly clean. This vomiting with clean tongue, however, is not an infallible indication for *Ipecacuanha,* for we sometimes find it in connection with worm symptoms, where *Cina* has it just as prominently, and is the remedy. *Digitalis* also has it in heart disease. *Ipecacuanha* affects the whole intestinal tract. One very characteristic symptom is that the stomach and bowels feel as if *relaxed* and *hanging down.*

There are three kinds of looseness of the bowels, or rather three characteristic stools:

1. Fermented stools—foamy, like yeast.
2. Grass-green stools—mucous or watery
3. Slimy stools—dysenteric, with more or less blood.

All these stools are found very often in children, especially in summer time, often as a consequence of overeating or wrong eating, when a dose of *Ipecacuanha* 200th will set matters to rights, and prevent the little patient from running into so-called cholera-infantum or entero-colitis, which often becomes a very serious and obstinate affection. The characteristic nausea is a sure indication.

We will also find this nausea present, where this remedy is the "proper caper," in *headaches.* Headache, as if bruised, all through the bones of the head, and down into the root of the tongue. This kind of headache may be of rheumatic origin, but the nausea is there just the same, if *Ipecacuanha* is to cure. Then we have a sick headache of gastric origin, the nausea beginning before the pain in the head, and continuing all through. In what seems to be hydrocephaloid with this nausea, *Ipecacuanha* has often cleared up the whole case in a few hours.

Again, we find the nausea accompanying the cough in the affections of the respiratory organs. Also in the hæmorrhages and in the fevers in which it is often indicated. In short, we cannot do better than to use Hering's expression: *"Nausea, distressing, constant, with almost all complaints, as if from the stomach, with empty eructations, accumulation of much saliva, qualmishness and efforts to vomit,"* **nothing relieves.**

During the nausea, the face is generally pale, eyes sunken, with blue margins, and often there is more or less twitching of face and lips, and sleepiness after vomiting. We have a great many remedies that are powerful emetics, like *Antimonium tartaricum, Zinc sulphate, Lobelia* and *Apomorphine;* but, so far as I know, the nausea is not so persistent, nor is it found in connection with so many other affections. Of course, no single symptom, however strong, would justify a prescription, if there were other symptoms just as strong in the same case.

For instance, if there were burning in the stomach, intense thirst, but could not drink, great restlessness and prostration, we would think of *Arsenicum album,* and it is often the best remedy to follow *Ipecac.,* if the case goes from bad to worse.

Ipecacuanha affects the mucous lining of the respiratory organs, almost as prominently as it does that of the alimentary tract.

There is a great accumulation of mucus, which loads up the air cells and bronchi, until there seems to be great danger of suffocation. Note the symptoms:

"Violent degree of dyspnœa, with wheezing and great weight and anxiety about the præcordia." (*Antimon. tart.,* coarse rattling.)

"Threatened suffocation from accumulation of mucus."

This excessive accumulation of mucus in the air passages seems to excite spasm like a foreign body, and an asthma, or spasmodic cough, or both together, ensue. But the spasmodic cough and asthma do not seem to all depend upon accumulation of mucus, for *Ipecacuanha* is often our best remedy in the first stage of both asthma and whooping cough, before the stage when the mucus is present.

Again, *"Suffocating cough, whereby the child becomes quite stiff and blue in the face."*

"Whooping cough, with nosebleed *(Indigo), bleeding from the mouth, vomiting, loses breath, turns pale or blue, and becomes rigid."*

Infantile pneumonia, with chest loaded with mucus, rapid, wheezing respiration, surface blue, face pale, finds a very effectual remedy in *Ipecacuanha.* Old people with emphysema from chronic asthma are also > by *Ipecac.* So that we might narrow down the respiratory troubles to two conditions:

1st. Those in which excessive accumulation of mucus characterized the case.

2d. Those in which spasm was the characteristic feature.

Of course, all the symptoms must be taken into consideration, in order to differentiate between *Ipecacuanha* and other remedies having the same objective states and conditions.

The control that this remedy has over hæmorrhages deserves honorable mention. It has hæmorrhages from the nose, stomach, rectum, womb, lungs and bladder; from all the orifices of the body. So does *Crotalus*, but the blood in *Ipecacuanha* is *bright red*, not decomposed. *Sulphuric acid* also has hæmorrhages from all the outlets of the body, but the other attending symptoms are different. With *Ipecacuanha*, the hæmorrhages are active, profuse, bright red. It is a better remedy than *Secale* ever was or can be, for post-partum hæmorrhages, and it is not necessary to use it in large and poisonous doses, for it will stop them in the 200th potency, and is quicker in its action than *Secale*. Let us notice a few remedies for hæmorrhages:

Ipecacuanha. Bright red, profuse, with heavy breathing and nausea.

Aconitum. Active, bright, with great fear and anxiety.

Arnica. From injuries, bodily fatigue, physical exertion.

Belladonna. Blood hot, throbbing carotid, congestion to head.

Carbo vegetabilis. Almost entire collapse, pale face, wants to be fanned.

China. Great loss of blood, ringing in ears, faintness.

Crocus. Blood clots, in long, dark strings.

Ferrum. Partly fluid, partly solid, very red face, or red and pale alternately.

Hyoscyamus. Delirium, and jerking, and twitching of muscles.

Lachesis. Blood decomposed, *sediment like charred straw.*

Crotalus, Elaps and *Sulphuric acid.* Black fluid blood, the first and last from all outlets.

Nitric acid. Active hæmorrhages of bright blood.

Phosphorus. Profuse and persistent, even from small wounds and tumors.

Platinum. Partly fluid, and partly hard black clots.

Pulsatilla. Intermittent hæmorrhages.

Secale. Passive flow in feeble, cachectic women.

Sulphur. In psoric constitutions; other remedies fail.

Other remedies and indications might be added here, but hæmorrhage is only one symptom, and never alone furnishes a reliable indication for any remedy. But *Ipecacuanha* is one of the best *if indicated.*

Ipecacuanha is a well-known intermittent fever remedy in our school. Jahr recommends it in the beginning of all cases, unless there are special indications for some other remedy, and says, "By pursuing this course I have cured many cases of fever and ague by the first prescription, thus saving myself a good deal of unnecessary seeking and comparing." Whatever may be said in condemnation of this loose prescribing, it is certainly preferable to the inevitable Quinine prescription of the old school, and some self-styled homœopaths, for the reason that it will *cure* more cases than Quinine, and do infinitely less harm. *Ipecac.* can cure more cases than Quinine, but both can cure the case to which they are homœopathic, and that in the potentized form of the drug. We have such clear-cut indications for the use of many remedies that we need not fail once where the allopaths do twenty times, with their indiscriminate Quinine treatment.

The whole case generally revolves around one to three guiding symptoms, for instance:

Ipecac. The persistent nausea in one or all stages.

Arsenicum alb. Irregularly developed paroxysm; thirst intense during heat, for small quantities.

Eupator. perf. Bone pains; vomits bile at end of chill; 7 to 9 A. M.

Ignatia. Chill, with red face, > by external heat; frequent sighing.

Capsicum. Chill begins between shoulder blades and spreads.

Nux vomica. During heat can't uncover in least, without chill.

Nat. Mur. Chill 10 to 11 A. M.; bursting headache during heat; sweat >; after Quinine.

Rhus tox. Cough in chill; restless and dry tongue in heat; tossing about.

Podophyllum. Great loquacity during chill and heat; jaundice.

Antimonium tart. Great sleepiness during heat and sweat, with pale face.

These characteristics are genuine and reliable, and many more might be added if we had time and space, but they can all be found in H. C. Allen's work on *Fevers.* They show how different the remedies, and how particular the true prescriber must be, when selecting his remedy for this, as well as other diseases. Remittents also often come under the control of this remedy.

ANTIMONIUM TARTARICUM.

Great accumulation of mucus in the air passages, with coarse rattling with inability to expectorate; impending paralysis of lungs.

Face very pale or cyanotic from unoxidized blood.

Great coma or sleepiness in most complaints.

Vomiting, intense nausea, with prostration; general coldness, cold sweat and sleepiness.

Trembling; internal, head and hands.

Thick eruptions like pocks, often pustular; as large as a pea.

Modalities: > from expectoration.

Both ends of life, childhood and old age; clings to those around; wants to be carried; cries and whines if any one touches it; will not let you feel the pulse.

* * * * *

Antimonium tartaricum is another powerful emetic. I can remember the time when the old allopaths used it almost as generally as the botanics did *Lobelia inflata,* to "*clean out the stomach.*" Now-a-days, washing out the stomach by lavage, and the rectum and colon by enemas, according to "Hall's method," is quite fashionable, and is withal much more sensible, inasmuch as they are so lame in their therapeutics.

Notwithstanding these improvements, there is still a great deal of "*gut scraping*" going on in the name of "cleaning out the system," as though the alimentary canal was not a self-cleaning institution, if kept, or put into a healthy condition, but must be regularly "gone through" once in about so often, on the "house cleaning" principle. To be sure it is folly, but they do the best they know. Neither *Antimonium tart.* nor any other emetic is used by us for emetic purposes from a therapeutic standpoint.

Our therapeutic uses of it are the same as those of any other remedy, on the principle of *similia similibus curantur.* The nausea of this remedy is as intense as that of *Ipecacuanha,* but not so persistent, and there is relief after vomiting. I have found it nearest a specific (of course we know there is no absolute specific for any disease) for cholera morbus of any remedy. For more than twenty-five years, I have seldom found it necessary to use any other, and then only when there were severe cramps in the stomach and bowels, when *Cuprum metallicum* relieved.

It has the nausea, vomiting, loose stools, prostration, cold sweat, and stupor or drowsiness found in almost all bad cases of this disease, and I have seldom been obliged to give more than two or three doses, one after each vomiting, before the case was relieved. It is not generally recommended in the text-books for this ailment, but is a gem, as I know from abundant experience and observation.

If *Antimonium tart.* possessed only the one power of curing, that it does upon the respiratory organs, it would be indispensable. No matter what the *name* of the trouble, whether it be bronchitis, pneumonia, whooping cough or asthma, if there is great accumulation of mucus with *coarse rattling,* or filling up with it, but, at the same time, there seems to be inability to raise it, *Tartar emetic* is the first remedy to be thought of. This is true in all ages and constitutions, but particularly so in children and old people.

There is one symptom that is very apt to be present in these cases, and that is, *great drowsiness* or sleepiness, sometimes amounting to coma. This is found, not only in diseases of the respiratory organs, but in cholera infantum, cholera morbus and intermittent fever. In pneumonia, both *Tartar emetic* and *Opium* may have great sleepiness; but there is no need for any confusion here as to choice, for in *Opium* the face is dark red or purple, and there may be sighing or stertorous respiration. With *Tartar emetic* the face is always pale, or cyanotic, with no redness, and the breathing is not stertorous.

Three remedies are remarkable for sleepiness, viz.: *Opium, Tartar emetic* and *Nux moschata,* but aside from this one symptom they are not alike. *Antimonium tart.* is also one of our best remedies for hepatization of lungs remaining after pneumonia. There is dullness on percussion, and lack, or absence of respiratory murmur, and shortness of breath, and patient continues pale, weak and sleepy.

If *Sulphur* should not promote absorption in such a case, *Tartar emetic* will often do it. I have used it from the 200th to the c. m. potencies with equally good results.

IRIS VERSICOLOR.

Burning of mouth, tongue, throat, clear down into stomach, and of anus if there is diarrhœa.

Vomiting of stringy, glairy, ropy mucus; hangs in strings down to receptacle on the floor.

Gastric or hepatic sick headaches with blur before the eyes at the beginning. Vomiting *sour,* or bitter.

* * * * *

Iris is another remedy which causes great nausea and vomiting. It is sometimes very serviceable in cholera infantum. The substance vomited is generally very *sour,* so sour that it excoriates the throat.

The gastric troubles of this remedy are often accompanied with a *burning of tongue, throat,* œsophagus and stomach, and, if diarrhœa is present, with burning of the anus. This burning of the alimentary canal is very characteristic of this drug.

The vomiting is *not* always sour, but may be bitter or sweetish. There is also profuse flow of saliva. I once had a case of stomach trouble in a middle-aged lady. She had frequent attacks of vomiting of a stringy, glairy mucus which was very ropy, would hang in strings from her mouth to the receptacle on the floor. Then the substance vomited became dark-colored; like coffee grounds. She became very weak, vomited all nourishment. She also had profuse secretion of ropy saliva. Thinking she had cancer of the stomach, she made her will and set her house in order, to die. *Kali bichromicum* was given with no benefit whatever, but *Iris* cured her completely in a short time and she remains well ten years since.

Iris is also one of our best remedies for sick headache. These headaches seem to be of gastric or hepatic origin, and often begin with a blur before the eyes. I used to give the remedy in the 3d; but of late years have given it in the 50m. and am better pleased with the result, because it is more prompt and lasting. It is recommended in sciatica, but I have had no experience with it in this affection. It seems to act most powerfully upon the alimentary tract. I have never used it in skin troubles.

SANGUINARIA CANADENSIS.

Pain beginning in occiput; spreads over the head and settles over the right eye, with nausea and vomiting. Sensitive to noise and light.

Loose cough with badly smelling sputa; the breath and sputa smell badly to the patient himself.

Pain in right arm and shoulder; worse at night in bed; cannot raise the arm. Also pain in places where the bones are the least covered.

Heat and tension behind sternum. Cough day and night with great emaciation.

Burning and pressing in breast, followed by heat through abdomen and diarrhœa. Acts intensely on right lung and chest.

* * * * *

Sick headache. Pain commences in the back of the head, rises and spreads over the head, and settles down over the right eye (left eye, *Spigelia),* with nausea and vomiting; patient wants to be in a dark room and perfectly quiet. I have made some fine cures in long-standing cases of habitual sick headaches of this kind with this remedy. It will probably cure, or greatly relieve, the ordinary American sick headache as often as any other remedy. I use the 200th. *Loose cough, with badly smelling sputa; the breath and sputa smelling badly to the patient himself.* There is sometimes a pain behind the sternum *(Kali hydroiod.).* This kind of cough usually comes on after a severe bronchitis or pneumonia, and it looks as though the patient were fast running into consumption. There may also be flushes of fever with circumscribed redness of the cheeks, like hectic fever. Many a case of this kind has been helped by this remedy. Dr. T. L. Brown used the first trituration of the alkaloid with fine effect. The 200th has made just as good cures. In typhoid pneumonia with great dyspnœa and circumscribed redness of the cheeks, *Sanguinaria* has, in my hands, done good service. The right lung seems to come markedly under its influence, either in acute or chronic troubles. *"Rheumatic pain in right arm and shoulder, worse at night in bed, cannot raise the arm."* This condition has often been relieved by this remedy in my hands and has won me much credit. I have seen *one dose* of the first trituration cure such cases of long standing. I have seen the c. m. do the same thing. Flashes of heat, with hot palms and soles, at the climacteric find a remedy in *Sanguinaria.* Sometimes indicated after *Sulphur* and *Lachesis* have failed, especially if the circumscribed redness of the cheeks appears.

PHOSPHORIC ACID.

Drowsy, apathetic; unconscious of all surroundings, but can be aroused to full consciousness.

Chronic effects of grief; hair turns gray; hopeless, haggard look.

Grows too fast and too tall; young persons with growing pains in bones.

Great physical and mental weakness from ovarian or sexual excesses.

Diarrhœa WHITE, watery, painless, with rumbling; meteorism; but not so much weakness as would be expected.

Very profuse, watery, or milky urine.

Modalities: < bad news, depressing emotions; masturbation or sexual excess; draft; wind; snowy air; > after short sleep.

Headache of school girls from eye strain, or overuse of eyes, occipital. Chest, weak from talking or coughing; cough, purulent, offensive expectoration, and pains in chest. Salty expectoration in proving.

* * * * *

The leading characteristic of this remedy lies in its effects upon the sensorium. *"He lies in a stupor or in a stupid sleep, unconscious of all that is going on around him, but when aroused is fully conscious."* This is *Phosphoric acid* in its intensest degree, as found in typhoid fever, in which it is one of our best remedies. But it is not alone here that the sensorial depression appears. It may be found in a lesser degree, in the results of depressing emotions, like grief at the loss of a friend, lover, property or position, and the effect seems to be even deeper rooted than in those cases which call for *Ignatia.* (See also *Lachesis.)* The subject seems **stupefied** with grief. There is not the nervous twitching of *Ignatia,* but a settled despair, general weakness or prostration. The hair turns gray, and a weary, worn and haggard, hopeless look obtains. I have succeeded in curing such a case when *Ignatia* failed. In such a case the patient sometimes complains of a pain like a *crushing weight on the vertex,* or, again, of pain in the occiput or nape of the neck, and with both they appear physically weak, or exhausted, want to lie down, don't want company, or to be noticed or spoken to. We often find this sensorial depression in connection with the effects of onanism or excessive coition. The patient is disturbed by the culpability of his indulgence, grieves over it, is inclined to sink into despair. This is true of both sexes, and the depression is much worse if the patient is *growing* too fast, or is overtaxed mentally or physically. With *Calcarea carb.* they grow too fat, with *Phosphoric acid* too fast and tall. We have in *Phosphoric acid* a remedy for the headache of students, especially of those who are growing too fast. It is a sin to keep such young people bowing down to hard study, and while it is true that youth is the time to get an education it is also true that it is the time when too great a strain in that direction may utterly wreck and forever incapacitate a mind which might, with more time and care, have been a blessing to the world.

Now *Phosphoric acid,* properly exhibited, may be of incalculable benefit in such cases. It will sometimes be a choice between *Phosphoric acid* and *Natrum muriaticum* or *Calcarea phos.,* the other symptoms must decide.

In regard to the use of *Phosphoric acid* in typhoids, there are no other remedies exactly like it in its depressing effect on the sensorium. *Arnica* has its apathy or indifference; but the *Arnica* depression is more profound, as is also that of *Baptisia,* for they both go to sleep while answering a question, showing how overpowering is the stupor. Then with the former we have petechiæ or ecchymosis, which is not found under *Phosphoric acid,* and under the latter the tendency to decomposition of the fluids as found in the terribly offensive stools and urine.

Opium surpasses them all in its stupefying powers, and the face, breathing and general appearance, is not at all like *Phosphoric acid.*

Rhus tox. and *Hyoscyamus* are very stupid also, but in other respects are very different. The description of these remedies is found under each, as we have written of their use in typhoids. *Nux moschata* ought also to be mentioned in this connection.

We must not forget the action of *Phosphoric acid* upon the bowels. It does not exhibit any peculiar characteristic action upon the stomach, but does in the abdominal region, as the following well-verified symptoms show: "*Meteoristic distention of the abdomen; rumbling and gurgling and noise as from watery, painless stools.*" "*Diarrhœa* **white,** *or yellow, watery, chronic or acute, without pain or any marked debility or exhaustion.*" Now, it seems very singular that, after so much talk about the general depression or weakness of this remedy, we should be obliged to record that the profuse and sometimes long-continued diarrhœa should *not* debilitate, as a characteristic symptom. Well, there are a good many unaccountable things, in both disease and therapeutics, and this is one of them, but the *fact* remains and we act upon it. Let us remember that the profound weakness and depression of *Phosphoric acid* is upon the *sensorium* and *nervous* system, and will be there whether diarrhœa is present or not. It is markedly so in typhoids, as I can fully attest from abundant observation. *China* debilitates by its diarrhœa or loss of fluids generally. *Phosphoric acid* attacks the nervous system primarily, even in onanism, and its results or effects are not so much the loss of semen as a vital fluid, as under *China,* the nervous system suffering very much, even though the emissions be neither very frequent nor profuse.

Young boys even suffer from the effects of the *orgasm* of onanism before there is much or any semen secreted. This is well to remember in a choice between these two remedies. There is a condition in which I have found this remedy very valuable, especially in men. The leading symptom is a "weak feeling in the chest from talking." You remember *Stannum* has this symptom very strongly (also *Sulphur)* and may lead us into a wrong prescription if only the one symptom were considered. If the patient is a young man, married or single; if, again, he seems weak in mind, listless, apathetic, reticent; if he is growing fast; all these things would indicate *Phosphoric acid,* and the proper use of it might save him from consumption, for many go into it in this way. If he has cough with expectoration, under *Phosphoric acid,* it will be copious, purulent, offensive; under *Stannum,* thick, heavy and of sweetish taste. All this condition of things may, when *Phosphoric acid* is the remedy, find its cause in one or both of two things: Onanism or sexual excess, and too rapid growth. *Phosphoric acid* has two very marked peculiarities in the urine, viz.: very profuse and *clear, watery,* or *milky urine.*

The first is found with general nervous depression, and if there is headache it is like *Gelsemium relieved* by the flow of urine. The other is from excess of phosphates in the urine, indicating nerve waste. We must distinguish between the profuse urine of *Ignatia* and *Phosphoric acid,* for the first is hysterical, the latter not at all so.

MURIATIC ACID.

Moaning or sliding down in bed from excessive weakness. (Typhoid.)

Tongue dry, leathery and shrunken; one-third its natural size. (Typhoid.)

Hæmorrhoids: Swollen and blue, and so *sensitive to touch* that they cannot bear the contact of the sheet.

Great debility; as soon as he sits down his eyes close; lower jaw hangs down; slides down in bed.

Malignant affections of mouth: Ulcers, deep, dark, base bluish, offensive, foul breath.

Diarrhœa: Stool involuntary while urinating. Cannot urinate without having bowels move at the same time.

* * * * *

This remedy, also one of our best remedies in typhoids, is found useful in cases of lower grade than in the *Phosphoric acid* case. It comes nearer to *Carbo vegetabilis* than any other remedy.

Its indications are given in "Hering's Guiding Symptoms" as well as anywhere. There is decomposition of fluids; the stools are involuntary while passing urine; stools dark, thin, or hæmorrhage of dark liquid blood. Mouth full of dark-bluish ulcers; unconscious. Moaning and *sliding down in the bed* from excessive weakness; lower jaw fallen, *tongue dry, leathery and shrunken to a third of its natural size,* and paralyzed; pulse weak and intermittent. It is hardly possible to draw a picture of a more desperate case of typhoid than this. It is not necessary to resort to quinine, brandy or any other fashionable so-called stimulants. Broth, milk or oatmeal gruel for nourishment, and *Muriatic acid* will do all that can be done for the saving of the life of such a patient, and will do it quicker and with less liability to relapse than any other course of treatment. Of course the friends are anxious, even desperate, and a show of *work* must be made. If much pressure is brought to bear in the way of suggestions or demands for counsel, all sorts of wonderful prescriptions that cured a great many cases like this, let *Sac. lac.* be given every five minutes. It is a wonderfully *quieting* medicine (to friends and meddlers) and should never be omitted. Send the most rampant howler off on horseback miles away, if you can, for something, no matter what. That is indispensable to the patient's recovery. The *greatest danger* to the patient is, that the physician losing his presence of mind, will suffer himself to be led or driven away from the only true helpful course. This advice is given only to those who need it. Many a patient has died because his physician "lost his head" under this kind of pressure.

Muriatic acid is very useful in hæmorrhoids, swollen and blue, and so **sensitive to touch** that they cannot bear the contact of the sheet.

Rectum prolapses easily *(Ignatia, Ruta),* cannot urinate without it coming down. Also when wind is passed or bowels move.

Bladder weak, urine passes slowly or must press until rectum protrudes.

Cannot bear the *least touch,* not even sheet on genitals *(Murex).*

NITRIC ACID.

Has a particular affinity for mucous outlets, where skin and membranes join; cracks; rhagades, fissures.

Pricking pains as of a splinter in the parts.

Urine strong smelling; like horse urine.

Hæmorrhages from all outlets of the body; blood bright red.

Pricking ulcers; excrescences; condylomata; figwarts (sycosis).

Nervous, irritable, dark complexioned persons.

Modalities: > riding in carriage.

* * * * *

Nitric acid is one of our most effective antidotes to the effects of allopathic dosing with mercury in syphilis. For the other bad effects of the abuse of mercury other remedies are better, notably, *Hepar sulphur. calc.* *Nitric acid* has a particular affinity for the outlets of mucous surfaces, where the skin and membrane join, such as the mouth (corners), nose and anus. In the mouth we find the corners cracked, ulcerated and scabby; also aphthæ, stomatitis with ptyalism, swelling of the gums, fœtor oris, etc.

If *Mercurius* has already been used without avail *Nitric acid* follows well and will often cure.

This ulcerated, swollen and spongy condition of the gums will extend into the throat, and if it is the result of combined syphilis and mercurialization of the old school *Nitric acid* is the first remedy. The action of this remedy is just as positive upon the other outlet of the alimentary canal.

The anus is cracked and fissured similarly *(Ratanhia)*,

and hæmorrhoids protrude, crack, bleed and are very sore. No remedy has more decided action upon the anus, and one very characteristic symptom is, "great pain after passage of stool, *even soft stool.*" He walks the floor in agony of pain for an hour or two after a stool *(Ratanhia).* In dysentery this symptom distinguishes this remedy from *Nux vomica,* which is *relieved* after stool and *Mercurius,* which has tenesmus *all the time,* or before, during and after stool.

Another very strong characteristic of this remedy in all these affections is, *"Pricking pain as of a splinter in the part."* *Nitric acid* has hæmorrhages from all outlets of the body, and the blood is generally bright red. It is especially so in typhoid and hæmorrhoids. *Nitric acid* is one of our best remedies in chronic diarrhœa. It is one of the celebrated trio, viz.: *Thuja, Staphisagria* and *Nitric acid* for condylomata. It is one of three remedies having very offensive odor to the urine, viz.:

Benzoic acid, Nitric acid and *Sepia.*

Benzoic acid, urine is very dark with very intense urinous odor.

Nitric acid, dark, smelling like horse urine.

Sepia, offensive and *sourish.*

SULPHURIC ACID.

Extreme weakness, with sense of *internal* trembling, which is not observable to others.

Hæmorrhages from every outlet of the body, with ecchymosed spots under the skin.

Child smells sour all over, despite the actual cleanliness. Sour, acid vomiting.

Adapted to the light haired, old people, especially women; flushes of heat in climacteric years.

Aphthæ, of mouth, gums, or entire buccal cavity, gums bleed readily; ulcers painful; offensive breath. Bad effects from mechanical injuries, with bruises, chafing and livid skin; prostration.

Sensation as if the brain was loose in forehead and falling from side to side *(Bell., Bry., Rhus, Spig.)*. Often very useful in the stomach troubles of old whiskey topers.

* * * * *

Sulphuric acid is another remedy of value in aphthous affections of the mouth. It is particularly efficacious in greatly debilitated subjects, and in children with marasmus with this kind of mouth. There is often present sour stomach *(Iris versicol.* and *Robinia,* sour eructations and vomiting) with sour vomiting, and *the child smells sour all over despite the greatest care in regard to cleanliness. (Rheum, Hepar* and *Magnesia.)* One of the strongest characteristics, perhaps *the* strongest, in weakened subjects in which this is the appropriate remedy, is a *sense of internal trembling.* This is a subjective symptom, for, notwithstanding this positive sensation, to a degree that is very distressing, there is no visible trembling. This symptom is frequently found in old topers (see *Ranunculus bulb.),* who are broken down or almost wrecked in health by strong drink. The symptom, however, is not confined to such subjects, but is often found in other cases when the debility is traceable to other causes; when markedly present from whatever cause, *Sulphuric acid* should never be forgotten. We have already spoken of the value of this remedy in purpura hæmorrhagica. Like *Crotalus,* it has hæmorrhages from every outlet of the body *(Acetic acid, Thlaspi)*, and the blood also settles in *ecchymosed spots under the skin.* This last symptom would indicate that *Sulphuric acid* might be useful in black and blue spots in the skin, as the result of bruising, and practice corroborates it, and it follows well after *Arnica*. *Ledum palustre* is also one of our best remedies for ecchymosis from bruises, "black eye," for instance; this is, of course, for bruises under the skin; while *Ruta* is just as efficacious for bruises of the periosteum. There is enough of the *Sulphur* element so that it may succeed in "flushes" of heat, after *Sulphur* has failed at the climacteric.

PICRIC ACID.

This is a comparatively new remedy, but has already developed some valuable therapeutic powers. In the first place, it attacks the vital force, as is manifested by an excessive languor or persistent **tired feeling** all over the body, which is generally accompanied with corresponding weakness of mind, indifference, and want of will power, and a desire to lie down. There is great heaviness of the legs, can hardly lift them from the ground, tired, aching feeling in the back with some burning *(Phosphorus* and *Zinc. met.)*, at times low down. Even the brain is fagged and the slightest exertion or mental effort brings on headache. This headache is oftenest found in students, overworked business men, and in persons depressed by grief or other emotions.

It oftenest locates in occipito-cervical region *(Nat. mur., Silicea)*. < especially by mental exertion. In short, this remedy presents a perfect picture of *nervous prostration.* I found this remedy very useful in apparent failure of brain power in an old man who had always been strong up to within a year or so of the time he called on me. He complained of heaviness in the occiput and inability to exert the mind to talk or think, and general tired "played-out" feeling. I feared brain softening but I gave him *Picric acid* 6th trit. and it promptly *cured* him. This remedy has strong points of resemblance to *Phosphoric acid* and *Phosphorus* in its effects upon the sexual organs, especially of the male. There is strong sexual desire with terrible erections, which is followed by corresponding weakness or complete impotence. There seems to be no doubt that it is destined to become one of our most valuable remedies for brain, spinal, and general nervous prostration, especially if connected with or arising from sexual excesses. It may be studied along with *Gelsemium, Phosphoric acid, Phosphorus, Argentum nitricum, Sulphur, Alumina* and *Silicea* and all those remedies affecting the brain, cord, and general nervous system.

CARBO ANIMALIS

Is another remedy whose great general characteristic is: **Great weakness,** *want of energy, prostration.* The subjects of it are often disposed to glandular swellings, indurations and suppurations.

Benignant suppurations are inclined to become ichorous. The swellings to become schirrous in character.

The swellings seem to have a choice for the *axillary,* inguinal or mammary regions. Then the sexual organs come markedly under its influence. Old suppurating, bluish colored (*Lach., Tarant. Cub.*), offensive buboes.

Menses too early and too long. Menorrhagia from chronic induration of the uterus; also in cachectic women with glandular swellings.

The flow **always weakens so that she can hardly speak.**

Mammary tumors in *hard nodules* in the breast.

Copper colored eruptions on the skin.

Weak ankles in children *(Nat. c., Sil.)*.

Easily sprained from lifting *(Calc. ost.)*.

GELSEMIUM NITIDUM.

Complete relaxation and prostration of the whole muscular system, with almost or entire motor paralysis. Eyelids droop; muscles refuse to obey the will.

Trembling of hands or lower extremities if he attempts to move; must lie still.

Mental faculties dull, cannot think; dowsy, with dull red face.

Susceptibility to mental disturbance, excitement or emotion; causes diarrhœa.

Dull, tired, prostrating headache at *base* of brain; wants head high, sometimes > by profuse urination.

Vertigo with blurred vision; dilated pupils; double sight; sense of intoxication.

Nervous chill, violent shaking with no sense of coldness.

Desire to be quiet; feels too weak to move.

Children: fear of falling, seize the nurse, grasp the crib, especially in intermittents.

Slow, weak pulse of old age.

Great heaviness of the eyelids; cannot keep them open.

Fears that unless constantly on the move, the heart will cease beating.

General deep-seated muscular pain with prostration (la grippe).

* * * * *

This remedy affects, primarily, the whole nervous system. The most prominent symptom, as we are in the habit of recording the effects of remedies, is *"complete relaxation and prostration of the whole muscular system, with almost or quite entire motor paralysis."* This muscular prostration seems to come through inability of the nerves to convey impressions; thus we have the symptom "muscles will not obey the will." This condition comes on gradually, the first symptom being a feeling of lassitude or general fatigue. He wants to lie down he feels *so weak (Picric acid),* and is inclined to drowsiness; the pulse becomes weak and slow, but is accelerated on the least motion. Then, if he attempts to walk, the *legs tremble,* or the *hands tremble* if he attempts to lift them, the *tongue trembles* if he attempts to protrude it; all this from *weakness,* both objective and subjective. If I were to put one adjective before this remedy to indicate its chief characteristic I would call it the *trembling* remedy. Sometimes this trembling is so severe as to actually *shake* the patient like a chill, but there is no chill, objective or subjective. This weakness may increase to the stage of complete paralysis, and such symptoms as these appear: The eyelids *droop (Sepia, Caust.)* until they are completely closed. The fingers become unmanageable, so that he can no longer guide them over the keys of the piano in playing; he cannot guide his feet where he wants to in trying to walk, notwithstanding the sensorium remains clear, with perhaps the exception of a little drowsiness. He knows perfectly well what he wants to do, but cannot do it.

Then, again, there may be neuralgia in various parts, and the pains may be a dull aching all over *(myalgia)*, or they may be sudden and darting, so acute as to cause sudden starting. Or, again, it may cause spasms or convulsions; but with all these there is the characteristic *prostration,* for instance, in prosopalgia the eyelids droop from weakness. So we repeat *Gelsemium is pre-eminently a nerve remedy.*

Having shown the central action of this great remedy as it manifests itself upon the nervous system, we will proceed to notice some of its local uses which will always be more or less associated with such action. Upon the mind it shows its depressing power, and is portrayed in such symptoms as these: *The Gelsemium subject is torpid, sleepy, and dreads movement. The mental faculties are dull, cannot think clearly or fix his attention;* "desires to be quiet; does not wish to speak or have any one near her for company, even if the person be silent." This condition of mind is in perfect accordance with the general nervous prostration already described. This condition of mind sometimes is temporarily suspended to give place to an alternate condition of excitement. But this is not the leading, characteristic, and legitimate effect of the drug, but is only the reaction; like a state of sleeplessness is to the characteristic sleepiness or stupor of *Opium.* I consider the large doses of either remedy used by some to quiet excited conditions, or to control spasms or convulsions by their toxic, depressing, or paralyzing action on the muscular system, antipathic, and in no way truly curative. There is an excessively sensitive condition of the nerves that is very peculiar, and that this remedy controls markedly, viz., *susceptibility to mental disturbance, such as sudden excitement or emotion, bad news or fright, the anticipation of an unusual ordeal.* One of the effects following these things is a diarrhœa. Many people are thus affected. *Gelsemium* not only cures the diarrhœa for the time being, but often cures the whole abnormal condition. I have never known the remedy to do much good in these conditions below the 30th potency, but often in the potencies much above that.

As would be naturally supposed from its general action upon the nervous system, this remedy exerts a decided influence upon the sensorium and brain. *Dizziness, with blurred vision, pupils dilated, double sight and sense of intoxication, show this influence.* One very characteristic symptom appears here which is found under only one other remedy with any prominence, viz., *"child starts and grasps the nurse and screams, as if afraid of falling."* If there is any difference between it and *Borax,* it is that in *Borax* the child manifests this fear only when it is being laid down in the cradle, or from *downward motion.*

The most characteristic headache of *Gelsemium* is a dull, tired headache at the *base of the brain.* The patient wants to lie with head raised upon a high pillow, and lie perfectly still. It is aggravated by mental labor, smoking tobacco, lying with the head low, and in the heat of the sun. *(Glonoine, Lachesis, Lyssin, Natrum carb.)* It is temporarily ameliorated by pressure and stimulants. Such headaches often follow a debauch. Sometimes we have a headache from passive congestion; then the pain begins in the occiput and spreads all over the head. The aggravations are about the same as in the other variety, or nervous headache. One notable characteristic is that sometimes the headache is *relieved by a profuse flow of urine.* (*Lac defloratum* has a profuse flow of urine *during* sick headache to which it is adapted, but the pain is not so markedly relieved by the flow.) *Gelsemium* has also a sick headache that is preceded by *blindness.* As the head begins to ache the blindness disappears. The sick headache of this remedy is not accompanied with much nausea and vomiting, as is that of *Sanguinaria, Iris versicolor* and *Lac defloratum,* but is accompanied by the characteristic weakness and trembling belonging to this remedy. *Gelsemium* is one of the so-called fever remedies. It is useful in the remittent fever of children. The fever is never of that active or violent form calling for *Aconite* or *Belladonna,* but of a milder form. The child lies drowsy, does not want to move, or, if it does, cannot move much on account of the weakness. One author says that *Gelsemium* stands midway between *Aconite* and *Veratrum viride.* I should rather place it between *Baptisia* and *Belladonna.* Like *Baptisia,* there is prostration, but the typhoid tongue and other symptoms are not so strong. There may be dark red face with both and a sort of besotted expression; but with *Baptisia* the sensorium comes more fully under the influence of the drug, so that the patient will fall asleep even when trying to answer questions. Then the offensive sweat, stool and urine of *Baptisia* are not found under *Gelsemium.* Like *Belladonna,* there is congestion to the brain and dilated pupils, but it is not so intense, accompanied by active or violent delirium as with *Belladonna.* *Gelsemium* is not a very great intermittent fever remedy; but is one of the best for nervous chill *(Gelsemium* chills run up and down the back in wave-like succession from sacrum to occiput; chill begins between scapulæ, *Capsic., Sepia;* chill begins in lumbar region, *Eupat. purp.* and *Nat. m.;* chill begins in dorsal region, *Eupat. perf., Lach.);* when there is great shaking and chattering of the teeth, with no objective, or even sense of coldness. *"Patient wants to be held because he shakes so."* This kind of chill is frequently found in hysterical, and heart diseases (organic). The pulse of *Gelsemium* is *slow* when quiet, but greatly accelerated on motion. For the weak, slow pulse of old age there is no remedy oftener useful. For the nervous prostration already described, just preceding typhoid, there is nothing like *Gelsemium.* I have aborted many cases of typhoid fever with this remedy—at least I think so.

BAPTISIA TINCTORIA.

Mind confused; as if drunk; cannot collect himself; feels scattered about, cannot get pieces together.

Face dark, dusky; eyes bleared, besotted expression.

Mouth ulcerated, with foul smell; or, dry, tongue dry in a streak down the centre.

Abdomen sensitive in right iliac region, with rumbling.

Stool loose, and urine with all other discharges; *very offensive.*

Awakes with oppressed feeling, must have more air.

Great prostration with aching and soreness all over. Great typhoid remedy.

Can swallow liquids only; least solid food gags.

In whatever position the patient lies the parts rested upon feel sore and bruised. *(Lach., Pry.)*

* * * * *

Baptisia tinctoria will quite naturally come in here, as it is often indicated after the *Gelsemium* stage is over in fevers. Typhoid fever can be aborted under proper homœopathic treatment, no matter what the old school says to the contrary. I have had but one case of typhoid fever run its full course in seven years, and that was a case of a young lady whose mother tried to treat her, until the disease was fully established. The symptoms indicating *Baptisia* are, in the first stage, great nervousness, chilliness, aching pains all over, but especially in head, back and limbs, and a sensation of *soreness all over;* feels as if bruised. Then the patient grows weak, prostrated, drowsy, becomes confused, the face and eyes suffused so as to give it a "besotted appearance;" the sensorium is so blunted that the patient falls asleep even before he can answer a question, or while he is in the middle of an answer. Then the tongue becomes streaked down the middle, at first white, even becomes brown in a well-defined streak down the middle, and as he comes more fully under the typhoid influence he mutters and reaches about the bed, tossing to and fro, and if he says anything he says he feel[s] *"scattered around the bed and is trying to get the piece[s] together."* Now the bowels begin to rumble, especially in the ilio-cœcal region, which is also sensitive to touch; later still the bowels begin to discharge, and all the discharges (stool, urine and sweat) are extremely offensive. This is a true picture of a *Baptisia* typhoid, and I have aborted in the first stage many cases and even checked their progress (in other cases) and cured them when they had been running eight to twelve days. I have used bot[h] the low and high preparations with equal success, but now use the 30th potency.

FERRUM PHOSPHORICUM.

This one of Schuessler's tissue remedies has proven a valuable remedy in some inflammatory diseases. In keeping with its element of *Iron,* it presents the *local congestion tendencies* of that remedy; and in its *Phosphorus* element its affinity for the lungs and stomach; and in its combination proves a great *hæmorrhage remedy.* The hæmorrhages are of bright blood, and may come from any outlet of the body. Further proving and clinical use will enable us to use it more scientifically than we now do. So far as I have observed, it is not adapted to the full-blooded, sanguine, arterial subjects, with an overplus of red blood that *Aconite* cures, but rather to pale, anæmic subjects, who with all their weaknesses are nevertheless subject to sudden and violent local congestions and inflammations, like pneumonia, or sudden congestions to head, bowels, or any other part, or to inflammatory affections of a rheumatic character. It is only useful in the first stage of such attacks, before the stage of exudation appears. It has been found useful also in the above-described weakened or anæmic subjects who have *sour eructations* occurring in stomach troubles, usually termed dyspeptic. In dysentery, in the first stage with a good deal of blood in the discharges, it is very valuable, and often cures in a very short time.

Again, it is often efficacious in the night sweats of the weak and anæmic. I am sorry not to be able to give characteristic indications for the use of this remedy, but I am fully persuaded that it is a very valuable one and ought to receive a thoroughly Hahnemannian proving.

VERATRUM VIRIDE.

A narrow, well developed red streak right through the middle of the tongue.

Intense fever, with twitching and tendency to spasms.

* * * * *

Veratrum viride is another remedy which at one time had a great reputation in the first or congestive stage of inflammatory diseases, and especially in those organs coming under the control of the pneumogastric nerve, viz., pharynx, œsophagus, stomach and heart. For a time the journals fairly bristled with reported cures of pneumonia, and its curative power was attributed to the influence of the remedy to control the action of heart and pulse. It was claimed that if we could control the quickened circulation so as to decrease the amount of blood forced into the congested lung, that you thereby gave the lung a chance to free itself of the existing engorgement.

It looked plausible, and certainly in many cases remarkable cures were effected, and that in a short time. I was a young physician and thought I had found a prize in this remedy. But one day I left a patient, relieved by this remedy of an acute and violent attack of pneumonia, to go to a town five miles distant, and when I returned found my patient dead. Then I watched others treated with this remedy, and found every little while a patient with pneumonia dropping out *suddenly* when they were reported better.

Now we don't hear so much of *Veratrum vir.* as the

greatest remedy for the first stage of this disease. What was the matter? 1st. It was (like other fads) used too indiscriminately. 2d. It is not desirable (it is wrong) to control or *depress the pulse,* regardless of all the other conditions. 3d. The patients, who had weak hearts, were killed by this powerful heart depressant. A quickened circulation is salutary, in all inflammatory diseases, and is evidence that the *Natural power* to resist disease is there, and at work. The pulse will come to its normality when the cause of its disturbance is removed and never should be forced to do so until then. Here is a common fault of the old school notwithstanding their cry of "*Tolle causam.*" So I find fault with Guernsey's keynote, "Great activity of the arterial system; very quick pulse." Next to *Digitalis, Veratrum viride* slows the pulse, as is abundantly shown in the provings. If quick pulse is ever a result of this remedy, it is a secondary or reactionary effect, like the sleeplessness of *Opium* or constipation of cathartics. So it seems to me that as an antiphlogistic (forgive me) it must go into the shade with the once vaunted *Digitalis.*

Then what is *Veratrum viride* good for? Well, I do not think that its sphere is yet fully defined, or can be without further provings and verification. The provings are already carried far enough to show that it must be a very powerful and useful remedy. That it inflames the œsophagus or stomach is well known, as is the fact that it congests the brain and lungs, but what are the characteristic symptoms that will enable us to prescribe this remedy in preference to the other remedies that do the same thing is not so well known. One peculiar symptom I believe to be characteristic, and which I have verified in a very severe case of erysipelas, which was accompanied by great delirium, is *"a narrow, well-defined red streak right through the middle of the tongue."* Again I believe *Veratrum viride* to be one of our best remedies for spasms, twitchings and convulsions, but do not know of any very reliable symptoms guiding us to its selection in the individual case. I once cured a man of a very severe and persistent attack of vomiting, which was aggravated on rising, with this remedy. He had suffered from several similar attacks before, but never any after this one, now several years ago.

VERATRUM ALBUM.

Collapse, with general coldness and cold sweat, especially on forehead; hippocratic face.

Mania, with desire to cut and tear things, with lewdness, lascivious talk, religious or amorous.

Disposed to silence, but if irritated gets mad. Scolds, calls names and talks of faults of others.

Rice water stools, profuse, exhausting, cramps in calves, coldness, collapse.

Rheumatic affections < in damp weather; drives patient out of bed.

The pains are maddening, driving the patient to delirium.

Copiousness of discharges: stools, vomiting, urine, saliva, sweat; craving for acids or refreshing things.

* * * * *

Here is a remedy that has a characteristic *"Cold sweat on the forehead."* It makes no difference whether it is cholera, cholera infantum, pneumonia, asthma, typhoid fever or constipation; if this symptom is prominently present, and the patient is in anything like a faint, collapse, or greatly prostrated condition, *Veratrum album* is the first remedy to think of. It is one of Hahnemann's trio of remedies for Asiatic cholera, *Camphor* and *Cuprum metallicum* being the other two; and today his indications for its use stand as true as when he first gave them to the profession. It abides the test because it is founded upon a natural law of cure, which is the same "yesterday, today, and forever."

Veratrum alb. has some very strong mind symptoms. "*Mania with desire to cut and tear things, especially clothes, with lewdness and lascivious talk, religious or amorous.*"

Here the choice will sometimes have to be made between this remedy and *Stramonium.* They are both very loquacious, and both strongly religious. Also both at times very violent; but the face of *Stramonium* is generally very red and bloated, while that of *Veratrum* is likely to be pale, sunken or hippocratic; again, there is greater general weakness with *Veratrum.* Sometimes the violent form of mania alternates with a "disposition to silence," but if irritated gets mad, scolds, calls names and talks of the faults of others. These forms of mania are often consequent upon suppressed menses or the puerperal state. They may be acute or become chronic. In either case we may find the cure in *Veratrum album.*

If we were to describe in *one word* the general condition, as near as possible, for which this remedy was best, it would be **collapse.** Let me quote: "Rapid sinking of forces; complete prostration; cold sweat and cold breath." "Skin blue, purple, cold, wrinkled, remaining in folds when pinched." "Face hippocratic; nose pointed."

"Whole body icy cold." "Cold skin, face cold, back cold." "Hands icy cold." "Feet and legs icy cold." (Icy coldness of surface, covered with cold sweat, *Tabacum.)* "Cramps in calves." All these are verified symptoms, and show to what an extreme degree of collapse a case may come and yet be cured. This condition may be found in rapidly progressing, acute cases like cholera, or it may be found in suppressed exanthemata; or, again, in the course of bronchitis, pneumonia, typhoid or intermittent fever. No matter where found, or in connection with whatever disease, if this collapse is present, and especially if the grand keynote, *"cold sweat on face and forehead,"* is present, we may give this remedy with full confidence that it will do all that *can be* done and much more than the old school system of stimulation with alcoholics. In choleraic diseases *Camphor* comes nearest to *Veratrum*, but with *Veratrum* the stools are profuse and like rice-water, while they are scanty or entirely absent with *Camphor*. The pains of *Veratrum* are very severe sometimes, driving the patient to delirium. It is said to be a good remedy for rheumatism, which is worse in wet weather and which drives the patient out of bed *(Ferrum met.)*. *Veratrum* is a remedy of wide range, because it covers a condition which may be found in so many different diseases.

HELLEBORUS NIGER.

Another remedy of not very wide range, so far as we have any clinical knowledge, but so far as we do know is invaluable.

We know of its use in the advanced stage of serious brain troubles, such as meningitis or any trouble of the brain where is threatened effusion, or effusion already present.

Symptoms: Head rolling from side to side on the pillow, with screams; great stupidity or soporous sleep; greedy drinking of water; wrinkled forehead with cold sweat; motion of jaws, as chewing something; dilated pupils, and often cannot be made to see or hear, or be made to sense anything at all; continual motion of one arm and leg, while the other lies as if paralyzed; *urine scanty or entirely suppressed,* sometimes sediment like coffee grounds. These symptoms indicate a desperate condition, and the patient will soon die comatose or in convulsions unless the proper remedy can be found.

Helleborus niger can often cure such cases, as I have often observed, not only in my own practice, but in that of others. I have sometimes observed that the first sign of improvement in such cases was a decided increase in the urine, and following it a general subsidence of all the other bad symptoms. I have used it with most prompt and satisfactory results in the 1000th (B. & T.) and 33m. (Fincke's) potencies.

Helleborus is also an excellent remedy in post-scarlatinal dropsies, which come on very rapidly. Here the coffee-grounds sediment may or may not be present. The choice is sometimes not easy between this remedy and *Apis mellifica.*

CUPRUM METALLICUM.

SPASM is the one word characterizing this remedy. Cramps or convulsions, in meningitis, cholera, cholera morbus, whooping cough, scarlatina, etc.

Spasms begin in fingers and toes and spreading from there become general.

Mental or bodily exhaustion from over-exertion of mind or loss of sleep.

Affections arising from suppressed skin troubles, especially from acute exanthemata.

* * * * *

The grand central characteristic symptom is expressed in one word—**spasms.** If in brain affections, congestions, meningitis or apoplexy *Cuprum* is to do any good, spasm will be present in some degree, at least, from a simple twitching of the fingers and toes to general convulsions. If in cardialgia, there is violent *spasmodic* griping and pressure, followed by vomiting. In cholera, cholera morbus, or cholera infantum the cramping pains are sometimes *terrible.* Dunham said: "In *Camphor* collapse is most prominent; in *Veratrum album,* the evacuation and vomiting; in *Cuprum,* the *cramps.*" In whooping cough *"children get stiff, breathing ceases, spasmodic twitchings; after a while consciousness returns,* they vomit and recover but slowly;" or the child coughs itself into a complete "cataleptic spasm with each paroxysm of cough." In all kinds of repercussed exanthematic spasms, *Cuprum* is the first remedy to be thought of (see comparison with *Zincum).*

These spasms may also be found in dysmenorrhœa, in child bed, or in after pains. Then, aside from any and all kinds of local affections, *Cuprum* may be found indicated in epilepsia, chorea, and other purely nervous spasmodic affections of a general nature. There is one thing peculiar in the spasms of *Cuprum* that I have often observed, and it is a strong indication for the remedy, viz.: The spasm begins by twitching in the *fingers and toes,* and, spreading from there, becomes general.

There is another symptom which Farrington thought very valuable, viz.: *"Mental and bodily exhaustion* from overexertion of mind, or loss of sleep." This is similar to *Cocculus* and *Nux vomica.* The other symptoms must decide between them. I have always used the metal instead of the acetate, because I used the potencies, and it acted promptly.

CICUTA VIROSA

Is another remedy which is characterized by its *excessively* **violent** convulsions. With this remedy the patient is thrown into all sorts of odd shapes and violent contortions, but one of the most invariable is the *bending* of the head, neck and spine backwards, opisthotonos. It is on this account that it was tried for cerebro-spinal meningitis. Dr. Baker, of Moravia, N. Y., cured, during an epidemic of this terrible disease, sixty cases of all degrees of malignancy without the loss of a single case. This is a wonderful record, and he thinks it is as near a specific for this disease as can be.

Cicuta is also one of our best remedies for convulsions during dentition or worms if *Cina* does not help. It is also a good remedy for the effects of concussion of the brain or spine, if spasms are in the train of chronic effects therefrom and *Arnica* does not relieve. In the affections for which *Cicuta* is useful the actions of the patient are as violent as are the spasms—moans and howls, makes gesticulations and odd motions, great agitation, etc.

All sorts of convulsions—tonic clonic, epileptic, cataleptic, worm, puerperal, etc.—if of a very violent character, should call to mind *Cicuta.*

It is also wonderful for skin affections, "pustules which

run together, forming thick, yellow scabs on face, head and other parts of the body." I once had a case of eczema capitis in a young woman—it was of long standing—which covered the whole scalp, solid, like a cap. I gave her *Cicuta* 200th and cured her completely in a very short time. She had used many local applications without benefit.

CAUSTICUM.

Great weakness, faint-like goneness, culminating in local paralysis (vocal organs, tongue, muscles of deglutition, eyelids, face, bladder and extremities).

Obstinate neuralgias, especially of psoric origin; pains of a cramping, drawing nature.

Sensation of *sore rawness* (scalp, throat, larynx and trachea, chest, rectum, anus, urethra and eruptions with burning).

Contractions of the ligaments (arthritis deformans).

Dry cough with pain in hip and involuntary urination. Soreness and rawness in air passages, cannot raise the mucus, < on expiration, > swallowing cold water.

Hæmorrhoids sore and raw < on walking. Constipation frequent, ineffectual desire for stool; passes better on standing.

Modalities: < dry weather, walking (piles), > wet weather, swallowing cold water (cough).

* * * * *

This is a very unique remedy, proven by Hahnemann and classed among the anti-psorics. Its exact chemical composition is not known but it is supposed to be a kind of potash preparation. It has quite a long list of peculiar symptoms, which are, nevertheless, very reliable. In the first place it has *great weakness,* such as characterizes the potash salts generally. It is with *Causticum "faint-like weakness, or sinking of strength, with trembling."* In this it resembles *Gelsemium,* and it has another symptom, in connection with its general weakness which resembles *Gelsemium,* viz.: *"Drooping of the lids." Sepia, Causticum* and *Gelsemium* is the trio having this peculiar symptom in a very marked degree. Now, the weakness of *Causticum* progresses until we have *"gradually appearing paralysis;"* indeed, *paralysis* is common with *Causticum* and attacks in a general way the right side *(Lachesis the left),* but it also has local paralysis; as, for instance, of the *vocal organs, muscles of deglutition, of tongue, eyelids, face, bladder* and *extremities.* On the other hand, it has all grades of nervous twitchings, chorea, convulsions and epileptic attacks, even progressive locomotor ataxia. I can only name these diseases here, but will notice further on the symptoms and conditions which appear in connection with them.

Neuralgic affections are also common with this remedy and are generally of an obstinate character. *Causticum* has helped me out in such cases when other seemingly indicated remedies failed. One of our oldest and most eminent writers on Materia Medica, Charles J. Hempel, sneered at the multiplicity of symptoms of this remedy, as found in the *"Chronic Diseases,"* but the clinical test has proven it to be a remedy of great use and wide range. On the mind it exerts a very depressing influence in keeping with its general action on the nervous system. *Melancholy mood; sadness,* hopelessness; is apt to look on the dark side of everything. This melancholy may come from care, grief or sorrow. It often comes from long-lasting brief or sorrow, and should be remembered here alongside *Ignatia, Natrum muriaticum* and *Phosphoric acid.*

This is the preponderant mood of *Causticum,* but it may alternate with an anxious, irritable or hysterical mood. We have already spoken of the paralysis of the eyelids. The vision is often affected; there is an appearance of gauze before the eyes, or as if a fog or cloud were there. This is often the case in incipient cataract, and *Causticum* often remedies it.

Upon the ears there is roaring, tinkling, humming and all sorts of noises. It is one of our best remedies in deafness with these noises. Reverberation of sounds, especially the patient's own voice, finds here a remedy. Then the ears (external) burn and are very red. *Sulphur* also has this symptom very prominently; and right here we may say that there are many resemblances between these two remedies, and they follow each other well, especially in chronic diseases.

Upon the face we have four prominent peculiar symptoms:

1st. Yellowness of the face; sickly yellow (not jaundice).

2d. Paralysis of a rheumatic or psoric origin.

3d. Prosopalgia of the same origin.

4th. Stiffness of the jaws; could not open the mouth.

This latter symptom also seems to be rheumatic and is in keeping with the arthritis deformans, of which we will say more further on.

Upon the tongue we have: 1st. Paralysis; or indistinct speech without complete paralysis *(Gels.).* 2d. Tongue coated white on the sides, red in the middle, but not so sharply defined as in *Veratrum viride.*

The throat comes strongly under the influence of *Causticum.*

"Burning pain in throat, not < by swallowing; pain is in both sides or seems to arise from chest."

"Rawness and tickling in throat with dry cough and some expectoration after long coughing."

This again is similar to *Sulphur,* which has burning in throat, more on right side. I have found that if *Sulphur* did not relieve, *Causticum* given after it, often would.

Intestinal Canal.—Sensation of lime being burned in the stomach, with rising of air. Guernsey praised this symptom and considered it reliable. I have not verified it. *Causticum* is one of our best remedies in anal troubles, and has very peculiar symptoms. *"Constipation, frequent but unsuccessful desire to stool." (Nux.)* "Frequent ineffectual desire to stool, with much pain and straining, *with redness of face."* "The stool passes better when standing. Hæmorrhoids impeding stool, swollen; itching; smarting; rawness; moist; stinging; burning; *raw and sore,* aggravated when **walking,** when thinking of them, from preaching or straining the voice." All these symptoms have been verified over and over again. There are other symptoms also in this region that are very valuable, but we are not writing a complete Materia Medica and will only say in addition that in all anal troubles we should let *Causticum* rank among the first in our mind when we are hunting for the simillimum. We do not know in what part the peculiar and characteristic symptom which leads to the simillimum will appear, but must be on the alert to recognize it promptly.

Causticum also has very marked action upon the urinary organs, as is shown by the following symptoms: "Itching of the orifice of the urethra." "Constant ineffectual desire to urinate, frequent evacuations of only a few drops, with spasms in the rectum and constipation."

This is like *Nux vomica* and *Cantharis,* and I once cured a chronic case of cystitis in a married woman, which had baffled the best efforts of several old school physicians, eminent for their skill, for years. There was another symptom in the case that was prominent, and that was a sensation of *soreness* or *rawness.* More will be said, when we come to write on *sensations,* of this last symptom. Again, "retention of urine, with frequent and urgent desire, occasionally a few drops dribble away."

"Involuntary passage of urine when *coughing,* sneezing, *blowing the nose;* at night *when asleep;* when walking." "He urinates so easily that he is not sensible of the stream, and scarcely believes in the dark that he is urinating at all, until he makes sure by sense of touch." I do not know of any remedy in which this weakness of the neck of the bladder is more prominent. *Causticum* also affects the urine itself. "The urine is loaded with lithic acid and lithates (Hughes), there are thick deposits or sediments of various colors from dark to light." These are a few of the leading urinary symptoms and show its importance here.

Respiratory Organs.—Hoarseness worse in the morning, with rawness and sudden loss of voice. Laryngeal muscles refuse to act; cannot speak a loud word. Chronic hoarseness remaining after acute laryngitis. Hoarseness with deep bass voice (like *Drosera*). These are all very reliable symptoms, and no remedy removes them oftener than *Causticum.* All this loss of voice may come from paresis of the vocal chords, or from catarrhal causes. Then following down the respiratory tract, we have great *rawness* and irritation of the trachea, cough dry, hollow; with sore or *raw* sensation in a streak down along the trachea. *Cough with pain in hip and involuntary urination.* Cough with sensation as if she could not cough deep enough to start the mucus. Coughs worse on expiration *(Acon.). Cough relieved by a swallow of cold water.* Cough with inability to raise the mucus, it must be swallowed; but the most characteristic symptom all through the cough and chest symptoms is the sensation of *soreness and rawness* accompanying them. Some will express this as a sensation of *burning,* if so we must remember *Iodine* and *Spongia.* In influenza or what is now called *La Grippe* it disputes for first place with *Eupatorium perf.* and *Rhus toxicod.* All three have a tired, sore, bruised sensation all over the body, and all have soreness in the chest when coughing, but if involuntary micturition is present *Causticum* wins. No homœopath can afford to be without an understanding of *Causticum* upon the respiratory organs.

Now upon the back and extremities we have—stiffness and pain in neck and throat, muscles feel as if bound, could scarce move the head. Painful stiffness of the back and sacrum, especially on rising from a chair. Paralysis of either or both lower and upper extremities. Dull drawing pain in hands and arms. Drawing and tearing in thighs and legs, knees and feet, worse in open air and better in bed. Weakness and trembling of the limbs. Rheumatic and arthritic inflammations with contractions of the flexors and stiffness of the joints. All these, and many more symptoms, show what a useful remedy this must be in its general action on the back and extremities, but right here I wish to say that if I were to select the three remedies to the exclusion of all others for the treatment of chronic rheumatism and paralysis *Causticum, Rhus tox.* and *Sulphur* would be the three. These three remedies studied in their correspondence and relation to each other will more than repay the careful student, and *Causticum* holds well its own in the comparison. You will remember that I have before alluded to the resemblances of *Causticum* and *Sulphur,* and may continue to do so further on. I wish here, although constitutionally opposed to making too much of complementaries and incompatibles (so-called), to state that there are no two remedies that are oftener indicated after each other, and work as well when so indicated, than these two. If Hahnemann had never given to the homœopathic school any remedy but *Causticum,* the world would still be to him under lasting obligations.

Sensations.—Tearing pains are characteristic of this remedy. They are often paroxysmal. This is often found in neuralgia of the face. Then again I wish to call particular attention to the sensation of **soreness** or **rawness.** This is found in scalp, throat, larynx and trachea, chest, rectum, anus, urethra and eruptions. We observe that the sensation of soreness is not like that of *Arnica,* which is a soreness as if bruised and mostly muscular, nor of *Rhus toxicodendron,* which is an aching soreness as if sprained and oftenest found in the tendons and sheaths of muscles, or areolar tissues; but it is a soreness mostly, if not altogether, of mucous surfaces as if the parts were *raw.* This is important and a very reliable sensation. Then again we have in *Causticum much burning.* These burnings are found almost everywhere, and in this we again see its resemblance to *Sulphur.* Now let it be remembered that the burnings of *Sulphur* are associated with *itching,* those of *Apis mellifica* with *stinging,* and those of *Causticum* with *soreness.* So we must always learn to differentiate, because it is only by so doing that we can select the one remedy out of a class, and sometimes a large class, having the same or similar symptoms. The *drawing pains* that in many cases result in forcing out of shape the extremities so as to cause that terrible affliction known as *arthritis deformans* are found as prominently under *Causticum* as under any other remedy, and it is one of the most useful agents for the relief or cure.

Causticum is classed among Hahnemann's anti-psorics. It is certainly one of the prominent remedies for affections arising from the suppression of itch or chronic skin troubles, like eczema. I was once called, in consultation, to a case of prosopalgia which had for a long time baffled the skill of a very good homœopathic practitioner. Not being able to relieve the case, he had become demoralized, and as the pain and suffering were very great he had resorted to anodynes, but with the usual result of making the patient worse, after the anodynes had worn out, than she was before. On looking over the case carefully, I found in addition to the emaciated and greatly debilitated condition of the patient, after so long suffering, that the pains came in paroxysms, that they were of a drawing nature, and that she had suffered from eczema for years, at different times, before this pain appeared. *Sulphur* had been given, but without relief. So I advised *Causticum.* It was given, in the 200th, and a rapid and a permanent cure was the result. Whether *Causticum* could be called an anti-sycotic as well as anti-psoric, or not, I do not know. Certain it is that it is one of our most successful remedies for warts. It stands next to *Thuja,* if not equal. It is also foremost in old sores originating in burns. I have given more space to *Causticum* than I otherwise would, for the reason that I am sure that this great remedy is not generally appreciated. I know of no remedy more positive and satisfactory in its action when indicated. Generally < *in clear fine weather* > *in damp wet weather.* (*Nux vom.,* asthma < in dry weather > in damp weather.)

HEPAR SULPHURIS CALCAREUM.

Hypersensitive to touch, pain, cold air; fainting with the pain.

General tendency to suppurations; even slight injuries or scratches on the skin suppurate.

Tendency to croupy exudations (larynx and kidneys; any mucous membrane).

Atony; stools passed with great difficulty, even when soft; urine flows slowly, must wait for it, then drops vertically down without force.

Sour diarrhœa; whole child smells sour.

Coughs; croup, bronchitis, consumption; < when exposed to least cold air.

Modalities: < exposure to dry cold air; > in moist wet weather.

Like *Sulphur, Hepar* is adapted to the psoric, scrofulous diathesis.

* * * * *

This remedy standing half-way between those two great anti-psorics, *Calcarea carb.* and *Sulphur,* has some very strong characteristics which guide to its use in a variety of ailments. Its strongest characteristic is its **hypersensitiveness** to *touch, pain* and *cold air.* The patient is so sensitive to pain that she faints away, even when it is slight. If there are inflammation or swelling in any locality, or even eruptions on the skin, they are so sensitive that she *cannot bear to have them touched,* or even to have the cold air to blow upon them. This is like *China off.,* only that while the latter is sensitive to the lightest touch it *can* bear hard pressure. (Remedies especially < in cold air are *Arsenicum alb., Calcarea ost., Hepar sul., Nux vomica, Psorinum, Silicea, Tuberculinum.)* This supersensitiveness to pain runs all through the drug. It is mental as well as physical, for the slightest cause irritates with hasty speech and vehemence. Next to this is the power of *Hepar sulph.* over the suppurative stage of local inflammations. It comes in only when pus is about to form, or is already formed. If given very high in the first case (that is before pus is formed), and not repeated too soon or often, we may prevent suppuration and check the whole inflammatory process. But if pus is already formed, it will hasten the pointing and discharge and help along the healing of the ulcer afterwards. I am not at all sure, as is generally taught, that it is necessary to give it low to hasten suppuration. The most rapid pointing, opening, and perfect healing I ever saw was in the case of a large glandular swelling on the neck of a child, under the action of the c. m. potency. *Hepar* has a general tendency to suppuration, for even the eruptions on the skin are liable to form matter, and slight injuries suppurate. *(Graphites, Mercurius, Petroleum.)* This remedy is also very valuable in diseases of the respiratory organs. I have found it very useful in cases of chronic catarrh, when the nose stopped up every time the patient went out into the cold air. He says it seems as if I get a new cold every time I get a breath of fresh air *(Tuberculinum)*. It is relieved in a warm room. In croup it has been, ever since Bœnninghausen prescribed his celebrated five powders, one of our standard remedies. We do not use the five powders as Bœnninghausen did in a certain order, but only use them according to indications. *Hepar* croup is accompanied with rather loose cough, with wheezing and rattling. Cough as if mucus would come up, but it does not. It is seldom indicated at first; but oftener comes in after *Aconite* or *Spongia.* Like *Aconite* it seems most effectual in those cases brought on by exposure to dry cold air; but the *Aconite croup comes on in the evening after first sleep* and *Hepar in the early morning hours.* This tendency to croupy exudations on mucous membranes seems characteristic of *Hepar* and is not confined to the respiratory organs. Kafka uses it on the ground of its ability to control such conditions in post-scarlatinal dropsy, to prevent or cure, and claims great success for it. I believe it to be one of the best prophylactics in such cases, for the reason that during and after the desquamative stage the skin is unusually susceptible to the effects of chill in cold air, and this is in accordance with the *leading* characteristic of this remedy. It *fortifies* the patient against such atmospheric influence.

In croup, as in other affections of *Hepar,* the cough, difficult breathing and all other symptoms are aggravated by the least breath of cold air, which the little patient must be carefully guarded against. Travelling downward the larynx is attacked, then the bronchia, and even the lungs, and the formation of croupy exudates will take place if not checked by the remedy. The breathing in all these cases becomes rattling, anxious, wheezing, even to threatened suffocation, so that the patient seems asthmatic. In these cases it is often able to relieve, especially if this condition follows a hard cold and the acute inflamamtory symptoms have been controlled by *Aconite* or some other indicated remedy.

In chronic asthma, *Hepar* often resembles *Natrum sulphuricum,* but there is this diagnostic difference, which is very valuable. The *Hepar* asthma is worse in *dry cold* air and better in damp, while *Natrum sulph.* is exactly the opposite, like *Dulcamara.* There is no other remedy that I know that has the amelioration so strongly in damp weather as *Hepar sulphur.* One characteristic must not be forgotten, viz.: *"Coughs when any part of the body becomes uncovered." (Baryta* and *Rhus tox.)* This is found in croup, laryngitis, bronchitis and consumption, and not only is the *cough* worse, but the whole case is aggravated. Then, again, it must be remembered that this is one of our strongest anti-psorics, and for that reason should be thought of for all respiratory ailments for which it has such a strong affinity, especially when such ailments have followed a suppressed or retrocedent eruption on the skin.

In accordance with its great power over all suppurative processes, it should come to mind in abscess of the lungs, of course in all cases when indicated by the symptoms *in toto.* Upon the throat we have 1st, "sticking in the throat, as from a splinter, on swallowing, extending to the ear, also on yawning." "Sensation as if a fish bone or splinter were sticking in the throat" *(Argentum nitricum, Dolichos* and *Nitric acid),* but probably the condition where *Hepar* is oftenest of use in throat trouble is in that distressing complaint, *quinsy.*

Here, as in croup, it is not generally indicated in the beginning. Having had much success and experience in this disease, I may here give the results of the application of several remedies and their indications:

Belladonna.—High fever, great swelling, and redness, headache, throbbing carotids.

Mercurius vivus.—Either side, fœtid breath, flabby, moist, indented tongue, and sweat without relief.

Mercurius proto-iodatus.—Same symptoms, but begins on right side, and tongue thickly coated *yellow* at the base.

Lachesis.—Left side extending to right, great sensitiveness to touch, and aggravation after sleep.

Lycopodium.—Begins right side, extends to left, with tongue swollen and inclined to protrude from the mouth, and stuffing up of nose.

Lac caninum.—Alternates sides, one day worse on one, and the next on the other.

Hepar sulph.—When notwithstanding all other remedies the case seems bound to suppurate and there is much *throbbing* pain. Now with each of these remedies I have aborted many cases in old quinsy subjects, who never expected to, and were told by old school physicians that they never could, get well, without suppuration, and in the end have cured them of all tendency thereto. I will add here that *Hepar sulphur.* is also a good remedy in chronic hypertrophy of tonsils, with hardness of hearing. In these cases which are generally very intractable, *Baryta carbonica, Lycopodium, Plumbum,* and others are also to be consulted according to indications.

Upon the alimentary canal *Hepar* has a decided influence. We have already noticed its action upon the throat. The stomach is inclined to be out of order, and there is a *"longing for acid things." (Veratrum alb.)* This is often the case in chronic dyspepsia and *Hepar* helps. This condition of the stomach is sometimes found in marasmus of children. It is often accompanied by diarrhœa, and a very important feature is that the diarrhœa is *sour;* indeed *the whole child seems to smell sour* no matter how much it is bathed. The sour stool is also very prominently under *Magnesia carbonica* and *Calcarea carbonica.* Then there is another condition of the bowels, namely, a kind of *atony.* The stools are passed with great difficulty, even though they are soft and clay-like, as they sometimes are under this remedy. This state of atony is also found in the bladder.

"Micturition impeded, he is obliged to wait awhile before the urine passes, and then it flows slowly for many days." "He is never able to finish urinating; it seems as if some urine always remains behind in the bladder." "Weakness of the bladder, the urine drops vertically down and he is obliged to wait awhile before any passes." This inability to expel makes one think of *Alumina* and *Veratrum album* and *Silicea.* Again, *Hepar sulph.* is a great "sweat" remedy, either partial or general. It may, for instance, come in after *Mercurius* in rheumatism, in which the patient *"sweats day and night without relief,"* and *Mercurius* does not help. So, too, with quinsy, and in large boils and swellings; and by the way *Hepar sulph.* is one of our best remedies after *Mercurius,* either in homœopathic practice, or as an antidote to old school poisoning. So also is it the leading antidote to Iodide of Potassa poisoning from the same source. We could not well do without this valuable remedy.

CALCAREA SULPHURICA.

One of Schuessler's so-called tissue remedies, not well understood as yet, but acting much along the line of *Hepar sulphur.* so far as we do know. I once had a case in which there was great pain in the region of the kidneys for a day and night. Then there was a great discharge of pus in the urine, which continued several days and weakened the patient very fast. A Chicago specialist had examined the urine a short time before, and had pronounced the case *Bright's disease.* I finally prescribed *Calcarea sulphurica* 12th and under its action she immediately improved and made a very rapid and permanent recovery. Since then I have found it a good remedy in profuse suppurations in different kinds of cases. This is all I know about the remedy.

CALCAREA HYPOPHOSPHORICA.

I once had a case like this: A boy eight years of age had several (four or five) abscesses in and around the knee joint. The ulceration had also attacked the tibia, which was half eaten off, so that the ragged necrosed bone protruded through the surface plainly in sight. The little fellow was greatly emaciated, and had no appetite, and was pale as a corpse. I told the mother that I thought this was a case for the surgeon, but I would try to get him in better condition for the operation. I remembered reading years before of the cures of abscesses by this remedy, made by Dr. Searles, of Albany, and empirically concluded to try it in this case.

I put him upon the first trituration, a grain a day. Called in a week and found a great change for the better. The mother exclaimed as I came in: "Ah, Doctor, the boy is eating us out of house and home." Under the continued use of the remedy he made a complete and rapid recovery, except that the tibia was a little bent. I have since used the remedy in some very large swellings where pus had formed, with the effect of complete absorption of the pus and no opening of the abscess on the surface. One was a case of hip disease which had been pronounced incurable by a *specialist on ulcerations.* (How is that for a specialist, *regular* at that.) The different combinations of the *Calcareas* ought to be so thoroughly proven as to enable us to put them each in their exact place. So, also, with the *Kalis, Magnesias, Natrums* and *Mercuries,* etc.

GRAPHITES.

Eruption on the skin, oozing out a thick, honey-like fluid.

Mucous outlets; eyelids inflamed, with pustules; ears discharge, moist sore places behind ears; mouth cracked in corners; anus, eruptions, itching, fissured.

Nails grow thick, cracked, out of shape.

Constipation; stools knotty, large lumps, united by mucous threads.

Diarrhœa; stools, brown fluid, mixed with undigested substances, and of an intolerably fœtid odor.

Sad and despondent; inclined to weep; thinks of nothing but death.

Especially adapted to persons inclined to obesity; particularly females who delay menstruation.

Hears better when in a noise; when riding in a carriage or car; when there is a rumbling sound.

Sensation of cobweb on forehead; tries hard to brush it off.

* * * * *

The chief leading characteristic of this remedy is found in its skin symptoms.

Hoyne had expressed it nearly right. "Eruptions oozing out a thick, honey-like fluid." It may be found on any part of the body, but is especially found on or behind the ears, on head, face, genitals, or eyelids. I once treated a case of eczema of the legs which was of twenty years' standing. It was in an old obese woman, and, by the way, that is the kind of subject in which this remedy is found most efficacious.

I gave her, on account of much burning of the feet, a dose of *Sulphur* c. m. In two or three weeks an eruption was developed all over the body which exuded a glutinous, sticky fluid. One dose of *Graphites* c. m., dry on the tongue, cured this as well as the eczema of the legs and left her skin as smooth as that of a child. This was years ago. Erysipelas sometimes takes this form, and in such cases recurs again and again. It will naturally occur to the physician that, because of this recurrence, there is some psoric taint which must be met by *Sulphur*. But we must not make the too common mistake of thinking that *Sulphur* is the remedy on account of its great antipsoric powers, or on the often misleading indication "when seemingly indicated remedies don't act," because *Sulphur* is not the only anti-psoric and where *Graphites* is indicated is not at all the anti-psoric for the case in hand. In short, we must not prescribe for psora (which is only a name after all) without indications any more than we would prescribe for the name scarlatina or diphtheria. *Graphites* is a powerful anti-psoric, as are also *Psorinum, Lycopodium, Causticum* and many others. Symptoms must decide here, as elsewhere. In order to still further show the wonderful anti-psoric powers of this remedy I will give another case from practice.

A child three years of age had eczema capitis. Under allopathic local treatment the eczema disappeared; but soon entero-colitis of a very obstinate character set in. Then the regulars could not "do" that as they had the eczema, and after they had given up the case, pronouncing it consumption of the bowels, the homœopath (myself) was called in on the ground that he could do no harm if he could do no good (so they said).

Case.—Child greatly emaciated, little or no appetite, very restless, and *"stools brown fluid mixed with undigested substances, and of an intolerably fœtid odor."* Taking into the account the history of the suppressed eczema I prescribed *Graphites* 6m. *(Jenichen)* and in a short time a perfect cure was the result. *Psorinum* has a similar stool as was present in this case, but the eruptions of the two remedies are different and this one corresponded to *Graphites,* hence *Psorinum* was ruled out. If this case of so long standing had not had the eruption I might have thought of *China* on account of the extreme weakness from long-continued drain or loss of fluid, for *China* is another remedy that has *brown, loose, fœtid stools.* So we must take into consideration *all the case,* psora and all. In chronic cases, in which *Graphites* is likely to be the remedy, we may look for affections of the *eyelids,* of the same eczematous character as that found on the head, behind the ears, etc.

Notice.—Eczema of lids, eruptions moist and fissured margins of lids covered with scales and crusts. In *Sulphur* lids the margins are *very red. All the orifices* under *Sulphur* are very red. *Graphites* leads all the remedies for eczematous affections of the lids, *Staphisagria* stands next, but of course special indications, local or general, or both, must decide.

Graphites is one of our best anal remedies. We have given the kind of loose stool characteristic of the drug. This is, however, exceptional, for it generally tends to constipation instead of diarrhœa. The *stools* are *knotty* and *large,* the lumps sometimes *united* by *mucous threads* and mucus often follows the stool. There is often eczema around the anus, and it is one of our best remedies for *fissura ani.* There is in these cases apt to be much pain after stool, and much soreness in anus on wiping it. Now if all this should occur in subjects of this tendency to sticky eruptions, we should not hesitate to give *Graphites* with expectations of success.

Another very characteristic calling for this remedy is found in the *nails.* Both finger and toe nails become thick, grow out of shape. Never forget *Graphites* when you find this state of nails present. Again, *Graphites* has cracks or fissures in the ends of the fingers *(Sarsaparilla),* nipples, labial commissures, of anus, and between toes *(Petroleum).* It is one of our best remedies for *wens* found in persons of herpetic dyscrasia. Old, hard cicatrices soften up and go away under its action, especially those left by abscesses of the mammæ. Lumps in the breast of suspicious appearance also go away under the action of this remedy. In menstrual troubles it resembles *Pulsatilla,* but there are plenty of points to differentiate them. In temperament it resembles *Calcarea ostrearum;* but in *Graphites* the menses are mostly scanty and delayed, in *Calcarea* too soon and too profuse; *Graphites* cures complaints of *many kinds* when you have present two things:

1st. The peculiar tendency to obesity.

2d. The characteristic glutinous eruptions.

PSORINUM.

Very sad, hopeless, despondent; "bluest of the blue."

Great debility; sweats on slightest movement; wants to give up and lie down.

Eruptions on the skin, dry, or moist; or skin scaly and dry as parchment; dirty, the great unwashed, unwashable.

Intense itching of skin < in warmth of bed.

Discharges and *exhalations* exceedingly offensive.

Very sensitive to cold air; wears a fur cap in summer.

Modalities: < in cold air, < in warmth of bed (itching); sitting up or motion; > bringing arms down close to the body, > lying down (even the dyspnœa); wrapping up warm; psoric manifestations.

Great weakness and debility; from loss of fluids; remaining after acute diseases; without any organic lesion or apparent cause.

Cough and dry, scaly eruptions return every winter.

Quinsy; to eradicate the tendency.

* * * * *

The disease products are powerful remedies, and when used in the potentized form have made many wonderful cures. It is believed by some that in the potentized form they are so changed that they become homœopathic to the disease which produced them, especially in any other person than the one in whom the original disease existed.

I have experimented more or less with these so-called nosodes, since they were so widely proclaimed by Dr. Swan. I never found them markedly efficacious in such cases, but I have seen remarkable results from them in cases resembling, for instance, gonorrhœal, syphilitic or psoric troubles, without any history of pre-existing trouble of the kind. I have cured eruptions on the skin resembling itch with *Psorinum,* rheumatic troubles that were very obstinate under our usual remedies with *Medorrhinum* and a long standing case of caries of the spine with *Syphilinum,* but in not one of these cases had the patient, that I could trace, itch, gonorrhœa or syphilis. The experience of many others seems to be different. I give only my own. That each nosode seems capable of producing the same or similar symptoms when given by mouth in proving as when inoculated the usual way seems well proven in the case of *Psorinum.* I do not see why the constitutional symptoms appearing after inoculations should not be considered a proving as well as those following a bee sting, cantharis blistering, or the local external poisoning of the varieties of *Rhus.* If *Rhus,* very high, will cure rhus poisoning, why should not *Syphilinum,* etc., cure syphilis? Who will answer?

All nosodes are as capable of curing as they are of poisoning. If not, why not? We must not let prejudice hinder honest investigation. As if in corroboration of the theory that the potentized disease product will cure the disease producing it, the *provings* of *Psorinum* indicate that the chief action and curative power of the poison is upon the skin. And is it not remarkable that *Psorinum* should so strongly resemble *Sulphur,* the old-time remedy for itch, and again that they follow or complement each other in curing skin troubles? Notice some of the leading skin symptoms.

"Itching when the body becomes warm."

"Itching, intolerable in warmth of bed." *(Merc. sol.)*

"Itching, scratches until it bleeds."

"Itching between fingers and in bends of joints." *(Sepia.)*

"Dry, scaly eruptions which disappear summers and return winters."

"Repeated outbreaks of eruptions."

"Skin has a dirty dingy look, as if the patient *never washed,* and the body has a *filthy smell* even after a bath."

These and many other symptoms, too numerous to mention here, show what an invaluable remedy this should be in skin troubles, and abundant experience and observation corroborate the truth of our law of cure in the curative power of disease poisons, as it also does in vegetable, and mineral, and insect or animal.

Psorinum is also found useful in the consequences of suppressed eruptions, and in such cases should never be forgotten when other anti-psorics fail. Dr. Wm. A. Hawley, of Syracuse, N. Y., once made a brilliant cure of a very bad case of dropsy in an old woman, being led to prescribe this remedy by the appearance of the skin. One dose of Fincke's 42m. potency, dry on the tongue, cured the whole case in a very short time. It was a case of long standing. Now, if we examine we will also find that this remedy resembles *Graphites* in many points. A close comparison will pay the earnest student of Materia Medica. *Psorinum* is *very depressed* in mind. "Greatest despondency, making his own life and that of those about him almost intolerable." This state of mind, following acute diseases, like typhus, is especially benefited by this remedy. When writing of *Graphites* we mentioned the resemblance of the two remedies in the *"stools, dark-brown, watery,* and of *intolerably* offensive odor." This is found in bad cases of cholera infantum or chronic diarrhœa. There is one valuable diagnostic difference between them, although the remedies are so much alike, and that is that the *Graphites* moisture from the eruption is *glutinous* or *sticky* and not markedly so with *Psorinum.*

Again, *Psorinum* is very useful for weakness or debility during convalescence from severe acute diseases. The patient *sweats profusely* when taking the least exercise. Notwithstanding, as a rule, the skin is generally *dry,* inactive, and rarely sweats. Here, again, as in the stool symptom, choice may have to be made between *Psorinum* and *China.* Loss of fluids, blood, suppuration, etc., would decide in favor of the latter and itching eruptions or tendency thereto, before or during the sickness, the former. One thing I forgot to mention in connection with the offensive stool. "All excretions, diarrhœa, leucorrhœa, menstrual flow and perspiration, have a carrion-like smell, even the body has a filthy smell, notwithstanding frequent bathing." The *Psorinum* subject is *very sensitive to cold air,* or change of weather *(Hepar),* wants to wear a fur cap, overcoat or shawl, even in the hottest weather.

Chronic complaints following or dating back for years to some imperfectly cured or suppressed acute disease. *(Carbo veg.)* I advise everyone to buy a copy of Allen's "key-notes," which has a very good rendering of the nosodes. So we see in *Psorinum* when *proven* a great remedy for very grave conditions. I have no doubt that all nosodes are equally valuable when as well understood.

AURUM METALLICUM.

Wants to commit suicide; thinks he is no good in the world.

Nodes and bone pains, caries and necrosis with great depression of mind.

Abuse of Mercury, in syphilis, in massive doses.

* * * * *

"Looks on the dark side, weeps, prays, thinks she is not fit for this world, longs for death, strong inclination to *commit suicide.*" Strange that this noble metal, for which mankind strives for its pecuniary value, should, when taken into the organism, cause the greatest unhappiness.

The *Aurum* patient is plunged into the deepest gloom and despair. Life is a burden, he *desires* death. Suicide dwells constantly in his mind. In men, I have observed it oftenest in connection with liver troubles. In women, with womb troubles, especially when enlarged, indurated or prolapsed. In both these cases, the result, so far as local conditions are concerned, seems to be from repeated attacks of congestion to the parts, which ends in hypertrophy. The liver is enlarged, the womb also, and prolapsus occurs from the very weight of the organs. These congestions, so characteristic of the remedy, take place also in head, heart, chest and kidneys; but, whenever they come, the peculiar mind symptoms are always present to furnish the chief indication for *Gold*. The *Gold* patient is also at times "peevish and vehement, the least contradiction excites his wrath." He will exhibit these outbreaks occasionally, even when the more characteristic depression and gloom greatly preponderate. Other remedies have a similar depression and tendency to suicide, like *Naja* and *Nux vomica*, but none in anything like the *degree* of *Aurum*. I once cured a young lady who tried to commit suicide by drowning. After she was cured she laughed at the occurrence, and said she could not help it. It seemed to her she was of no use in the world. She *felt* so.

Aurum has been found efficacious in curing some bone affections of syphilitic origin, especially if such cases had been the subjects of old school dosing with Mercury. *There would be a great falling off of business for physicians if the old school could learn to cure their patients without poisoning them with their drugs.* The locality where *Aurum* has made its best record in these syphilitico-mercurial affections is in caries of the bones (caries of long bones, *Fluoric acid, Angustura)*, of the nose and palate, also of the mastoid process. In these nasal troubles it is sometimes of great use in the catarrh, or ozæna, before the trouble has progressed to actual caries. The nostrils are agglutinated, ulcerated, and nose obstructed and filled with crusts, or there are excessively fœtid discharges, and the patient is melancholy and disposed to suicide. *Aurum* is one of the few remedies that has hemiopia or half-sight, and has cured it even in the 200th potency. *Lycopodium* and *Lithium carbonicum* also have half-sight, but *Aurum* sees only the lower, while the other two see only the left half of objects.

Aurum not only causes and cures indurations of the womb in the female, but indurations also of the testicles in the male, and in both cases the ever-present mental symptoms of *Aurum* or the syphilitico-mercurial history furnish the chief indications for its use. In fatty heart, in ruddy, corpulent, old people it is one of our best remedies. In these cases there is much vascular disturbance. "Violent palpitation, with anxiety and congestion to the chest, and visible beating of the cartoids and temporal arteries."

Belladonna may relieve the attack, but *Aurum* goes deeper and is more lasting in its effect. *Aurum* is one of our best remedies for *bone pains.* Never forget it. It ranks with *Kali iodide, Asafœtida* and the *Mercuries* in periosteal affections.

ARGENTUM NITRICUM.

Impulsive; time goes too slow; must walk fast.

Apprehension, on getting ready for church, opera, etc.; has an attack of diarrhœa.

Vertigo, with buzzing in the ears, and weakness and trembling.

Canthi, as red as blood; swollen, standing out like a lump of red flesh.

Irresistible desire for sugar; gastric ailments, with violent loud belchings.

Stool; green, mucous, like chopped spinach in flakes; turns green on remaining on diaper; expelled with much spluttering.

Profuse, sometimes purulent, discharges from mucous membranes, generally.

Dried-up, withered patients, made so by disease.

Craves fresh air.

* * * * *

Guernsey says: "We think of this remedy on seeing a withered and dried up person, *made so by disease.*" This especially in children. "He looks like a little withered old man." (*Fluoric acid,* young people look old.) *Argentum* like *Gold* profoundly affects the mind. Like *Gold* it is one of the best remedies for hypochondriasis. The symptoms are so many in this trouble that we can only call attention to them as found in *Guiding Symptoms.* I will only mention a few more prominent and peculiar symptoms that have been frequently verified. "The sight of high houses makes him dizzy and causes him to stagger. It seemed as if the houses on both sides of the street would approach and crush him."

"When walking in the street he dreads to pass a street corner, because the corner of the house seems to project and he is afraid he will run against it." "Impulsive, must walk very fast, always hurried." (*Lilium tigrinum.*) "Apprehension when ready to go to church or opera; brings on diarrhœa." (*Gelsemium.*)

The hurried feeling of both *Argentum nitricum* and *Lilium tigrinum* have occurred mostly in uterine troubles; while the diarrhœa on excitement seems to depend upon a general nervous condition. Unless the indications pointed strongly to one in preference to the other remedy it might be well to try the vegetable first. The minerals are generally longer and deeper in their action, and would perhaps be preferable the more chronic the case.

Some of the very curious symptoms found under this and other remedies are not found in everyday practice, but when found are all the more valuable because the cases presenting them are rare and not easily understood or cured by the ordinary remedies. Some of our most brilliant cures have been made in just such cases, and they are very gratifying to both physician and patient.

Argentum nitricum is sometimes the best remedy for hemicrania; this kind of headache is often very distressing and hard to cure. One peculiar symptom belonging to *Argentum nitricum* in headache is a feeling of *expansion,* feels as though head were enormously enlarged, and like *Pulsatilla* and *Apis,* feels better when *tied up tight.* This feeling of expansion is also a general symptom, feels as though the whole body or part of it were expanding, some express it as a feeling of fullness. (*Æsculus hippocastanum.*) It is found under other remedies also, but very prominently under this.

Argentum nitricum has a great deal of *vertigo,* which is often accompanied with buzzing in the ears, general debility and trembling. Cannot walk with the eyes closed; the sight of high houses makes him dizzy. These symptoms call to remembrance *Gelsemium.* Both remedies have much vertigo; great tremulous weakness, accompanied with general debility, actual trembling and tremulous sensation, and both have been found useful in locomotor ataxia. I should, other things being equal, give the preference to *Gelsemium* in recent cases, or in the beginning, and *Argentum nitricum* further along. But there are generally diagnostic indications which enable us to choose between them. In eye affections *Argentum* is one of our most valuable remedies, and like all remedies which are very valuable for anything has been woefully abused by the old school. It is a pity that they do not know enough to get the good and to avoid the bad effects of such valuable agents, for many times the disastrous results of their misuse brings the remedies into such disrepute that others are afraid to use them at all. It was for this reason that the old botanics rejected all mineral remedies. Mercury had so scared them. It falls to the Homœopath to teach how to use all in such a way as to get the good, while avoiding the bad effects. In eye troubles Allen & Norton write as follows: "The greatest service that *Argentum nitricum* performs is in purulent ophthalmia. With large experience, in both hospital and private practice, we have not lost a single eye from this disease, and every one has been treated with *internal remedies,* most of them with *Argentum nitricum* of a high potency, 30th or 200th. We have witnessed the most intense chemosis, with strangulated vessels, most profuse purulent discharge, even the cornea beginning to get hazy and looking as though it would slough, subside rapidly under *Argentum nitricum* internally. The subjective symptoms are almost none. Their very absence, with the *profuse purulent* discharge, and the swollen lids from a collection of pus in the eye, or swelling of the sub-conjunctival tissue of the lids themselves, indicates the drug. *(Apis; Rhus.)*" Later Norton writes: "I do believe that there is no need of cauterization with it except in the *gonorrhœal* form of purulent conjunctivitis." Such testimony from such sources ought to shame the abuse of this agent in the hands of old school physicians, and sometimes bogus Homœopaths. In ophthalmia neonatorum in my own practice as a general practitioner I have had very often better success with *Mercurius solubilis,* especially where there was much purulent matter pouring out on opening the eyes. In blepharitis *Graphites* and *Staphisagria* have served me oftener than *Argentum nitricum,* but this may not be the experience of others, for in eye troubles, as in all others, the indications are to be studied and carefully recognized in their entirety. (*Borax* must not be forgotten in blepharitis.) Specialists are apt to lose sight of this and be led to local treatment when constitutional would be infinitely better. The symptom, "red, painful tip of the tongue, papillæ erect, prominent," has guided to the cure of many different kinds of cases. There are also some valuable symptoms in the digestive organs; for instance, "*Irresistible desire for sugar;* fluids go right through him; most gastric ailments are accompanied by belching; belching after every meal, stomach as if it would burst with wind, belching difficult; finally air rushes out *with great noise and violence.*" All of these are characteristic, and there is no doubt that this remedy is sometimes indicated when *Carbo veg.*, *China* or *Lycopodium* are given because they are generally so much better understood. Dyspepsia, gastralgia and even gastric ulcer have sometimes found a powerful remedy in *Argentum,* and it has also done great good in very obstinate cases of diarrhœa of various kinds.

"Green mucus *like chopped spinach in flakes.*"

"Stool turning green after remaining in diaper."

"Stool expelled with much spluttering."

"Stool shreddy, red, green muco-lymph, epithelial substance." "During stool emission of much noisy flatus." Now there are other remedies which have some of these symptoms in a marked degree, notably: *Calcarea phos.*, which has the spluttering stool with much noisy flatus, and it is also a fact that both remedies are very valuable ones in hydrocephaloid consequent on the long-continued drain from intractable cases of entero-colitis. If the bone development should be slow with open fontanelles and sweaty head of course *Calcarea phos.* would win. Then in *Calcarea phos.* the child wishes smoked meats, bacon, etc., in *Argentum nitricum* sugar or sweets. Yet both have great emaciation, the child looking old and wrinkled, and it will sometimes be close individualizing to choose between them. *Argentum nitricum* has its place in the treatment of throat affections. There is thick, tenacious mucus in the throat obliging him to hawk and causing slight hoarseness. Rawness, soreness, scraping in throat, causing hawking and cough. Sensation as of a splinter lodged in the throat *(Nitric ac., Hepar sulph., Dolichos),* and wartlike excrescences, which feel like pointed bodies when swallowing. This kind of throat may extend downward until it involves the larynx, especially in singers, clergymen, or lawyers who are using their voice very much. Then it is doubly indicated. When we come to the back and extremities we again find our remedy in the field for a share of the honors. "Pain in the back (small of) relieved when standing or walking, but severe when rising from a seat," is a condition often found in practice. I have often relieved it with *Sulphur* or *Causticum,* but remember also *Argentum nitricum.* If in back troubles we find great *lassitude (Kali carbonicum),* with weariness, especially in forearms and lower legs, especially calves, or if in addition to this we find vertigo and trembling of the extremities, we may be sure *Argentum nitricum* will do us good. In paraplegia from debilitating causes or paralysis after diphtheria we may find this remedy indicated. Also in epilepsy or convulsions; in the former (epilepsy) one characteristic symptom is that for hours or days *before the attack* the pupils are dilated; in the latter the convulsions are preceded for a short time by great restlessness.

Cuprum metallicum has great restlessness *between* the attacks. Finally *Natrum muriaticum* is the best antidote for the abuse of *Argentum nit.*, especially upon mucous surfaces.

FERRUM METALLICUM or ACETICUM.

Anæmia with great paleness of all the mucous membranes; with sudden fiery-red flushing of the face.

Profuse hæmorrhages from any organ; hæmorrhagic diathesis; blood light with dark clots; coagulates easily.

Local congestions and inflammations, with hammering, pulsating pains; veins full, flushed face, alternates with paleness.

Canine hunger, alternates with complete loss of appetite.

Regurgitations or eructations, or vomiting of food at night that has stayed in the stomach all day; undigested painless diarrhœa.

Red face during chill.

Modalities: < after eating and drinking; while at rest, especially sitting still; > *walking slowly around.*

* * * * *

This is another one of the abused remedies. It stands with the old school for anæmia, as does *Quinine* for malaria. Each can and does cure its kind of both conditions, but can cure no other; and each, when it is the true curative, is capable of doing its best work in the potentized form. Dr. Hughes writes: "The treatment of anæmia by *Iron* is one of the few satisfactory and certain things in modern medicine. From whatever cause this condition may arise, whether it be the chlorosis of defective menstruation, or the simple poverty of blood induced by hæmorrhages, deficiency of air, light, and suitable food, or by exhausting diseases, *Iron* is the one great remedy." I must say that I think that a man who would write like that of any remedy is not to be blamed for talking of the few satisfactory and certain things in modern medicine. *Iron* is no more of a panacea for anæmia than is *Quinine* for malaria or *Phosphate of Lime* for deficient bone development. My experience has taught me that there are several other equally efficient remedies for these conditions and that when they are not indicated they not only cannot cure but do injure every time they are prescribed, especially in the material doses in which they are generally recommended by such teachers. I must here state my experience founded on abundant practice and observation that such prescribing is not only un-Hahnemannian, but in every sense un-homœopathic, and I warn all beginners not to practice along that line or they too will come to talk of the few satisfactory and certain things in modern medicine. Now we have given this quotation from Dr. Hughes, it is only fair to him to quote him again, inasmuch as he, in this latter quotation, talks more sensibly. Talking about anæmia, he says: "The malady does not ordinarily arise from any failure of the quantity of iron supplied in the food. If the element is deficient in the blood the fault lies in the assimilative processes. But Reveil has ascertained that in anæmia there is no change whatever in the amount of iron present in the blood. However few the corpuscles they contain within them the full proportion of the metal normal to health, and though under the influence of iron itself they increase to double and triple their number they yield no more iron." Then Cowperthwaite adds: "It is also true that when iron is introduced into the system in large quantities with a view to supplying a deficiency of iron in the blood that it is not assimilated, but may be almost entirely obtained from the fæces, having been eliminated by the intestines. It is evident, therefore, that iron does not act as a curative agent by virtue of its absorption as a constituent of the blood, but rather, as we are led to conclude, from its physiological effects upon the organs and tissues of the body, that it owes its therapeutic virtues to the same essential dynamic agency possessed by other drugs, and its application is subject to the same therapeutic law." Sound words, these; then let no man prescribe *Iron* or any other remedy for anæmia, or any other disease, without *indications* according to our therapeutic law of cure. I have seen better cures of bad cases of anæmia by *Natrum muriaticum* in potentized form than I ever did from *Iron* in any form, although *Iron* has its cases, as have also *Pulsatilla, Cyclamen, Calcarea phos., Carbo veg., China* and many other remedies. We will now call attention to the symptoms that indicate *Iron* in anæmia or any other condition where *Iron* is the remedy.

"Ashy, pale or greenish face, with pain or other symptoms the face becomes bright red." (Raue.) *"The least emotion or exertion causes a red, flushed face."* (Guernsey.) *"Rush of blood to head; veins of head swollen; flushes of heat in the face." "Hammering, beating, pul-*

sating pains in the head." (*Bell., China, Natrum mur., Glon.*)

"Great paleness of mucous membranes, especially that of the cavity of the mouth." (Raue.)

"Always better from walking about, notwithstanding weakness obliges patient to lie down." (Guernsey.) *"Menses too soon, too profuse, too long lasting, with fiery red face, ringing in the ears (China), flow pale, watery and debilitating."* Now if in addition to these symptoms you have, notwithstanding the general anæmic condition of the patient, frequent rushes of blood to the head, chest, face, or other local congestions you have a typical *Iron* case and may confidently expect a cure if given in potency and at proper intervals. But if your patient has been already "loaded up" with *Iron* on the theory that the blood must be "fed" with it, the fact is, generally, that she is suffering from the over-dosing more than from the original disease and you will proceed to find the best antidote, guided by the symptoms here as elsewhere, and, in adapting such remedy to the case as it *is,* will often be able to cure both the natural and drug disease together.

It is a blessed thing that this is so, for if the *Quinine, Iron* and other medicinal cachexia stalking about in our midst were not curable, we would be a sorry spectacle as human beings if allopathic dosing were allowed to go on. Now while we are talking about this so-called blood remedy we will speak about its general hæmorrhagic tendencies.

These local congestions so characteristic of *Iron* are attended by hæmorrhages from nose, lungs, womb, kidneys, etc., hence it becomes one of our best remedies for hæmorrhages in anæmia or debilitated subjects with the peculiar symptoms before mentioned. In the form of *Ferrum phos.*, of which we have already written, taking the fact that both remedies entering into the combination have decided hæmorrhagic tendencies, it becomes doubly effective in this sphere.

But *Iron* is not by any means confined in its usefulness to blood troubles, and we will notice briefly some other uses of this valuable curative agent. In disorders of stomach and bowels it becomes sometimes the only remedy, and has some peculiar and characteristic symptoms indicating it here.

"Canine hunger (China), alternating with complete loss of appetite." "Regurgitation of food, or eructations after eating." "Wants bread and butter; meat disagrees (opposite *Natrum mur.). Beer or tea also disagrees. Food lies in the stomach all day and is vomited at night." "Bowels feel sore as if they had been bruised, or as if he had taken cathartics; undigested, painless stools at night, or while eating or drinking." (Croton tig., China.)* These and many other symptoms show its value here, and it is noticeable, the resemblances of this remedy to *China*. There is sometimes difficulty in choosing between them, but there is more *flatulence* with *China*. Both remedies have, markedly, lienteria and painless diarrhœa. These two remedies both antidote and complement each other under certain circumstances. They should be studied in comparison as *debility* remedies.

Next to the easily flushed and red face as a characteristic symptom stands this—*"Walking slowly about relieves."* (One other remedy has this general characteristic almost, if not equally strong, viz., *Pulsatilla.)* This is true of the general restlessness, of the great weakness also; he feels better walking slowly about, even though he is so weak he has to sit down every little while to rest; pain in the hip joint drives out of bed and is only relieved while walking slowly. I once had a rather pale lady come to me for treatment for pains in the forearms; after prescribing for her for a week, she let drop this symptom, that the only way in which she could get relief nights (when the pain was almost unbearable) was by getting right up out of bed and walking slowly about the room. *Ferrum metal.* 1000th cured her promptly and she never had a return. Some people think that metals cannot be potentized, but when I make numerous cures like this with *Iron, Stannum, Zinc* and *Platina* I don't believe it. Palpitation of the heart, hæmoptysis and asthma are also relieved in the same way by walking slowly about. It would seem hardly possible that such complaints could be so relieved, but there are many such curious and unaccountable symptoms in our Materia Medica which have become reliable leaders to the prescription of certain remedies.

Ferrum is one of our best remedies for cough with vomiting of food. It is also one of the very few remedies having a *red face during chill,* and has more than once led to the cure of intermittent fever on that symptom. Again it is one of the remedies found in intermittents that have been abused by *Quinine.* In these cases we often find the splenic region sore on pressure and much swollen.

PLUMBUM METALLICUM or ACETICUM.

Abdomen retracted toward the spine, as if drawn in by a string; both objective and subjective.

Distinct blue line along margin of the gums.

"Wrist-drop" paralysis of the extensor muscles.

* * * * *

Notwithstanding the very extensive provings, this remedy has not been so useful as it would seem it should be. One symptom has proved to be very characteristic and has led to its successful administration in different diseases, viz.: *"Abdomen retracted to the spine as if drawn in by a string."* In this symptom there is both, or either, actual retraction and *sensation* of retraction in the abdomen. Excessive pain in abdomen radiating to all parts of the body *(Dioscorea)*. It is found mostly in colic, but may be found in uterine troubles, such as menorrhagia, etc. Also in constipation. H. N. Guernsey claimed great powers for it in jaundice; whites of eyes, skin, stool and urine all are very yellow, and I have prescribed it with success. Its power to produce paralysis is well known, and it is owing to this power that lead colic is induced, which is one of the most distressing and dangerous of diseases. I cured one case of post diphtheritic paralysis with it. It was a very severe case in a middle-aged man. His lower limbs were entirely paralyzed, and there was at the same time a symptom which I never met before, nor have I since, in such a case, viz., excessive hyperæsthesia of the skin. He could not bear to be touched anywhere, it hurt him so. After much hunting I found this hyperæsthesia perfectly pictured in Allen's Encyclopædia, and that, taken together with the paralysis, seemed to me good reason for prescribing *Plumbum,* which I did in one dose of Fincke's 40m., with the result of bringing about rapid and continuous improvement until a perfect cure was reached. He took only the one dose, for a repetition was not necessary.

The father-in-law of Dr. T. L. Brown, over seventy years of age, was attacked with a severe pain in the abdomen. Finally, a large, hard swelling developed in the ileo-cæcal region very sensitive to contact or to the least motion It began to assume a bluish color, and on account of his age and extreme weakness it was thought that he must die. His daughter, however, studied up the case, and found in Raue's Pathology the indications for *Plumbum* as given in therapeutic hints for typhlitis. It was administered in the 200th potency, which was followed by relief and perfect recovery.

Plumbum has *excessive and rapid emaciation;* general or partial paralysis; "wrist drop." *Distinct blue line along margin of gums.*

CHELIDONIUM MAJUS.

Fixed pain (dull or sharp) under the lower inner angle of the *right shoulder blade.*

Yellow eyes, face, skin, hands, stool clay colored or *yellow as gold;* urine yellow. *Tongue thickly coated yellow,* with red edges.

Right-sided remedy; supra-orbital; hypochondriac; lungs; hip; foot cold as ice, etc.

* * * * *

The center of action of this remarkable remedy is in the liver, and its most characteristic symptom is a *fixed pain* (dull or sharp) *under the lower inner angle of the right shoulder blade.* This very characteristic symptom may be found in connection with general jaundice, cough, diarrhœa, pneumonia, menses, loss of milk, exhaustion, etc., in fact, no matter what the name of the disease this symptom present should always bring to mind *Chelidonium* and close scouting will generally reveal hepatic troubles or complications as would be naturally expected with such a remedy. *Chelidonium* is like *Lycopodium,* by preference, a right-sided remedy, right supra-orbital neuralgia, right hypochondrium and scorbiculum cordis tense and painful to pressure; right-sided pneumonia and shoulder painful; shooting pain in right hip extending into abdomen; drawing pain in hips, thighs, legs, or feet, more right-sided; right foot cold as ice, left natural. Further study will show that *Chelidonium* not only is a right-sided remedy, but in many other points stands close to *Lycopodium,* and in my experience one is often found indicated after the other. Although this characteristic infra-scapular pain is as reliable as any in the Materia Medica, there may be cases in which it does not appear at all, which can only be cured by *Chelidonium,* especially liver and lung trouble. If we should find pressive pain in the region of the liver, whether it be enlarged and sensitive to pressure or not, bitter taste in the mouth, tongue *coated thickly yellow, with red margins showing imprint of the teeth,* yellowness of whites of eyes, face, hands and skin; stools gray, clay colored, or *yellow as gold,* urine also yellow as gold, lemon colored or dark brown, leaving a yellow color on vessel when emptied out, loss of appetite, disgust and nausea, or vomiting of bilious matter, and especially if patient could retain nothing but hot drinks on the stomach, we would have a clear case for *Chelidonium* even though the infra-scapular pain were absent. All these symptoms might be found in either a chronic or acute case. If in a chronic case, some anti-psoric like *Lycopodium* might have to be called in, according to indications, of course, to help complete a cure, but *Chelidonium* would be the chief reliance.

These liver troubles range from simple congestion and inflammation of the organ, to the more severe and deep-seated affections like fatty liver, gall stones, etc. *Chelidonium* is one of the leading remedies in pneumonia, which is complicated with liver symptoms. Sometimes in coughs which are persistent with much pain through right side of chest and into shoulder, *Chelidonium* helps us out and saves the patient from what might easily terminate in consumption.

AURUM MURIATICUM NATRONATUM.

When writing of *Aurum metallicum* we might have said something of this combination as a remedy for jaundice or liver troubles. Several years ago I was troubled with frequent attacks of derangement of the liver characterized by, first, a white fæcal stool for several days in succession, with dullness of the head, bad tasting mouth, coated tongue, fullness and pain in right side and shoulder, and jaundiced skin. This would either culminate in an attack of bilious vomiting and diarrhœa, or in fæcal stools as black as tar, for several days in succession, with gradual relief of the general bilious symptoms. I tried various remedies, as well as I was able to choose them, among which were *Mercurius*, *Leptandra*,

Podophyllum, Lycopodium and others, with nothing more than temporary relief, and sometimes not even that. While on a visit to New York City, I called upon Dr. M. Baruch, partly to see the man who had been reported to me as both very skillful as a prescriber and eccentric as a man. During my call I stated to him my case. He prescribed for me a dose of *Aurum muriaticum natronatum* 1000th, followed by a powder each of *Veronica officinalis* 500th, 200th and 30th, and directed me to take them in the order named once in sixty hours and said: "In three months you will be well." I took the powders as directed and have never been troubled in that way since. Since then I have prescribed the *Aurum muriaticum natronatum* for some obstinate cases of jaundice, with the alternating white and black stools, and have been successful in relieving them.

LEPTANDRA VIRGINICA.

While writing on *Aurum muriaticum natronatum* I mentioned *Veronica* with which Dr. Baruch followed that remedy in the cure of my own case. After returning home I tried to find the two remedies. Found *Aurum muriaticum natronatum* in Hering's Guiding Symptoms, and, although meager, had something to go by in treating other cases, with the result there mentioned. But I could find no *Veronica* proven unless it was the *Leptandra,* which is one of the *Veronica* tribe. So the next time I saw Dr. Baruch I asked him if it was the *Leptandra* that he gave me, and he said, "No, it was the *Veronica officinalis*" (common Speedwell). It is not found in our Materia Medica as yet. There is no doubt the *Veronicas* and especially the *Leptandra* are good liver remedies, but aside from the alternate ashy and black stools we have nothing very definite to guide us to their selection. The only two provings made were with the alkaloid, and that in too low preparations to be of much value. I once succeeded with *Leptandra* in curing, or at least she improved until she was well, a lady very sick with what was called by her former physician typhoid fever. The following indications which I found in Jahr's Clinical Guide (by Lilienthal, first edition) led to its prescription. Symptoms:—"Great prostration, stupor, heat and dryness of skin, calor mordax or coldness of the extremities, *dark, fœtid, tarry,* or watery stools mixed with bloody mucus, and a jaundiced skin." Otherwise I have never seen any marked benefit from this remedy in any case. Still I believe it to be capable, with scientific proving, in potency, of developing great curative powers. If I might, in this short notice, inspire some young physicians to thoroughly prove it I should not have written in vain.

BERBERIS VULGARIS.

Bruised pain, with numbness, stiffness and lameness in region of kidneys < in bed in the morning.

Soreness in the region of the kidneys; *bubbling* sensation, < stepping or jarring motion.

Rheumatism or pains, like gouty pains in the joints; the pains radiate from a center.

* * * * *

"Bruised pain, with stiffness and lameness in the small of the back." "Rise from a seat with difficulty." "Backache worse when sitting or lying, especially when lying in bed in the morning." "Sensation of *numbness, stiff-*

ness and *lameness,* with painful pressure in lumbar and renal regions." These pains sometimes extend all through the hips. Guernsey says: "A great many old troubles in the back. *Sufferings in the back aggravated by fatigue."* One might say all these symptoms are found under *Rhus tox.* True, but in the *Berberis* cases they all come from or are in connection with kidney or urinary troubles, *Rhus tox.* seldom so. The pains extend often into the bladder and urethra, and the urine itself is changed. It may have a turbid, flocculent, clay-like, copious, mucous sediment, or a reddish, mealy sediment, or be blood-red, but the persistent pains in the back are the leading indications. It is especially to be thought of in arthritic and rheumatic affections, when these back symptoms connected with urinary alterations are present. One very characteristic symptom is a *bubbling sensation* in the region of the kidneys. Another is *soreness* in region of kidneys when jumping out of a wagon or stepping hard downstairs or from any jarring movement. There is almost always, in the back troubles of *Berberis,* a great deal of prostration or a sense of weakness across the back, and the face looks pale, earthy complexion, with sunken cheeks and hollow eyes, with blue circles under them. No matter what ails the patient, if he has persistent pain as above described in the region of the kidneys do not forget *Berberis.*

TEREBINTHINA.

Burning and smarting on passing urine; urine red, brown, black or *smoky* in appearance.

Tongue smooth, glossy, red, with excessive tympanites (typhoid).

Hæmorrhages from all outlets, especially in connection with urinary or kidney troubles.

* * * * *

Terebinthina ought to come in here, because it, like *Berberis,* has much pain in the back with kidney and bladder troubles. Painters working under the smell of *Turpentine* are often seriously affected by it. Some are unable to work in it. In the *Turpentine* kidney troubles there is apt to be more strangury than with *Berberis* and more blood in the urine. The urine becomes brown, black, or *smoky* in appearance from more or less admixture of blood. For burning and smarting on passing urine, *Turpentine* stands nearer to *Cantharis* or *Cannabis sativa* than it does to *Berberis.* All four may be found useful in the first stage of albuminuria, *Turpentine* taking the lead, and it may sometimes require considerable study to choose between them. *Mercurius corrosivus* generally comes in a little later. *Terebinth.* is one of our best anti-hæmorrhagic remedies. Hæmaturia, hæmoptysis, and hæmorrhage from the bowels, especially in typhoid, and even in purpura hæmorrhagica it may do splendid work. One of the chief characteristics for its use is the *smooth, glossy, red tongue (Crotalus, Pyrogen);* another is *excessive tympanites.* These two symptoms are often found in typhoids, and then *Terebinth.* is the remedy. Dropsy after scarlatina, with smoky urine, may find its remedy here, but *Lachesis, Apis, Helleborus niger,* or *Colchicum* will often dispute claims with it. The old school make great use of it in many other affections as a local application. I have seen some bad effects from its use in that way for the chest in pneumonia in their hands. I would not recommend it.

CANNABIS SATIVA

Is another remedy having a strong action on the urinary organs, particularly upon the urinary tract or urethra. It is the remedy par excellence with which to begin the treatment of gonorrhœa, unless some other remedy is particularly indicated, and such cases are very few. The most characteristic symptom is *that the urethra is very sensitive to touch or external pressure.* The patient cannot walk with his legs close together because any pressure along the tract hurts him so. If the disease has extended up the urethra, or into the bladder, tnere will often be severe pains in the back every few minutes and the urine may be bloody. I used in my early practice to put five drops mother tincture into four ounces of water (in a four-ounce vial) and let the patient take a teaspoonful three times a day. After about four days the inflammatory symptoms would have subsided, and the thin discharge have thickened and become greenish in appearance. Then *Mercurius solubilis* 3d trituration, a powder three times a day, would often finish the case. Or if a little, thin, gleety discharge remained, I cured that with *Sulphur, Capsicum* or *Kali iodide.* I have cured many cases in from one to two weeks this way. Later I have used the c. m. potency in the first stage, and sometimes never have to use the second remedy. If I do, *Mercurius corrosivus* c. m. is generally the remedy. Sometimes *Pulsatilla, Sulphur* or *Sepia* to finish up the case. There are exceptions, but the rule is that cases get well promptly under this treatment. After *Cannabis sativa, Mercurius corrosivus,* if the discharge is thick and green, if the burning continues. *Pulsatilla* or *Sepia* if the discharge is thick and bland. *Sulphur* for gleet. Of course I have not mentioned all of the remedies that are necessary in this disease. I used them all in the c. m., and I know, having tried both, that they cure better than the low potencies. There is one curious symptom I have several times removed by this remedy, namely, a sense of dropping, around, or in the region of the heart. I do not know its pathological signification, but it is very annoying and the patient is very grateful to be rid of it.

BENZOIC ACID.

The grand central characteristic of this remedy is found in the urine, which is scanty, of a *dark brown color* (like French brandy), *the urinous odor being highly intensified.* This odor comes at the *time of passing* and remains afterward. One need not wait on a long-standing specimen to find it. It is found in connection with rheumatism, quinsy, dropsy, diarrhœa, headache and other diseases. Of course many other remedies have offensive urine, like *Nitric acid* urine offensive like *horse* urine, *Berberis,* but the deposit is tűrbid, *Calcarea ostrearum,* but the deposit is white. *Benzoic acid* often smells horribly, with no deposit at all. Both *Benzoic acid* and *Berberis* are great remedies for arthritic troubles with the urinary symptoms. *Lycopodium* and *Lithium carb.* also claim attention in this affection, the concomitants deciding the choice. I have seen wonderful relief from *Benzoic acid* in nephritic colic with the characteristic offensive urine. In dribbling of urine of old men with enlarged prostate it has also done good service. The urine in the clothing scents the whole room. Menstrual difficulties and prolapsus uteri with the characteristic urinary symptoms are also relieved by it. Heart troubles of rheumatic origin also. So we have a widely diversified list of diseases in which this remedy is *the one*, and all seem to be connected with this one strong characteristic symptom.

SARSAPARILLA.

White sand in urine; also slimy or flaky urine.

Much pain at the conclusion of passing urine; almost unbearable.

Marasmus; neck emaciates and skin lies in folds.

* * * * *

Sarsaparilla is another remedy which has excruciating neuralgia of the kidneys. Renal colic and passage of gravel and formation of vesicle calculi. Dr. Hering gives many testimonials to the efficacy of this remedy to relieve the sufferings attendant on gravel, especially with rheumatic symptoms. *Lycopodium* has *red sand with clear urine; Sarsaparilla* white sand with scanty, slimy or flaky urine. They may both be very useful in chronic rheumatic troubles, with these urinary complications. The most characteristic symptom of *Sarsaparilla* is "*much pain at the conclusion of passing* urine; almost unbearable." *(Berberis, Equisetum, Medorrhinum, Thuja.)* There is often in this case great tenesmus of the bladder at the same time. No remedy has this symptom so strongly as *Sarsaparilla. Pulsatilla* has something similar, so far as tenesmus is concerned, in connection with *enlarged prostate. Natrum muriaticum* has also,—"After urination burning and cutting in the urethra; spasmodic contraction in abdomen, etc." So we must be careful about prescribing on one symptom alone, be it ever so prominent. In marasmus *Sarsaparilla* stands alongside of *Iodine, Natrum mur.,* and *Abrotanum.* In *Sarsaparilla* the neck emaciates and skin (in general) lies in folds. *(Sanicula, Natrum mur.* and *Lycopodium* emaciate from above downward. *Abrotanum* from below upward.) *Iodine,* general emaciation, wishes to eat all the time. *Natrum mur.* eats and emaciates all of the time, *neck particularly. Abrotanum,* general marasmus, *legs* most. *Argentum nitricum,* child looks old, dried up, like a mummy. *Sarsaparilla* is one of the best remedies for headache or periosteal pains generally, from suppressed gonorrhœa. I have seen great results from the 200th. It is also a good remedy for syphilitic eruptions, with great emaciation; cracks on hands and feet, especially on sides of fingers and toes.

Retractions of nipple *(Silicea).*

PODOPHYLLUM PELTATUM.

Diarrhœa; stools profuse (drain the patient dry), offensive, < morning and during dentition.

Persistent *gagging,* without vomiting; rolling the head and moaning with half-closed eyes.

Great *loquacity* during the fever stage, especially with jaundiced skin.

Prolapsus of uteri; prolapse of rectum.

* * * * *

There are many remedies that are powerful cathartics, and this is one of them. A superficial understanding of our law of cure would lead a novice to conclude that all one would have to do for a case of diarrhœa would be to prescribe *Podophyllum*. Of course failure would often be the result. The simple fact of diarrhœa is only a factor in the case, where the selection of a remedy for its cure is concerned; for each cathartic has not only a diarrhœa, but a peculiar kind of diarrhœa which no other remedy has. The diarrhœa of *Podophyllum* is characterized by:

1st. The *profuseness* of the stool. 2d. The *offensiveness* of the stool. 3d. The aggravations *in the morning, hot weather,* and *during dentition.* Then again the concomitants are very peculiar. There is often present prolapsus ani, sleep with eyes half closed and rolling the head from side to side and moaning; frequent gagging or empty retching. These symptoms present have often led to the administration of this great remedy with very gratifying results. In regard to the profuse stools, they are so much so that they seem to drain the patient dry at every one. They may be yellow or greenish watery, and when watery, always profuse. Then again they may be pappy and profuse (*Gambogia*), or mucous and scanty, but always with *Podophyllum* very offensive. I have cured these cases in all stages. In the first onset of the disease, as well as in the very far advanced and apparently hopeless cases of cholera infantum, the 1000th potency (B. & T.) has done the best for me. Notwithstanding the fact that this remedy is one of quite a list set down for liver troubles, both with looseness of the bowels and constipation, I have not found it very efficacious in the latter. I can readily see how it might be, however, in liver troubles with constipation which had followed a preceding diarrhœa, just as *Opium* might cure the sleeplessness that followed preceding stupor, and *Coffea* sleepiness which followed preceding excitement. All drugs have their double action, or what is *called* primary and secondary action. But the surest and most lasting curative action of any drug is that in which the condition to be cured simulates the primary action of the drug. For, as I have held elsewhere, I think that what is called secondary action is really not the legitimate action of the *drug,* but the aroused powers of the organism *against* the drug. So the alternate diarrhœa and constipation in disease is a fight, for instance, between the disease (diarrhœa) and the natural powers resisting it. It is of considerable importance then to be able to recognize in such a case whether it is the diarrhœa or constipation that is the disease, against which the alternate condition is the effort of the vital force to establish health. Yet such an understanding is not always absolutely imperative, for in either case there are generally enough concomitant symptoms to decide the choice of the remedy. Indeed, the choice must always rest upon either the peculiar and characteristic symptoms appearing in the case or the *totality* of them. None but the true homœopathist learns to appreciate this. Here is where what is called pathological prescribing often fails, for the *choice of the remedy may depend upon symptoms entirely outside of the symptoms which go to make up the pathology* of the case, at least so far as we as yet understand pathology.

Podophyllum has a great desire to press the gums together during dentition. When this symptom is prominent, the choice will have to be made between this remedy and *Phytolacca,* both being great remedies for cholera infantum. In the nausea of *Podophyllum* vomiting is not so prominent as with *Ipecac,* but the *gagging* without vomiting is very marked, as it is also under *Secale cornutum.* Rumbling in the abdomen, especially in the ascending colon, is strong indication for this remedy even in chronic bowel troubles. Prolapsus ani is also a prominent symptom of this remedy, so also is prolapsus of the uterus, especially after straining, over-lifting or parturition. Here the choice will often be between *Podophyllum, Rhus tox.* and *Nux vomica.*

Podophyllum seems also to have a strong affinity for the ovaries, and some remarkable cures have been made on the symptom,—"Pain in right ovary, running down thigh of that side." *(Lilium tig.)* Sometimes there is also numbness attending. Ovarian tumors have disappeared under the action of this remedy, when this symptom was present. I once made a brilliant cure of an obstinate case of intermittent fever with this remedy. The chills were very violent and were followed by intense fever with *great loquacity.* There was also great jaundice present. When the fever was past the patient fell asleep, and on awakening did not remember what he had said in his loquacious delirium. The range of this remedy does not seem very wide, but within its range its action is surprisingly prompt and radical.

ALOE SOCOTRINA.

Insecurity of rectum; rectum feels full of heavy fluid, which will fall out, and does, if he does not go to stool immediately. Diarrhœa.

Solid stool, passing (in large balls) away involuntarily and unnoticed.

Great fullness and weight in whole abdomen, with feeling of weight in rectum and hæmorrhoids protruding like a bunch of grapes; > by cold water applied.

* * * * *

This remedy should be considered alongside of *Podophyllum,* because it is one of the so-called cathartics. Although one is as decided a cathartic as the other the characteristics which guide to their choice are very different.

Both are apt to be worse during hot weather.

Both are apt to be worse in the morning.

Both are often well supplemented with *Sulphur.*

But now let us look at some of the more marked and peculiar symptoms of *Aloe.* Stools yellow, fæcal, bloody or transparent jelly-like mucus. Sometimes this jelly-like mucus *(Kali bich.)* comes in great masses, or "gobs," and drops out of the rectum almost unnoticed. Again the stools are often passed involuntarily when expelling flatus or passing urine. There seems to be not only an actual weakness in the sphincter ani, but a distressing *sense* of weakness. The rectum feels as if full of heavy fluid which will fall out or escape from the patient, and in fact does so if he doesn't "git there, Eli." This escape of stool with flatus in *Aloe* finds its counterpart in *Oleander.* No two remedies are more alike in this respect, though *Muriatic acid* is also similar. Again a very characteristic symptom in the *Aloe* diarrhœa is "Great rumbling in the abdomen just before stool," and the feeling of weight in the rectum already mentioned is not always confined to the rectum, but is also felt through the whole pelvis and abdomen. Again, the rectum protrudes in *Aloe* like a bunch of grapes, and is relieved by the application of *cold water*. *Muriatic acid* is relieved by hot applications. Both of these remedies have blue hæmorrhoids; the *Aloe* itching intensely, while those of *Muriatic acid* are very sore and sensitive to touch, even of the bed clothes. In addition to the aggravations already mentioned, the diarrhœa of *Aloe* is aggravated by walking or standing, after eating or drinking. In dysentery there is violent tenesmus, heat in the rectum, prostration even to fainting and profuse clammy sweats. The weakness of the sphincter ani is also found in constipation. It is a curious symptom, and I would not believe it until I had seen it with my own eyes. "Solid stool passing involuntarily, passing away unnoticed." I was called to treat a child five years of age suffering from birth with a most obstinate form of constipation. He had to be forced and held to the stool crying and screaming all the while being totally unable to pass any fæces even after an enema. After trying several remedies in vain, I asked the mother to turn the child over (he was in bed) to let me examine the anus and rectum. As she turned down the bed clothes to do so, a large chunk of solid fæces appeared in the bed. "There," she said, "that is the way it is. Notwithstanding his inability to pass stool when he tries, we often find these things in the bed, and he does not know when they pass, nor do we." I then gave a few doses of *Aloe* 200th and cured the whole trouble quickly and permanently. *Aloe* like *Podophyllum* has also prolapsus uteri, and the feeling of heat, heaviness and fullness in the abdomen, pelvis and rectum guides to its selection. Like *Podophyllum,* also, its range of action is not wide, but positive, reliable and satisfactory.

CROTON TIGLIUM.

Stool yellow, watery, coming out like a shot, **all at once**; < after least food or drink.

Excruciating pain, running from nipple to scapula; of same side when child nurses.

Eczema, especially of the scrotum; itches intensely, **but is so sensitive to touch and sore that he cannot scratch.**

* * * * *

When the Allopaths, in any case where they considered *an operation of the bowels* imperative, had exhausted all other resources, *Croton tiglium* was their "biggest gun for the last broadside." In other words, this is a most violent cathartic. Now if Similia, etc., is not true, *Croton tig.* ought utterly to fail to cure diarrhœa; but it is true, and notwithstanding this remedy has proven its truth over and over again the Allopaths deny and reject Homœopathy. As in *Podophyllum* and *Aloe, Croton tig.* cures its kind and no other. Its guiding symptoms are:

First: "Yellow watery stool."

Second: "Sudden expulsion, coming out like a shot, all at once."

Third: "Aggravation from the least food or drink."

In this combination *Croton tig.* leads all of the remedies. The first symptom is found notably under *Apis mel., Calcarea ost., China, Gratiola, Hyoscyamus, Natrum sulph.*, and *Thuja.* The second under *Jatropha, Gratiola, Podophyllum* and *Thuja.* The third under *Argentum nit.* and *Arsenicum alb.* The *Calcarea ost.* is found in the *Calcarea* temperament and *China* in cases weakened by loss of fluids, and all the others have strongly marked symptoms which distinguish them from *Croton tiglium.* For want of space we cannot give them here. *Aloe* has rumbling before the stool, while *Croton tig.* has swashing in the intestines as from water. Both of these remedies having aggravation after eating or drinking, we would have to look further for the symptoms deciding between them. Another symptom that has frequently been verified in this remedy is—"Excruciating pain running from nipple to back (scapula) of the same side when the child nurses." I have cured bad cases of mastitis guided by this one symptom. *Croton tig.* cures eczema especially of the scrotum, where the eruption itches intensely, but is so sensitive and sore to touch that he cannot scratch. This comprehends the main uses of this valuable remedy.

NATRUM SULPHURICUM.

Diarrhœa, acute or chronic < in the morning on beginning to move *(Bry.)*, with much flatulence *(Aloe* and *Calc. phos.)*, and rumbling in abdomen, especially right ileo-cæcal region.

Loose cough, with great *pain* in the chest; < in *lower left* chest (right, *Chel.)*.

Modalities: < in cold, wet weather; damp cellars; hydrogenoid (diarrhœa, rheumatism, asthma).

Mental effects from injuries to head.

Chronic effects of blows, falls.

Toothache > by cold water, cool air *(Coff., Puls.)*.

Gonorrhœa; greenish-yellow, painless, thick discharge (*Puls.*).

* * * * *

Natrum sulphuricum is also one of our armamentarium

for diarrhœa, both acute and chronic. Like *Podophyllum, Sulphur, Nuphar* and *Rumex,* the diarrhœa is aggravated in the morning. *Sulphur* drives the patient out of bed, but *Natrum sulph.,* like *Bryonia,* is worse only after beginning to move. Then again *Natrum sulph.* has, like *Aloe,* much rumbling in the bowels as of flatulence. This rumbling of flatus is often with *Natrum sulph.* located in the right side of the abdomen in the ileo-cæcal region.

Again the *Natrum sulphuricum* stool is, like *China, Argentum nit., Calcarea phos., Agaricus* and *Aloe,* accompanied by a profuse emission of flatus. This flatulence is not always present, but is often so. In chronic diarrhœa there is almost always some trouble with the liver, evidenced by soreness in right hypochondrium, which is sensitive to touch, and hurts on walking or any jar. One very strong characteristic for this remedy in this trouble is aggravation of the diarrhœa, pain, etc., in damp weather. In this it resembles *Dulcamara* and *Rhododendron.* The *Dulcamara* has the aggravation in change from warm to cold weather, whether damp or dry. This aggravation in damp weather is not confined to diarrhœa in *Natrum sulph.,* but is especially present in cases of chronic asthma. I have seen very great benefit in such cases of this very troublesome and obstinate disease, and as aggravation in damp weather very commonly occurs in cases of old asthma this remedy is often indicated. I have not observed much benefit from this remedy in runarounds, for which it is highly recommended; but have seen nice results from it in very obstinate cases of gonorrhœa, when the discharge was thick and greenish and little pain. *Loose cough, with soreness and pain through the left chest, is very characteristic.* This is one of the chief diagnostic points of difference between *Bryonia* and *Natrum sulphuricum,* that while with both there is great soreness of the chest with the cough, with *Bryonia* the cough is dry, while with *Natrum sulph.* it is loose. The patient springs right up in bed, the cough hurts him so.

There is as much soreness as there is with *Bryonia,* and when the patient coughs he springs up in bed and holds the painful side in his hand to ease the hurt. This symptom may be found in chronic affections of the respiratory organs, such as asthma, phthisis, etc., and I have several times seen remarkably prompt relief and cure follow its administration in pneumonia when this symptom was present. This pain through the lower left chest is as characteristic for *Natrum sulph.* as is that of pain running through right lower chest for *Kali carbonicum.*

NATRUM MURIATICUM.

Melancholy, depressed, sad and weeping; consolation aggravates.

Great emaciation, even while living well; shows most in the neck.

Anæmia with bursting headaches, especially at the menses; also school girls' headache.

Great dryness of mucous membranes from lips to anus; lips dry and *cracked,* especially in the middle; anus dry, cracked, fissured; constipation.

Heart palpitates, flutters, intermits, pulsates violently, shaking the whole body; < lying on left side.

Itching eruptions, dry or moist; < at the margins of the hair.

Modalities: < 10 to 11 A. M. (many complaints), especially malarial affections; lying down, especially on left side; heat of sun or heat in general; abuse of Quinine, relieved by sweat.

Tongue; mapped with red insular patches.

For bad effects; of anger, nitrate of silver; too much salt; craves salt and salty things.

Hang nails; skin around the nails dry and cracked; herpes about the anus, in border of hair.

Warts on palms of hands (sore to touch, *Nat.)*

* * * * *

Now that we have introduced the *Natrums,* we will continue them. Common salt. A gentleman once said to me when I prescribed a dose of *Sulphur* 30th, "Pshaw, I get more sulphur than that in every egg I eat. How can that do me any good?" My answer was, wait and see. And he was cured of both doubts and disease. There is no remedy in the Materia Medica, I think, that so disgusts the advocates of the low potency, and low only, as this one. The unquestionable cure of the most obstinate cases of intermittent fever with the 200th and higher potencies demoralizes them. That people eating salt in appreciable quantities right along and can't live without it, don't get well on it, and *do* get well on the same thing potentized, does not hold to reason, the microscope, molecular theory, spectrum analysis, or anything else scientific (so called) not being able to discover any material in the dose. But there stand the cures, like the blind man whom Jesus healed. It is a hard thing to be confronted by such facts against our prejudices. "Oh, well," said one of these doubters, "people sometimes get well without medicine." So they do with, I replied.

Isn't it curious how some physicians will hoot at a potency and fly like a frightened crow from a bacillus varying in size from 0.004 millimeters to 0.006 m.m. They can hardly eat, drink or sleep for fear a little microbe of the fifteenth culture will light on them somewhere, but there is nothing in a potency above the 12th. Oh, consistency! When prejudice gives way to honest, earnest investigation for truth, the world may be better for it. *Natrum mur.* is one of our best remedies for anæmia. It does not seem to make much difference whether the anæmia is caused by loss of fluids *(China, Kali carb.)*, menstrual irregularities *(Puls)*, loss of semen *(Phos. acid, China)*, grief or other mental diseases. In these cases of anæmia, to which *Natrum* is adapted, we may, in addition to the general paleness, have emaciation, notwithstanding the patient eats well. Severe attacks of throbbing headache; shortness of breath, especially on going upstairs, or other physical exertion; scanty menstruation; more or less constipation and generally great depression of spirits. In fact, depression of spirits is characteristic of this drug; the patient weeps much, like *Pulsatilla,* the difference being that the *Pulsatilla* patient is soothed and comforted by consolation, while the *Natrum mur.* patient is aggravated.

There is almost always in these anæmic cases a great deal of fluttering, palpitation, and even intermittent action of the heart. I have helped many such cases with this remedy high, in single doses, only repeating when improvement lagged. I have seen a patient who had lost 40 pounds of flesh (weight, 160 lbs.), though eating well all of the time, under one dose of *Natrum mur.*, tip the scales at 200 lbs. within three months from the time of taking. He was very hypochondriac at the time of the beginning of treatment. I cannot speak too highly of *Natrum mur.* in these affections. *Natrum mur.* is one of our best remedies for chronic headaches. They come in paroxysms and would, by their intense throbbing nature, cause one to think of *Belladonna,* only that they occur mostly in the anæmic, and the face is pale, or at least slightly flushed. If the face is red and burning, eyes injected, and pain of beating or throbbing nature, we would immediately think of such remedies as *Melilotus, Belladonna,* or *Nux vom.,* and then look for concomitant symptoms to decide between them The headaches of *Natrum mur.* are very apt to occur after the menstrual period, as if caused by loss of blood, and you know that *China* also has throbbing headache in such cases. With *Natrum* the throbbing headache occurs whether the menses be scanty or profuse. *Natrum mur.* also cures the headaches of school girls, and here it may be difficult to choose between it and *Calcarea phos.,* both remedies also being particularly adapted to anæmic states. Indeed, I have sometimes missed and had to give *Calcarea phos.* when *Natrum* failed and vice versa, because I could not make the choice. These headaches are often brought on by eye-strain, as in long-continued study, close sewing, etc. Then we have asthenopia with the headache, and must study also *Argentum nit.* and *Ruta graveolens.* In actual practice such cases do sometimes occur, where the case in hand is not far enough developed in symptomatic indications to enable one to choose between two about equally indicated remedies. If a man hits it well without ever having to try but twice I can forgive him for failing the first time, and am willing to be forgiven myself. In these cases, however, let the physician be blamed, and not Homœopathy, for that never fails. So-called sick headaches often find their simillimum in *Natrum mur.* For want of space we cannot give all of the symptoms which might indicate it. *Natrum mur.* acts upon the whole alimentary tract, from mouth to anus, and has very characteristic symptoms guiding to its administration. The lips and corners of the mouth are dry, ulcerated, or cracked *(Condurango).* In this it resembles *Nitric acid,* as it also does at the other end of the alimentary canal; for with both remedies the anus is fissured, sore, painful and sometimes bleeding. *Antimonium crudum* and *Graphites* are also to be remembered in this connection; but while *Graphites* has the affection of both mouth and anus, it is more of an eczematous or eruptive character than either of the other remedies. *Natrum* has great *sense* of dryness in the mouth without actual dryness. Now *Mercury* has thirst with moist mouth, but there is with this remedy swollen tongue, or flabby tongue, with indentations or prints of the teeth upon it, and very offensive breath, all of which is not markedly so of *Natrum mur.,* so there is no danger of confounding the two. You will remember that although alike or similar in their mind symptoms *Pulsatilla* has the exact opposite as regards this symptom, viz., *dry mouth with no thirst,* furnishing a very marked contrast where a choice is necessary. *Natrum* has another similarity to *Pulsatilla,* in that it has bitter taste, and loss of taste. Again *Natrum* has a sensation upon the tongue similar to *Silicea,* viz., sensation of a hair upon the tongue (also *Kali bich.).* Deep painful fissure in middle upper lip is given in Guiding Symptoms, but I have found it in the lower lip and believe it to be just as characteristic. I made a splendid cure, being led to examination of the remedy by this symptom.

Blisters like pearls around the mouth are found in *Natrum mur.*, especially in intermittents. If the upper lip is much thickened or swollen, not of an erysipelatous character, we would think of three remedies, all of which have it, *Belladonna, Calcarea ost., Natrum mur.* Alone, of course, this symptom would not amount to much but is strongly corroborative if found in connection with other symptoms of any of these remedies. The symptoms of the gums may be summed up in one word, scorbutic. Now study also *Mercurius, Carbo veg., Muriatic acid,* etc.

There is another curious symptom in which I was helped by the elder Lippe to prescribe *Natrum mur.* with success in a case that had baffled me for a long time, viz., numbness and tingling of tongue, lips and nose. This came in connection with a chronic soreness of the liver, derangement of digestion, such as is often found in a condition which is popularly termed biliousness. This condition *Natrum mur.*, given very high (said Lippe) c. m., clears up the case in a very short time. *Map tongue* is found under *Natrum mur., Arsenicum alb., Lachesis, Nitric acid,* and *Taraxacum.* I have used *Natrum* with success oftener than the others. I have not found *Natrum mur.* a great throat remedy, except in follicular pharyngitis, which had been abused with local applications of Nitrate of Silver. In post-diphtheritic paralysis of the muscles of deglutition *Lachesis* or *Causticum* have served me much better. Salivation profuse, watery and salty, is the reactionary or secondary action of *Natrum* and may find its remedy here. But this is not so often found as the other condition of dryness. *Natrum mur.* has some strong characteristics under the head of appetite, thirst, desires and aversions. No remedy is more hungry, yet he loses flesh while eating well. *(Acetic acid, Abrotanum, Iodine, Sanicula* and *Tuberculinum.) Iodine* has this canine hunger with emaciation; but after eating the *Natrum* patient feels weary and sleepy, while the *Iodine* one feels better. The *Natrum* patient after eating feels dull, with heavy aching and sense of fullness and discomfort in the region of the stomach and liver, which is relieved as digestion advances (see *China*); but the *Iodine* patient wishes to eat all of the time and feels comfortable only when the stomach is full or being filled. There are several remedies which are either hungry or relieved by eating, notably *Anacardium, Chelidonium* and *Petroleum,* as well as *Natrum mur.* and *Iodine.* One might add also as hungry remedies *China* and *Lycopodium.* The *Anacardium* has pain in the stomach which extends to the spine, and an *all gone* sensation which must be relieved by eating, and after two hours returns and he must eat again. *Chelidonium* hunger is accompanied with the characteristic liver symptoms. (See *Chelidonium.)* In *China, Natrum mur.* and *Lycopodium* hunger, patient *fills up quickly* and fullness, flatulence and distress follow until the process of digestion is well advanced, when they are relieved. Again, *Natrum mur.* is a very useful remedy for an abnormal craving for salt. Patient salts everything he eats. A dose of the c. m. corrects this craving and often cures other symptoms accompanying. *Causticum* also has this symptom, and if the other symptoms indicate must take the preference.

Of course the intense thirst of salt is well known, and keeps pace with the hunger. Now this is the case with diabetes, for which *Natrum* is a curative if otherwise indicated. In all of these cases, of course, it must be used high, for we get the low in our food.

Under the head of stool and rectum few remedies have stronger symptoms. I quote verbatim from "Guiding Symptoms:"—"*Constipation; obstinate retention of stool; stools irregular, hard, unsatisfactory; during menses; stools in large masses; stools like sheep dung; from inactivity of rectum; anus contracted, or torn, bleeding, smarting, or burning afterwards; stitches in the rectum causing hypochondriasis or ill humor; great torpor without pain; from want of moisture, dryness of mucous linings, with watery secretions in other parts; difficult expulsion, fissuring anus with flow of blood, leaving sensation of much soreness; with uterine displacements; hæmorrhoidal; in Addison's Disease.*" Now to read this rightly we must entirely separate these symptoms, here separated by the semi-colon, and put the word constipation before each one. That saves the error of supposing that all the symptoms here quoted must be present in a single case of constipation to make *Natrum muriaticum* the proper remedy.

One of the best possible exercises for a student of Materia Medica is to compare these different symptoms, as follows: Stools dry, crumbling, is also found under *Ammonium muriaticum* and *Magnesia muriatica.* Constipation from inactivity of the rectum, *Alumina, Veratrum album, Silicea,* etc. Anus contracted, torn, bleeding, smarting and pain after stool, *Nitric acid.* From want of moisture, dryness of mucous linings,

Bryonia and *Opium.* Leaving sensation of much soreness, *Ignatia, Nitric acid, Alumen.* Then again *Natrum mur.* may become the only curative for cholera infantum, chronic diarrhœa, and other conditions where *loose stools* predominate. I will not wait to specify all the symptoms. Emaciation, hunger and thirst are present, especially in cholera infantum, emaciation being most noticeable in the neck. *(Abrotanum* in the legs, also *Ammon. mur.* and *Argent. nit.)* Emaciation, *Natrum, Sarsaparilla* and *Iodine.* On the urinary organs I will only call attention to the increased secretion already spoken of, and the involuntary escape of urine, which is also found under *Causticum, Pulsatilla, Zincum* and others, and a burning and cutting in the urethra *after* urination. *Sarsaparilla* has the nearest to this last symptom, and we remember here the resemblance of these two remedies as to emaciation in cholera infantum. This cutting in the urethra may be found in chronic cases of gleet, and in these cases the discharge is almost always, as it is under *Natrum mur.* in all mucous membranes, clear and watery. This remedy is one of the best for bearing-down pains in women, which are worse in the morning. The patient feels as if she must sit down to prevent prolapsus. This is like the pains of the *Sepia* patient, who feels as if she must cross her legs for the same purpose. Now if we had the stool and anal symptoms of *Natrum* present, and especially the hypochondriasis, we would have almost a sure thing in *Natrum.* These uterine symptoms of *Natrum* are often accompanied by back pains, which are relieved by lying upon back, like *Rhus.* I have already spoken of the headaches accompanying, and especially following the menses. They are throbbing and accompanied by great soreness of the eyes, especially on turning them. I have a patient now who has these headaches occasionally. She is inclined to anæmia. Was, when young, very anæmic. She is always relieved by this remedy in the 250m. potency, and under it is regaining her color and general health.

Natrum mur. has strong action upon the heart and circulation, as the following marked symptoms indicate: "*Fluttering of the heart with weak faint feeling, worse lying down. Irregular intermission of beats of heart and pulse, worse on lying on left side. Violent pulsations of the heart which shake the body.*" *(Spigelia.)* All these symptoms are more markedly present in anæmic subjects, with constitution generally weakened by grief, sexual excess, loss of blood and other debilitating causes. It is especially efficacious in subjects suffering from abuse of *Quinine*. In fevers it is among Hahnemannians too well known to need much space here. In intermittents it is especially useful in cases suppressed, not cured, by *Quinine*, and its leading characteristic is in the *time* of the appearance of the chill.

Natrum appears characteristically at 10 to 11 A. M.

Eupatorium perfoliatum at 7 A. M.

Apis mellifica at 3 P. M.

Lycopodium at 4 P. M.

Arsenicum alb. at 1 to 2 P. M. or A. M.

Without fixing the time just to the hour, there are many remedies which have chills in the morning or in the evening, etc. Now in regard to the time of aggravation in fevers, they occur quite as characteristically in other than intermittents. For instance the *Natrum* at 10 A. M., the *Arsenic* at 1 P. M. or A. M., etc.

The fever, headache and all other symptoms of *Natrum* are *relieved by sweating,* as are those of *Arsenicum* also. There are some strong symptoms found in the extremities. *"Hang nails."* The *Natrum* subject is always having them. Again, *numbness and tingling in fingers and toes,* like that also found in the lips and tongue, should make one think of *Natrum.* The ankles are weak and turn easily, especially in children who are late in learning to walk. *Painful tension in the bends of the limbs,* as if the cords were too short. This may amount to actual deformity, like *Causticum, Guaiacum* and *Cimex.* Then the spine is very irritable, sensitive to touch, yet relieved *by hard pressure,* with weakness of the limbs, fluttering of the heart, even half paralyzed extremities. As far as this spinal weakness is concerned, it may take on a form of general debility, for which there is no better remedy than *Natrum mur.* The mental and physical powers seem greatly relaxed, and physical and mental labor equally prostrating. This condition may gradually progress to paralysis, and may be the result of badly treated intermittents, sexual excesses, diphtheria, depressing emotions or other causes of nervous exhaustion. The action of *Natrum* upon the skin must not be overlooked. First and foremost is its eczema, which is raw, inflamed, and *especially worse at the edges of the hair.* Next for tetters at the bends of the joints. They crack and crust over and ooze an acrid fluid. Finally in urticaria it ranks with *Apis, Hepar sulphur.* and *Calcarea ost.* I have used more space for this remedy, as I did for *Lachesis* and *Causticum,* than for most other remedies, for the following reasons: First, they are all remedies more efficient in high potencies. Second, they are not appreciated by the general profession. Third, I hope to induce those who do not use them to investigate them. I have found that those who highly value these three remedies are generally good Homœopathic prescribers.

NATRUM CARBONICUM.

One of the most frequently corroborated symptoms of this remedy is the modality—*aggravated by mental exertion.* The patient is unable to think or perform any mental labor without headache *(Argentum nit., Sabadilla)* vertigo or a sense of stupefaction. This symptom alone makes it an invaluable remedy, as we often come across that kind of patient. At least I have, and have frequently gained great credit by relieving them. I generally use the 30th potency here. Again this kind of headache is apt to be worse on exposure to the sun's rays or under gaslight. Persons suffering from over-heating from the sun may find relief from *Natrum carb., Glonoine, Lachesis* or *Lyssin.* Like the other *Natrums,* the carbonate is *greatly depressed in spirits,* wholly occupied with sad thoughts. It is one of our best remedies for chronic catarrh of the nose, which extends to the posterior nares and throat. There is violent hawking and spitting of thick mucus that constantly collects again. *(Corallium.)* Although never produced in the proving, clinical use has proved it a great remedy for "bearing down" pains. Here the concomitant symptoms of mind, sadness, over-sensitiveness to noise, especially music, etc., will confirm its choice. Weakness of the ankles from childhood finds a good remedy in *Natrum carb.* I cured a very bad case in a young man who was very fleshy and walked on the inside of his ankles, feet bending outward, from such weakness, his ankles refusing to support him, especially when a little over-fatigued. Those are the only uses of *Natrum carb.* that I know from personal experience or observation.

MAGNESIA CARBONICA.

Stools green and frothy, like the scum of a frog pond; doubling up colic $>$ after stool.

Toothache in decayed teeth, worse at night; must get up and walk about for relief (especially during pregnancy).

To exhausted nerves in worn-out women what *China* is for loss of blood.

Menses; flow only at night or when lying, and in absence of uterine pains.

* * * * *

The salts of *Magnesia* are not new to the medical profession as remedies. Especially is the one under consideration so well known in its action upon the intestinal canal that it has for a long time been "my lady's" habitual resort for sour stomach and constipated bowels. Of course, then it should become a very useful remedy for diarrhœa in the hands of a Homœopathist, and so it is. The kind of diarrhœa to which it is most applicable is—*"Stools green and frothy like the scum of a frog pond."* All of the *Magnesias* are great pain producers, consequently pain relievers, and, as might be expected, the stools of *Magnesia carb.* are preceded by *griping, doubling-up colic.* So far as colic is concerned, sometimes it might be difficult to choose between *Magnesia carb.* and *Colocynth,* but the stools are not alike. *Rheum* comes nearest to *Magnesia carb.,* in that both have colic before stool, *sour stool and sour smell of the whole body;* but with *Magnesia* the *green stool* stands first and with *Rheum* the *sourness.* The stool of *Rheum* is oftener *dark brownish* than green. *Chamomilla* has green stool with much pain, but the stool is watery, while *Magnesia carb.* is more slimy. *Mercury* has the slimy stool which may be green also; but with *Mercury* tenesmus is the leading symptom, and the mouth symptoms and sweat without relief under it are not like the other remedies. *Magnesia carb.* has toothache which at first sight seems to simulate that of *Mercury.* It comes in decayed teeth and is worse at night. There is a finer shade of difference, however, that distinguishes them. *Mercury* is worse from the *warmth of the bed* (a general characteristic of *Mercury),* while *Magnesia carb.* is worse quiet. The patient is obliged *to walk about* for relief. This kind of toothache is common among pregnant women, and I have often cured it. *(Ratanhia.)* I have used it in the 200th potency for this trouble. Have used it lower in diarrhœas. I once cured a severe case of coccydynia, a case of long standing. The pains were sudden, piercing, causing the patient to almost faint away. *Magnesia carb.* 200th cured promptly. *Lobelia inflata* has *extreme sensitiveness;* sits leaned forward to avoid contact of even soft pillow.

MAGNESIA MURIATICA.

Constipation; stools knotty or lumpy, like sheep dung; crumbling at the verge of the anus.

Nervous headache, > from pressure *(Puls.);* on wrapping the head up warmly *(Sil.).*

Palpitation of heart when the patient is quiet, > when moving about.

Urine; pale yellow; can only be passed by bearing down with abdominal muscles; weakness of bladder.

Adapted to nervous, hysterical women inclined to spasms.

* * * * *

This salt of *Magnesia* seems to act differently from the *Magnesia carb.*, for while the latter most characteristically produces diarrhœa, and we find it oftenest useful there, the former constipates. It has a peculiar form of constipation. The stools are hard, difficult, slow, insufficient, knotty, like sheep's dung, and *crumble at the verge of the anus.* Sometimes can only be passed by *bearing down with the abdominal muscles.* The remedies most resembling it in this form of constipation are *Natrum mur.* and *Ammonium mur.* and now that I think of it I might as well mention here another similarity between *Ammonium mur.* and *Magnesia carb.* which is characteristic, viz.: The menstrual flow is worse at night. I forgot this when writing of *Magnesia carb.* Perhaps it will be all the better remembered for this interruption. With the *Magnesia mur.* menstruation is very painful, accompanied with severe cramps, which may increase to general spasms of a hysterical nature. This nervous condition, if found coupled with the peculiar constipation above described, will be a sure indication for the use of this remedy. Again it has a peculiar nervous headache, which is better from strong pressure *(Pulsatilla),* or wrapping head up warmly *(Silicea).* This headache also is often hysterical. The spasms in connection with uterine troubles may find rival remedies in *Actæa race-*

mosa and *Caulophyllum,* the *tout ensemble* must decide. *Magnesia mur.* is a liver remedy, and in some symptoms resembles *Mercurius,* notably, the tongue *takes imprint of the teeth and the aggravation from lying on the right side.* But the stools of these remedies are characteristically very different. Again, while *Mercurius* is best adapted to acute affections of this organ, *Magnesia mur.* is more so to the chronic. *Ptelea,* liver troubles are *worse when lying on the left side.* A very peculiar symptom of *Magnesia mur.,* often confirmed is: Palpitation of the heart when the *patient is quiet, relieved* when moving about.

Children *cannot digest milk* during dentition *(Sepia).*

MAGNESIA PHOSPHORICA.

Cramping pains everywhere, also lightning-like in coming and going.

Spasmodic affections without febrile symptoms. Colic, whooping cough, cramps in calves, etc.

Modalities: < cold air, cold water, touch, > heat warmth, pressure, bending double.

* * * * *

Now we come to the prince of the *Magnesias.* It is comparatively new and has never been accorded a place in our Materia Medica according to its importance and merits. Dr. H. C. Allen gives the best rendering of it in the transactions of the International Hahnemannian Association for 1889. *Magnesia phos.* takes first rank among our very best neuralgia or pain remedies. None has a greater variety of pains. They are sharp, cutting, piercing, stabbing, knife-like, shooting, stitching, lightning-like in coming and going *(Belladonna)*, intermittent, the paroxysms becoming almost intolerable, often rapidly changing place and **cramping.** This last is in my opinion *most characteristic*, and is oftenest found in stomach, abdomen and pelvis. For colic of infants it ranks with *Chamomilla* and *Colocynth* and for dysmenorrhœa of the neuralgic variety, with the characteristic crampy pains, I have found no remedy equal to it. In this last affection I habitually prescribe the 55m. made by myself upon the gravity potentizer, so that I know exactly what it is. So often are we confronted with the question when we report cures with the high potencies, where do we get them, and are you sure they are what they purport to be? Now let me say right here, if I have not done so before, that we have potencies as high as th m. m., made by ourselves upon this accurately self-registering potentizer, that are marvelous for their curing powers. We (Dr. Santee and myself) invented the machine for our own individual use and have never yet offered the potencies for sale. So we can hardly be accused of mercenary motives in reporting cures, from them. Alongside the characteristic cramping pains of this remedy is its characteristic *modality—relief from hot applications.* No remedy has this more prominently than *Arsenicum alb.*, but you will notice that among all the various kinds of pain we have mentioned as belonging to *Magnesia phos.* the one conspicuous for its absence is the one most characteristic of *Arsenicum*, viz.—*burning* pains. I watched this difference and found that if burning pains were relieved by heat, *Arsenicum* was almost sure to relieve, while those pains not burning but also relieved by heat were cured by *Magnesia phos.* I think that this will be found a valuable diagnostic between the two remedies. At least I have found it so. During painful menstruation *Magnesia phos.* is quicker in its action than *Pulsatilla, Caulophyllum, Cimicifuga,* or any other remedy that I know. The *Cimicifuga* seems to me to cover better, cases of a rheumatic character, or in a rheumatic subject, while *Magnesia phos.* cures those of a purely neuralgic character. The pains cease when the flow begins, for *Magnesia phos.* In facial neuralgia this remedy has made many cures. In fact, it seems to be applicable to neuralgic pains anywhere if the proper conditions are present. So far as its power to control spasms or convulsions is concerned, I have no experience that proves it unless its power over cramping pains is proof. I have no faith in the Schuesslerian theory in regard to it. Similia similibus curantur has stood the test with other remedies and will with the so-called tissues remedies regardless of theories.

Now in regard to the **cramping pains** so characteristic of *Magnesia phos.;* when such a symptom stands out so prominently, it is a great *leader,* and narrows down the choice to a *class of* remedies having the same. Let me illustrate.

Cramping pains. *Cuprum, Colocynth, Magnesia phos.*

Burning. *Arsenic, Canthar., Capsic., Phosphorus, Sulph. ac.*

Coldness (sensation). *Calc. ost., Arsenic. alb., Cistus, Helod.*

Coldness (objective). *Camphora, Secale, Veratrum alb., Heloderma.*

Fullness (sensation). *Æsculus hip., China, Lycopod.*

Emptiness (sensation). *Cocculus, Phos., Sepia.*

Bearing-down. *Belladonna, Lilium tig., Sepia,* etc.

Bruised soreness. *Arnica, Baptisia, Eupatorium perf., Pyrogen, Ruta.*

Constriction. *Cactus grand., Colocynth, Anacard.*

Prostration or weariness. *Gelsemium, Picrid acid, Phos. ac.*

Numbness. *Aconite, Chamomilla, Platina, Rhus toxicod.*

Erratic pains. *Lac caninum, Pulsatilla, Tuberculinum.*

Sensitiveness to pain. *Aconite, Chamomilla, Coffea.*

Sensitive to touch. *China, Hepar sul., Lachesis.*

Bone pains. *Aurum, Asafœtida, Eupat. perf., Mercurius.*

Sticking or stitching pains. *Bryonia, Kali carb., Squilla.*

Pulsation or throbbing. *Belladonna, Glonoine, Melilotus.*

Hæmorrhages (passive). *Hamamelis, Secale, Crotal., Elaps.*

Hæmorrhages (active). *Ferrum phos., Ipecac., Phosphorus.*

Emaciation. *Iodine, Natrum mur., Lycopod., Sarsapar.*, etc.

Leucophlegmasia. *Calc. ost., Graphites, Capsicum.*

Constitutions (psoric). *Sulphur, Psorinum,* etc.

Constitutions (sycotic). *Thuja, Nitric acid, Medorrhinum,* etc.

Constitutions (syphilitic). *Mercury, Iodide potassium, Syphilinum,* etc.

Blue swellings. *Lachesis, Pulsatilla, Tarantula Cub.*

So we might go on and indicate from one to three or more remedies having characteristic power over certain symptoms or conditions, and it is well to have them in mind, for with this start we will be very apt to have, or seek to find out, the diagnostic difference between them. Such knowledge forearms a man, preparing him for emergencies, and often enables the prescriber to make those wonderful *snap-shot cures* that astonish the patient and all beholders.

OPIUM.

Abnormal painlessness.

Want of susceptibility, trembling, lack of vital reaction. Blunted morals, worst liars in the world.

Reversed peristalsis and fæcal vomiting.

Fright; the fear of the fright remaining.

Sleepy but cannot sleep. Hears sounds not ordinarily noticed.

Very hot skin with sweating; perspiration.

Profound stupor with dark-red face and stertorous breathing.

Bed feels so hot she cannot lie on it; moves often in search of a cool place; must be uncovered.

* * * * *

One of the worst abused, because frequently used, remedies of all schools of medicine. I must explain. I said all schools. The true Homœopath does not abuse it, but many members of the school calling themselves homœopathic do. A teacher in one of the homœopathic colleges defended its use in narcotic doses in many cases to produce sleep and relief from pain. I will say just here that any homœopathic physician that feels obliged to use *Opium* or its alkaloid in this way and for this purpose does not understand his business and had better study his Materia Medica, and the principles of applying it according to Hahnemann, or else go over to the old school where they make no pretensions to have any law of cure. In the first place *Opium* in narcotic doses does not produce sleep, but stupor, and it only relieves pain by rendering the patient unconscious to it. How many cases have been so masked by such treatment, that the disease progressed until there was no chance for cure? Pain, fever and all other symptoms are the voice of the disease, telling where is the trouble and guiding us to the remedy. The true curative often relieves pain even more quickly than *Opium,* and does so by curing the condition upon which it depends. And even in cases where it does not so quickly stop the pain, it is often far better to suffer awhile until the curative can get in its work. Probably ninety-nine in a hundred of those suffering from the terrible habit of morphine eating are first led into it by physicians who prescribe morphine to "relieve pain and procure rest and sleep." And when we take into this account the abuse of stimulants, under the name of tonics, habitually prescribed by the same class of physicians it is no wonder that they are often heard to say, I don't know whether I have done more good or harm.

It is this very narcosis which presents the leading characteristic indication for the Homœopathic use of this drug. No remedy produces such profound stupor, and it is expressed in our Materia Medica as follows: *"Stupid, comatose sleep, with rattling, stertorous breathing."* In addition to this the face is red and bloated, the eyes bloodshot and half open and the skin covered with hot sweat. Now this condition, which is nothing more or less than such a fullness of the vessels of the brain or head that, from pressure, a paralysis or semi-paralysis of the nerves which carry on the act of breathing, keep the lower jaw up (which drops), and close the sweat glands, takes place. There are many diseases in which this state of things may appear, such as typhoid fever, where the patient becomes totally unconscious and oblivious to all around. There is no response to light, touch, noise or anything else, except the indicated remedy, which is *Opium*. So in pneumonia, where *Opium* has made remarkable cures in Homœopathic hands; while in massive, or what they like to call heroic, doses of the old school (given to stop pain and procure sleep) it has sent many a poor victim to his long resting place. In many other diseases, in fact in any disease where these symptoms are found, we may confidently expect *Opium* either to cure the case or to so change the condition that other remedies will follow it to a perfect cure. Other remedies may vie with it, for instance in typhoids, such as *Lachesis* or *Hyoscyamus*. These two remedies will often claim attention in typhoid pneumonia. It often requires close discrimination to choose between them. Apoplexy often calls for *Opium*, but here as elsewhere the symptoms must decide.

The fact that *Opium* is capable of banishing pain, or, rather, I should say, rendering the organism incapable of sensing pain, is one of the chief indications for its use in homœopathic therapeutics. There is not only complete absence from pain, but as complete unsusceptibility to general drug action. You know that we are told that when the seemingly indicated remedy does not act give *Sulphur*. Now it may be that *Opium* is a better remedy to give, if all there is of the case is that there seems to be no vital reaction. *Sulphur* would be likely to be the best remedy if the lack of reaction were due to some psoric taint; but even here all the symptoms must be taken into account. *Laurocerasus* is another remedy to arouse reaction when it seems to depend upon excessively low vitality. *Psorinum* may succeed in psoric obstructions to vital reactions when *Sulphur* fails. There is nothing to be more condemned in homœopathic prescribing than *routinism.* This same paralyzing effect of *Opium* is seen in the intestines. Their irritability is lost. Peristaltic action is entirely suspended. There is no *desire* even for movement. The fæces lie there in the convolutions of the intestines, form into hard, black balls, which must be removed by enemas or purgatives. Again, the urinary organs come under the same action. The urine is retained from paralysis of the fundus of the bladder; can't pass water from blunting of the sensitiveness of the walls of the bladder, etc. Or the other extreme, involuntary urination or stool from paralysis of the sphincters. Everywhere *Opium* is a producer of *insensibility* and partial or complete paralysis and, other things being equal, is homœopathically indicated there.

Now we find an exactly opposite state of things under *Opium* to that we have been describing as indicated by the following symptoms: "Delirious, eyes wide open, glistening; face red, puffed up." "Vivid imagination, exaltation of the mind." "Nervous and irritable, easily frightened." "Twitching, trembling of head, arms, hands; jerking of the flexors, even convulsions." "Sleeplessness *(Cimicifuga, Coffea)*, with acuteness of hearing; clock striking and cocks crowing at a great distance keep her awake." These are the secondary or reactionary symptoms of *Opium.* Nature has been pushed like a pendulum, clear to one side of the perpendicular or normal condition. Now, nature endeavoring to undo this mischief, like the law of gravity with the pendulum, pulls back with such force that the pendulum swings not only to its normal state, but clear over to the other extreme, and then if left to herself will continue to oscillate back and forth until the normal place is found and natural law again reigns supreme. It must be remembered here that the first class of symptoms are *drug action,* the later action nature's efforts against the drug; so that such excitement, irritability and spasms never come under the homœopathic action of *Opium* as a remedy unless this state has been preceded by drowsiness, stupor and insensibility, etc. It cannot be the homœopathic remedy to the case without this, for its perfect similarity is not to be found there. This is the reason why the Homœopath can make his sleepless patient sleep a natural sleep with *Opium* in the little dose, while the allopath forces his patient into a stupor (not a sleep) with his big dose. The one is curative, the other poisonous.

NUX MOSCHATA.

Stupor, insensibility, *unconquerable sleep;* sleepy with most all complaints.

Excessive dryness of the tongue, mouth, lips and throat; no thirst.

And < cold damp weather, getting wet, or washing; after eating (bloating); > in room, dry weather.

Changeable humor; one moment laughing, the next crying.

* * * * *

The nutmeg, though frequently used for its peculiar flavor in common cookery, is nevertheless a powerful poison, hence a valuable remedy. The mind and sensorium are profoundly affected by it, as shown by the following characteristic symptoms: "Stupor and insensibility, and unconquerable sleep." Again, "Vanishing of thought while talking, reading, or writing." Again, "Weakness or loss of memory." Again, "Fitful mood, changing from deepest sorrow to frolicsome behavior; now grave, now gay." Again, "Absence of mind, cannot think; has to collect his thoughts before he can answer simple questions." Many more symptoms appear among the provings that show the action of this drug upon the brain. The effect upon the brain, while producing a sleepiness and dulness almost equal to that of *Opium,* is of an entirely different character, the *Opium* being seemingly due to fullness of the blood-vessels and pressure, while that of *Nux moschata* seems to be a benumbing of the very nerve substance itself. It is interesting to notice the sleepiness of *Opium, Nux mos.* and *Tartar emetic,* and to study these drugs in comparison. *Opium* and *Tartar emetic* are often remedies for pneumonia, but the concomitant symptoms are very different. *Opium* and *Nux vom.* in typhoid fever, but the choice, notwithstanding this symptom of stupor common to both, is not at all difficult. All three of these remedies in bowel complaints of children have this symptom in common, but it is not hard to choose between them. Another very characteristic symptom of this remedy is *excessive dryness of the mouth.* Mouth so dry that the tongue sticks to the roof, yet no thirst. *The tongue, lips and throat are all dry.* Of course, there are other remedies having this dryness without thirst, such as *Apis, Pulsatilla* and *Lachesis,* but in this respect *Nux moschata* is the strongest. Then again *Nux moschata* is greatly troubled with flatulence. The abdomen is enormously distended, especially after meals. There are two remedies which have pain and distress in the stomach *immediately* after eating, even when the patient is still at the table. They are *Nux mos.* and *Kali bichromicum.* With *Nux vomica* and *Anacardium* the pain comes on an hour or two after eating. With *Nux mos.,* everything they eat seems to turn to wind *(Kali carb., Iodine),* and fills the stomach and abdomen so full as to cause pressure upon all of the organs of the chest and abdomen. Again there is diarrhœa with this remedy. It is very efficacious in cholera infantum, when the above mentioned sensorial symptoms are present. I once had a very severe case of typhoid fever of the *nervous stupida* variety. On account of the stupidity, the yellow watery diarrhœa, and rumbling and bloating of the abdomen, I thought surely *Phosphoric acid* must help; but it did not. I finally discovered the excessive dryness of the mouth, which had escaped my attention before. This completed the picture for *Nux moschata.* Under the action of the 200th potency, the patient rapidly improved unto complete recovery. So we must "watch out" when the seemingly indicated remedy does not cure, for it may not be *Sulphur, Opium, Laurocerasus* or *Psorinum* that will have to be given, as we said when writing on *Opium* and *Sulphur;* but we have not, no matter what the "seemings," chosen the homœopathic remedy at all, and, as in this case, some symptom may appear that will change the prescription entirely.

Now we will notice in detail the mind and sensorium

symptoms that we have given, by way of comparison. I will add to the comparison made between this remedy and *Antimonium tart.* and *Opium, Apis mellifica,* which has soporous sleep; but it is interrupted by *piercing screams,* especially in brain diseases, where the sopor is generally found. None of the other remedies have these screams (cri encephalique) so prominently. "Vanishing of thought while talking, reading or writing" may find their similar under *Camphor, Cannabis Indica* and *Lachesis.* "Loss of memory" under many remedies, but notably under *Anacardium, Lycopodium, Bryonia alb., Sulphur* and *Natrum muriaticum.* The "fitful, changing moods and disposition" is found under *Aconite, Ignatia, Crocus* and *Platina.* "Absence of mind," *Anacardium, Kreosote, Lachesis, Natrum mur.* and *Mercurius.* I notice that those remedies that are oftenest similar to *Nux moschata* in its mind and other symptoms are often found among the so-called hysteric remedies. And why not? For *Nux moschata* is one of our best in this hydra-headed complaint. Taking together all of the symptoms we have been over, and adding to them that other one, "easy fainting," where can you find a more complete general picture of the average hysteric? I will not use more space here for this remedy, but recommend to every careful student, and practitioner, who does not already understand it, a careful study of this certainly valuable drug. That it has not received the use in practice that it should is due, I have no doubt, to the fact that it is used so frequently in foods, that many think it cannot be much of a remedy.

BARYTA CARBONICA.

Mental and physical weakness; both ends of life; don't grow. Almost imbecile (children) feeble and tottering; childish and thoughtless (old age); loss of memory.

Tonsils inflame, swell and suppurate repeatedly, on every cold exposure; chronic hypertrophy afterwards.

Glands swell, infiltrate, *hypertrophy;* neck, parotids, submaxillary, groin, lymphatics, in the abdomen; hypertrophy, sometimes suppuration.

Offensive foot-sweats; toes and soles get sore; throat affections after checked foot-sweat.

Great sensitiveness to cold.

* * * * *

This is one of the leading so-called anti-scrofulous remedies. Please refer to what I said on this subject (scrofula) while writing on *Sulphur*. This is also one of the remedies which has one of its leading indications, like *Calcarea ost.*, in the constitution of the patient. Complaints of *dwarfish children; mind and body weak; don't grow; inclined to glandular swellings. The defective growth is both mental and physical. The weakness of the mind may amount almost to idiocy or imbecility. Then again it is equally adapted to old age, with mental and physical weakness; feeble and tottering; childishness and thoughtless behavior.* It is especially adapted to apoplexy of old people, or a tendency thereto. For loss of memory in such subjects it stands equal to *Anacardium.* Now we see that if all this is true, *Baryta carb.* becomes a valuable remedy at both ends of life. *Marasmus, infantile or senile,* comes equally within its range. In the marasmus of children we may have to choose from among other remedies such as *Silicea, Abrotanum, Natrum muriaticum, Sulphur, Calcarea* and *Iodine.* Under all these remedies we may find emaciation of the rest of the body, while the abdomen is greatly enlarged. Again under every one of them, the child may have a voracious appetite; eat enough, but grow poor all of the time. *It is defective assimilation.* There are some strong points of resemblance between *Baryta carb.* and *Silicea,* namely: *Offensive sweat on the feet. The head is disproportionately large for the body. Both suffer from damp changes in the weather and both are sensitive to cold about the head.* But *Silicea* has the important diagnostic difference —*profuse sweat on the head* equal to that of *Calcarea ost.,* which *Baryta* has not. And there is not that weakness of mind in *Silicea* that is found in *Bryonia;* on the contrary the child is self-willed and contrary.

The resemblances to the other remedies, other than those we have mentioned, are so many that we will not undertake to compare them here, but will proceed to notice some of the other strong points of *Baryta.*

Besides the strong action of *Baryta* upon the glandular system generally, it seems to have a peculiarly strong affinity for the throat, *especially the tonsils, which become greatly inflamed, swollen and suppurate as a consequence of the least exposure to cold.* Thus it becomes one of our most valuable therapeutic agents in old quinsy subjects. Alone it is often sufficient to abort an attack of quinsy and with an occasional dose at long intervals with a high potency, to overcome the tendency thereto. *(Psorinum.)* But like *Lachesis, Lycopodium, Phytolacca* and other remedies, it must be chosen according to all the indications. *Baryta* is really fully as useful to change the constitutional tendencies to quinsy, as it is in the acute attack. You will find occasionally a case of *chronic cough in children with enlarged* tonsils, reported in the journals as cured by this remedy. The cure of the cough depends evidently upon the power of the remedy over the condition which produced the enlarged tonsils, for aside from this, I have never found it to be a great cough remedy. In tonsilitis acute or chronic which seems to have come as the result of a *suppressed foot-sweat,* we would immediately think of *Baryta,* notwithstanding *Silicea* has more troubles arising from such suppression than any other remedy, but *Silicea* has not nearly the same affinity for the throat that *Baryta* has.

Here we will close *Baryta,* for while it is a remedy of the greatest value, its range is not a wide one. Some of the remedies of this kind make up for the lack of range by a positiveness within their range, and this is one of them.

IODIUM.

Always hungry; eats or wants to all the time, yet emaciates; > while eating.

Hypertrophy of all glands except mammary, which dwindle; while body withers glands enlarge.

Mentally anxious, anguish, wants to move, do something, hurry, kill somebody, etc. *(Arsen.)*

Warm blooded notwithstanding emaciation: wants a cool place to move, think, or work in.

Pulsations all over, stomach, back, even arms, fingers and toes. *(Bell.)*

Especially suitable to dark haired, dark eyed, dark skinned persons of scrofulous habit.

Modalities: < fasting, in warm air or room; > while eating; moving, and cold air.

Great weakness and loss of breath on going up stairs.

Hard goitre in dark haired persons; also tumors in the breast.

Sensation as if the heart was squeezed together; as if grasped with an iron band. *(Sulph.)*

Croup; membranous; in scrofulous children; child grasps the larynx; face pale and cold; in fleshy children.

* * * * *

This is another so-called anti-scrofulous remedy. Here are a few characteristic indications:

First: "Scrofulous diathesis; low cachectic condition, with profound debility and great emaciation."

Second: "There is a remarkable and unaccountable sense of weakness and loss of breath on going up stairs."

Third: "Ravenous hunger; eats often and much, but loses flesh all of the time."

Fourth: "Feels relieved after eating or while eating."

Fifth: "Dwindling of the mammæ and soreness."

Sixth: "Profuse uterine hæmorrhages; cancer of uterus."

Seventh: "Chronic leucorrhœa, which is abundant and so corrosive as to eat holes in the linen."

Eighth: "Swelling of glands, especially mesenteric and thyroid."

Ninth: "Membranous croup, wheezing, sawing respiration, dry, barking cough, especially in children with dark eyes and hair; child grasps the throat with the hand when coughing."

Tenth: "Aggravations in general from warm room." Here is *Iodine* in a nutshell. *The remarkable hunger relieved by eating, with progressive emaciation, is the first in importance.* This relief by eating is not only of the sensation of hunger, but his sufferings in general; *he only feels well while eating,* or always feels best while eating. It makes no difference whether it is phthisis pulmonalis, mesenteric, or general, that this symptom well developed rules out everything but *Iodine* in almost every case and it has made many remarkable cures. I have cured many cases of goitre with *Iodine* c. m., when indicated, giving a powder every night for four nights, after the moon fulled and was waning.

I have only failed in one case either to check the further development or cure. ·Some will sneer at this, but the *cured ones* do not. The local application for glandular enlargement is foolish and dangerous.

BROMINE.

An element proven and arranged by Hering and an important remedy in laryngeal affections. Also in scrofulous and tubercular affections of the glands. It is well known to act best on persons with *light blue eyes, flaxen hair, light eye-brows, fair, delicate skins, red cheeked scrofulous girls.* It will be remembered how almost exactly opposite, so far as temperament is concerned, is *Iodine,* which is also one of our chief anti-scrofulous remedies. In glandular affections, three remedies that are not as often thought of as they perhaps should be, are *Carbo animalis, Conium* and *Bromine;* in all three the glands are *stony hard with a cancerous tendency.* In *Bromine* the pains are not characteristic, but with *Conium* and *Carbo animalis* they are lancinating, cutting or burning, more like cancer pains.

In diphtheria, where it has done some wonderful work, the membrane first forms in the bronchi, trachea or larynx, running upward, just the opposite of *Lycopodium*, which often forms first in the nose and runs downward.

In membranous croup, there is great rattling of mucus like *Hepar*, but no expectoration. There seems to be great danger of suffocation from accumulation of mucus in larynx (in bronchi, *Ant. tart.*).

Sensation of cobweb in face (*Bar., Graph.* and *Borax*).

Fan-like motion of alæ nasi (*Ant. t., Lycop.*).

Hypertrophy of heart from gymnastics (*Caust.*).

Membranous dysmenorrhœa (*Lac can.*).

CINA.

The child is cross and ugly, kicks and strikes; wants to be carried or rocked or don't want to be touched or looked at; wants things and pushes them away when offered.

Frequently boring the nose with the fingers.

Pale sickly look about the eyes, or white and blue about the mouth.

Frequent swallowing as if something came up in the throat.

Alternate canine hunger or no appetite at all.

Urine turns milky on standing.

Frequent sudden attacks of very high fever, with glowing red hot face, with paleness around mouth and lips, or sometimes alternates with pale face with dark bluish ring around the eyes.

* * * * *

Here is a truly unique remedy that none but the homœopathist knows how to use. The old school chagrined at our success with it, and not willing to resort to our small doses, have bungled with its alkaloid, doing more harm than good, and at last have come to sneer at the idea of children being troubled with worms at all. I have known of several instances of the kind and it has become so common in the region where I practice that the people often ask me—"Doctor, do you believe in worms? Old school doctors don't. I have found several worms that my child has passed, and have come to you to see if you can do anything for them." It is of great advantage to us Homœopaths to *cure the little patients*, whether we *believe in worms* or not. But *Cina* is not always the remedy for worms. But it is perhaps the oftenest indicated remedy for complaints arising from lumbricoides, or children infested with the animal. Another thing I have proven to my entire satisfaction, and that is, that it is more efficacious for these cases in the 200th or highest potencies than in the alkaloid or lower potencies. Now I say this in order to induce those who have lost faith in the remedy to try it high, according to well-known indications as laid down in our Materia Medica. So many "lose the good they oft might win by fearing to attempt." Let us look at a few of the leading symptoms. The wormy child will be very restless nights, "*screams out sharply* in its sleep," making one think of *Apis*, but other symptoms appear which rule *Apis* out. *The child is cross* and *ugly* like *Chamomilla, kicks and strikes the nurse, wants to be carried (Chamomilla) or rocked, or don't want to be touched or looked at (Antimonium crud.), desires things and then refuses them when offered (Bry.* and *Staphisagria)*, or, unlike *Chamomilla*, it cries if any one tries to take hold of or carry it. Isn't that a perfect picture of the mind of a wormy child? When these symptoms appear in a child we may sometimes be at a stand between *Cina* and *Chamomilla,* but close watching will generally decide. For instance, if you watch or inquire of the nurse you will find that it *alternates between a red-hot face, glowing with a bright redness of both cheeks, and a pale, sickly face, with dark rings or circles around the eyes; or, again, red face with great paleness around the mouth and nose.* This is *Cina.* If the face is frequently red and hot on one side and pale and cold on the other, it is *Chamomilla.* Then again, on inquiry, or we may observe ourselves, the child is *boring or picking its nose* a great deal of the time, *grinds its teeth when asleep,* and jumps and jerks in its sleep, *frequently swallowing* as if something came up into the throat, or even *choking and coughing* for the same cause. Such a combination is not found under any other remedy. Both *Chamomilla* and *Cina* have profuse and pale urine, but *Cina* urine becomes *milky* after standing awhile. *Cina* has alternating *canine hunger and no appetite at all. Cina* is one of our best remedies for whooping cough, also jerking, trembling, twitching and even convulsions; but in all these affections I have found it efficacious when the aforementioned *worm symptoms* were present. I once had, at one time, and in one family, five cases of typhoid fever, and they were all very sick. There was no mistake about the diagnosis, and I speak thus positively, because some think that a child under the age of six years cannot have this disease. This child, five years of age, was the last one of the family attacked with the disease, and it pursued the same course as the others in its regular rise and fall of temperature, bloating of abdomen, diarrhœa and other symptoms common to this disease. This being in the earlier years of my practice, and *Cina* not being set down in the text-books as a remedy for typhoid, I selected as well as I could from the usual remedies for typhoid. I knew perfectly that she had *Cina* symptoms all mixed in with those already mentioned, and as the case "got no better fast," I resolved to give a few doses of *Cina* anyway, and to my surprise I found my patient much better every way at my next visit and the improvement progressed right along to complete recovery. I had to learn several such lessons as that was in my "kittenhood" of homœopathic practice before I learned for good, that, for purposes of prescribing, the *name* of the disease was of little account. Since I settled that question, I have had frequent opportunities to help my younger brethren out of difficulties along the same line, and they have been as much astonished as I was.

DULCAMARA.

Affections caused by taking cold when the air changes suddenly from dry and warm to *wet* and *cold*.

Tongue and jaws become lame, if cold air or water chills them; neck stiff, back painful, loins lame, after taking cold.

Colic as if diarrhœa would occur, from *taking* cold.

Yellow watery diarrhœa with cutting colic before every stool, or dysentery from taking cold.

Most catarrhal states, with secretion of much mucus, caused by exposure to damp cold.

Dropsical swelling after suppressed sweat, or paralysis and other troubles from suppressed eruptions, after taking cold.

Modalities: < from wet, cold weather after warm, dry; at nights and when at rest; > rising from a seat; motion; warmth in general, and dry weather.

Glands; swell and hypertrophy on repeated exposures to cold, damp air, also acute and chronic tonsilitis.

* * * * *

This remedy, like many others, finds its chief characteristic in its modality. "Complaints caused or aggravated by *change of weather from warm* to cold." Of course all kinds of inflammatory and rheumatic diseases may spring from such a cause and so *Dulcamara* comes to be indicated in a long list of them. For instance: *After taking cold the neck gets stiff, back painful, and limbs lame, or the throat gets sore and quinsy results, with stiff tongue and jaws; the tongue may even become paralyzed.* We see here a resemblance to *Baryta carb.*, and indeed the two remedies complement each other nicely. If we had present in a sore throat the above mentioned stiffness and lameness, *Dulcamara* would be preferred. This cold in throat may travel downward and invade the bronchi and lungs, and cough and bloody expectoration result. It is especially apt to occur in children or old people this way, and then there is apt to be much mucous secretion, hard to raise, with threatened paralysis of the vagi. Here it again resembles *Baryta carb.* It also resembles it in the tendency to get these colds. Asthma humidum, loose cough and rattling of mucus is another affection, and the choice here may lie between *Dulcamara* and *Natrum sulphuricum,* which is another *wet cold weather* remedy. Colic and diarrhœa, from cold exposure, are often quickly relieved by *Dulcamara,* especially if taking place in hot weather, when the days or nights become suddenly cold; also dysentery. Let me repeat that it is a great remedy for *back troubles* from taking cold. I have made particular mention of these affections because such marked relief has followed its administration; but we need not by any means stop here. The bladder, skin or any other part of the body comes in for the beneficial action of this remedy, when we have present its characteristic modality. *Dulcamara* is for affections from *damp cold,* what *Aconite* is for the same from *dry cold.*

RHODODENDRON

Will naturally come in for notice while we are upon *weather* remedies. Like *Dulcamara,* its strongest characteristic is in its modality, *"aggravation in wet stormy weather;"* but *Rhododendron* is particularly worse *before* the storm, especially a thunder storm; after the storm breaks the patient feels better. The aggravation before the thunder storm does not at all seem to depend on the coldness or dampness, but partially at least on the electric conditions of the atmosphere. This is like *Phosphorus, Natrum carb.* and *Silicea. Rhododendron* resembles *Rhus toxicod.* in that it is worse during rest and better during motion. Again, the pains of *Rhododendron,* which are aggravated in damp weather, differ from those of *Rhus toxicod.* in that they seem to be deeper seated and are felt in the periosteum, as in the teeth, and in the bones of the forearm and tibia. These pains are not, however, *confined* to periosteal membranes, but attack also muscles and ligaments, so as to make it difficult to choose between these remedies.

So we have quite a list of marked wet weather remedies in *Dulcamara, Natrum sulphuricum, Rhododendron, Rhus toxicodendron* and *Nux moschata.* (*Calcarea phosphorica,* wet cold, especially melting snow.)

Rhododendron seems to have an especial affinity for the testicles. They are swollen, with drawing contusive pains, which sometimes extend to abdomen and thighs, and they are very sensitive to touch. The remedies most like it are *Aurum metall., Clematis erecta, Pulsatilla, Argentum metall.* and *Spongia.* If the affection was of syphilitic origin we would prefer *Aurum,* especially if the case had been abused by old school mercurialization. If it came from suppressed gonorrhœa, *Clematis* or *Pulsatilla;* if of rheumatic origin, *Rhododendron.* Of course all the case would come into the calculation when making up the perfect picture.

RUTA.

This remedy, which has already been mentioned as to its prominent action in the periosteum, especially in injuries and effects therefrom, also, like *Arnica,* has a "*bruised,* lame sensation all over as after a fall; worse in limbs and joints," and also "all parts of the body upon which he lies are painful, as if bruised." Like *Rhus tox.,* the *Ruta* patient wants to change position frequently. The pains and lameness of *Ruta* seem to have a particular liking for the *wrists.* Here also must *Eupat. perf.* be remembered.

These pains in the wrists of *Ruta* are, like *Rhus tox-*

icod., < in cold, wet weather, and > on motion. **There** is no remedy oftener useful for *eye-strain* from **close** study, sewing, etc., than *Ruta.* The *eyes feel weary and ache as if strained,* or they burn like balls of fire. Two other remedies must be remembered for eye-strain, viz.: *Natrum muriaticum* and *Senega.* An understanding of these three remedies may save many cases of asthenopia or weakness of accommodation from the abuse of spectacles. *Ruta* is also one of our best remedies for **prolapsus of the rectum.**

Ignatia stands closest here. Both are < on stooping, lifting, or at stool. *Muriatic acid* and *Podophyllum* should also be *remembered;* with the former the prolapsed organ is very *sore and sensitive* to the least touch, even of the sheet on which he lies, and the rectum comes down even when urinating *(Aloe).* The prolapse of *Podophyllum* is almost always accompanied by the characteristic diarrhœa, but may be the result of strain by lifting, when the uterus may also prolapse. These uses of *Ruta* make it a very valuable remedy.

LEDUM PALUSTRE.

Rheumatism begins in feet and travels upward *(Kalmia* opposite).

The swellings are pale, sometimes œdematous, and < at night, in the heat of the bed; uncovering or cold water relieves.

Ecchymosis; "black eye" from a blow or contusion; better than *Arnica.*

Rheumatism and rheumatic gout; joints become the seat of nodosities and "gout stones," which are painful.

Complaints of people who are cold all the time; lack of animal or vital heat; parts cold to touch, but not cold subjectively to patient.

Punctured wounds by sharp-pointed instruments, rat bites, stings of insects, especially mosquitoes.

* * * * *

Ledum is a very valuable remedy for rheumatism. This complaint is confessedly a very difficult disease to cure by old school treatment. Seldom is a case of the inflammatory form completely cured by them. The great majority of their cases run from the acute into the chronic form, and last for life. They are often drawn all out of shape (their patients), or left with incurable valvular heart trouble. This is not the case under homœopathic treatment. On the contrary the patients treated homœopathically are generally *cured,* and very seldom left with any heart trouble, even if the disease commenced there, as it sometimes does. Oftener, of course, it begins in the back, extremities or joints generally, and then if treated allopathically with local applications it is *driven* to the heart, which cannot be reached with local applications, hence stays there until exudations occur and hardened deposits form upon the valves. Any homœopathic physician guilty of treating a case this way, with such results, ought to lose his practice and his diploma.

I do not say this inadvisedly, for I have lived and practiced for thirty years past in a decidedly rheumatic district and know whereof I affirm. When we homœopaths of the East condemn those of the West for the Quinine (in material doses) treatment of intermittents, we are reminded that we do not live in miasmatic districts so we are not authority and we can only reply that we know many physicians who do live there who cure their patients without the abuse of Quinine. But in this verdict of mine on rheumatism I cannot be turned off that way. Rheumatism is one of those diseases that presents plenty of symptoms and modalities to guide to the choice from a long list of remedies of the *one appropriate* to the case in hand. There is such a great difference in the results of applying the remedy according to symptomatic indications, and those arising from simply pathological prescribing, that one does not need long to experiment to be convinced. Indeed the pathological condition in this complaint does not figure largely in the account, for purposes of prescribing. But sensations and modalities do.

The *Ledum* rheumatism begins in the feet and travels upward. This is the opposite of *Kalmia,* which goes the other way. *Ledum* may be indicated in both acute and chronic forms of this complaint. In the acute form the joints are swollen and hot, but not red. The swellings are pale and the pains are *worse at night* and from the *heat of the bed,* wants them uncovered. This is like *Mercurius,* but with *Mercury* the profuse *sweat without relief,* and especially the characteristic mouth and tongue symptoms will decide. I have seen wonderful benefit from *Ledum* in such cases.

In the chronic form of the disease this remedy is equally efficacious. Here also we have the joints swollen and painful, especially in the heat of the bed, and painful, hard nodes and concretions form in the joints of feet first, then hands. The periosteum of the phalanges is painful on pressure. The ankles are swollen and the soles are painful and sensitive; can hardly step on them. This painful and sensitive soles of feet is also found under *Antimonium crud.*, *Lycopodium* and *Silicea,* and I have relieved it, other symptoms agreeing, with each and every one of these remedies. In these cases of rheumatic troubles the *Ledum* patient is unnaturally cold. "Lacks vital or animal heat," in this, again, resembling *Silicea;* but although the *Silicea* patient has chronic rheumatism of the feet, ankles and soles similar to *Ledum,* aggravated also at night, the warmth of the *bed* does *not* aggravate, but on the contrary he wants to be covered warmly. Under *Ledum* the relief from cold is so prominent that sometimes the only amelioration is from putting the feet into cold water. It is well to think of *Ledum* in all cases of rheumatism of the feet and *study it up.*

We must not leave this remedy without calling attention to its virtues as a remedy for injuries. We are apt to think of *Arnica* first, for bruises and the results therefrom, and, on account of its well deserved reputation, to forget that there are sometimes other remedies equally valuable. *Ledum* sometimes comes in to finish up a work that *Arnica* began well, but could not complete, even when *Arnica was* best at first, for it often removes the ecchymosis and discoloration more rapidly and perfectly. For black and blue spots from blows or bruises there is no better remedy than *Ledum.*

Then, again, we have *Sulphuric acid,* which is very useful in ecchymosis from the same cause, especially if occurring in cachectic or weakened constitutions, with tendency to purpura, or breaking down of the blood. This pathological condition would be attended with the characteristic symptoms of the drug. We often have ecchymosis into the conjunctiva or sclerotica, for which *Nux vomica* is specific, but for "black eye" from a blow of the fist no remedy equals *Ledum* in the 2c potency. *Ledum* is a good remedy for punctured wounds, such as the sticking of a nail into the foot, or an awl into the hand, etc.; also, for stings of insects, especially mosquitoes, but this also needs modification. It makes some difference what kind of tissue is wounded by this kind of wound. If a nerve, for instance, *Hypericum* would be preferable; if the periosteum, *Ruta;* if the bone, *Calcarea phos.,* or *Symphytum* to promote re-union or repair. We must not forget to mention in connection with what has been said of *Ledum* in injuries of the eye that if there is great pain in the eyeball itself from the blow, *Symphytum* may have to be used. For all these affections I believe the 200th potency better than the lower preparations.

BISMUTH.

Diarrhœa; stools *watery, profuse,* painless and offensive or cadaverously smelling.

Vomiting of large quantities and *intense thirst; water* is vomited the *moment* it reaches the stomach; food is retained a little longer.

Restlessness, anguish, great prostration; pale with blue rings around the eyes; surface covered with sweat, but it is *warm sweat.*

* * * * *

Bismuth is one of our best remedies for cholera infantum; genuine cholera infantum, where the disease is sudden in its onset, and rapid in its course. Such cases die in a night or even a few hours, unless *Bismuth, Veratrum, Kreosote* or some remedy of such rapid action saves them. With *Bismuth* the stools are *watery, profuse,* painless and very offensive; cadaverous smelling. There is also vomiting of large quantities and the *intense thirst* is accompanied with vomiting of the water drunk the **moment** it touches the stomach. Water *only* is so vomited. Food is retained a little longer (with *Arsenicum* both water and food are vomited). There is prostration equal to that of *Arsenicum* or *Veratrum album,* but the surface is warm and often covered with warm sweat. The face is deathly pale, with rings around the eyes. This is a perfect picture of *Bismuth,* and no other remedy need be confounded with it.

Again, *Bismuth* is a remedy for purely nervous gastralgia. The pain is of a pressing nature, sometimes pressing between the shoulders and sometimes there is much burning in the stomach *(Arsenicum).* It is also often of benefit in cancer of the stomach, when there is at times vomiting of enormous quantities of food that seems to have lain in the stomach for days. In such cases there is much burning and pain. It has a restlessness and anguish, similar to *Arsenic,* wants to move around, can't stay long in one place. In the neuralgic form of gastralgia the lower triturations have served me best, but in cholera infantum I never use lower than the 200th and have seen remarkable results. Solitude is unbearable, child wants mother to hold its hand for company *(Stramonium).*

KREOSOTUM.

Cholera infantum; profuse vomiting; cadaverous smelling stools.

Hæmorrhagic diathesis; small wound bleeds profusely *(Phos.)*.

Acrid, fœtid, decomposed, mucous secretions; sometimes ulcerating, bleeding, malignant.

Gums painful, dark red or blue; teeth decay as soon as they come.

Sudden urging to urinate or during first sleep, which is very profound.

* * * * *

This curious substance seems to act chiefly upon the mucous membranes, producing profuse and offensive secretions and ulcerations, with greatly depressed vitality. This is especially true of the genital organs of the female. Leucorrhœa is putrid, acrid, corrosive, staining the linen yellow. The parts with which the discharge comes in contact itch and burn, while scratching does not relieve but inflames the parts. This remedy has a **tendency to hæmorrhages,** which are often very obstinate. The hæmorrhages occur with leucorrhœal trouble; they are intermittent, will almost stop, then freshen up again and again. This is often the case with the lochia after confinement, when the choice may lie between these three remedies, *Kreosote, Rhus tox.* and *Sulphur.* The other symptoms must decide between them. This ulceration may be found in cancer of the uterus, and then *Kreosote* will often be of great value. I have no doubt that many cases which degenerate into cancer might be prevented by its timely use. In some cases there is awful burning in the pelvis, as of red-hot coals, with discharge of clots in foul smelling blood. I see that Guernsey recommends it in cancer of the mammæ, saying it is hard, bluish-red and covered with scurvy protuberances. I have never so used it, but in corrosive leucorrhœas and ulcerations I have with great satisfaction. I generally use it in the 200th, with simply tepid water injections for cleanliness.

There is perhaps no remedy that has a more decided action upon the gums (not even *Mercury*) than this one. It is not used often enough in painful dentition. The gums are *very painful*, swell, look dark-red or blue, and the teeth *decay almost as soon as they are born*. A child that has a mouth full of decayed teeth, with spongy, painful gums, will find its best friend in *Kreosote*. Cholera infantum in such children is of common occurrence, and is of a very severe type, for the vomiting is incessant and the stools cadaverous smelling. Never forget *Kreosote* in cholera infantum, which seems to arise from painful dentition, or in connection with it, for I have seen some of the finest effects ever witnessed from any remedy from this one.

I have used it here also in the 200th. *Kreosote* is also one of our best remedies in other kinds of vomiting; in the vomiting of pregnancy and in that other intractable disease of the stomach, known as gastromalacia. I do not know any characteristic indication for it here; but should I find the troubles before mentioned, in part or whole, such as corrosive leucorrhœa, or the hæmorrhages, or a general hæmorrhagic tendency, *small wounds inclined to bleed profusely* (like *Lachesis* and *Phosphorus*), I would feel confident of *Kreosote*.

Kreosote has strong characteristics in regard to urination.

First, it has copious pale urine.

Second, they can't go *quick* enough, the *urging* is so great or sudden. *(Petroselinum.)*

Third, the child wets the bed during first sleep, which is *very profound,* can hardly wake it. *(Sepia.)*

Can only urinate when lying. *(Zinc. met.,* only when sitting bent back.)

To recapitulate. *Bad teeth and gums* "from way back," *fœtid corrosive discharges; great debility* and *hæmorrhagic tendency,* should always call to mind this remedy.

LAC CANINUM.

Inflammatory affections travel crosswise, from side to side, back and forth (rheumatism, sore throat, etc.).

Breasts and throat get sore at every menstrual period.

Mastitis; breasts very sore and tender; cannot bear a jar of the bed; on stepping has to hold them up, on going down stairs.

* * * * *

At one time I would not have admitted this substance into my list of remedies, for I thought it a disgrace to try to foist dogs' milk upon the profession as a homœopathic remedy. But after accumulated evidence in its favor, and the rule that I had adopted early in my professional life, "to prove all things and hold fast that which was good," I concluded to try it, and my first trial was in a case of inflammatory rheumatism which had withstood my best efforts to relieve for two weeks.

The pain travelled from joint to joint, but *Pulsatilla* utterly failed. I noticed, after awhile, that it not only travelled from joint to joint, but crosswise; one day in the right knee, the next day or two in the left, and then back again, etc. *Lac caninum* cured the case very quickly. Not long after I had a very severe case of scarlatina. The throat was swollen full, and the restlessness was so marked with pains in the limbs which left the patient tossing from side to side that I thought surely *Rhus tox.* must be the remedy. But it failed to relieve. Then I discovered that the soreness of the throat and the pains alternated sides. This called my mind to the remedy, which was given with prompt relief. I used the c. m. in both these cases.

Two cases of tonsilitis in one house in separate families. I was called to treat one of them, and a very excellent Allopathic physician the other. Of course there was close watching to see which case would get well the quickest, and especially if either could be cured without suppuration taking place. They were both very bad cases. Both progressed rapidly for forty-eight hours. In my case the swelling began on one side; the next day was even worse on the other side, so I told them that as the first side was better I thought the last one would be better tomorrow; but alas the next day number one was worse again, the patient could not swallow, food and drinks came back by the nose. It was with much difficulty, choking and struggling that even a spoonful of medicine could be taken. I hesitated no longer, but gave *Lac caninum* c. m. at noon, and when I visited her in the evening found her taking oyster broth and she could speak distinctly, whereas she could not articulate a word in the morning. In another day the patient was well except some weakness. The other case went on to suppuration and was over a week longer in getting around. So another victory was scored for Homœopathy, and I have continued to verify this characteristic of erratic pains, alternating sides, until I consider it as reliable as the key-note of any other remedy.

The curative power of this remedy being settled in my mind, I determined to test it by a proving. I induced three clerks in a dry goods store to take pills (No. 35) of the 200th (B. & T.), once in two hours. They would not consent to do it until I told them what they were to take, and one of them, a well-read young man, remarked with a laugh that if wolf's milk would not kill Romulus and Remus it would not them. The result was that within three days they had sore throats, and the young man mentioned had on both tonsils distinct patches as large as a thumb nail. The other young man was frightened and would not continue the proving, and the young lady's sore throat was followed by a severe cough with soreness of the chest for over a week.

I have found *Lac caninum* a very useful remedy in mastitis, the chief indication being great tenderness and soreness which cannot bear the least jar of the bed or stepping on the floor. Again, if the breasts and throat get sore during menstruation, especially if the menses flow in gushes instead of continuously, *Lac caninum* is the remedy.

KALI SULPHURICUM.

Yellow or greenish discharges from mucous membranes; cough loose and rattling.

Rheumatic pains in joints; moving from joint to joint.

Modalities: < in warm room; in the evening, > in open air.

The chronic of *Pulsatilla*.

* * * * *

When writing upon the *Kalis* I left this one out. There is no proving (deserving the name) of this drug, but like some other remedies in our Materia Medica clinical use on the theory of Schuessler has developed some valuable guides to its homœopathic uses. It resembles *Pulsatilla* in a number of its symptoms, and being a deeper acting remedy is sometimes useful to complement that remedy. But first let us note the similarities:

1st. Yellow or greenish discharges from mucous membranes.

2d. Evening aggravation of fever symptoms.

3d. Amelioration (general) in open air.

4th. Rheumatic pains in joints, or any part of the body, of a shifting, *wandering* nature.

5th. Aggravation in a heated room.

6th. Loose cough, with *rattling* of mucus.

These are all very similar to *Pulsatilla,* and I have frequently verified them, in cases of catarrh of mucous membranes, whether acute or chronic, but especially chronic, or after the failure of *Pulsatilla.*

I once *produced* rheumatism of the joints with *Kali sulph.,* and it was of the above described kind, thus proving the symptom genuine, though up to that time it was only clinical. I always use it in the 30th, and I think that any after-cured symptom from a potency as high as the 30th will be found in accordance with our law of similia when thorough proving of the drug is made.

ANACARDIUM ORIENTALE.

Pain in stomach when it is empty, > by eating.

Frequent ineffectual desire for stool, from insufficiency

or paralytic state of rectum; with sense of *lump* or plug in anus; with the effort the desire vanishes.

Loss of memory; irresistible desire to curse and swear; feels as if he had two wills, one commanding, the other forbidding, to do things.

Pain and sensation as of a blunt plug in different parts.

Suspects every one and everything around him; when walking he felt anxious, as if some one were pursuing him; weakness of all the senses.

* * * * *

Anacardium orientale is a very valuable remedy, but is not, I think, generally appreciated by our school. It ought often to be used in that hydraheaded complaint called dyspepsia, for which *Nux vomica* is so indiscriminately used. Both are excellent remedies, and it is only necessary to know the difference to make the choice between them easy. *Anacardium* has a pain in the stomach, which comes on *only* when the stomach is empty and is *relieved by eating,* while *Nux vomica* is relieved after the process of digestion is over. The pain of *Nux vomica* is worst two or three hours after meals, but lasts only until digestion is accomplished, and then comes relief, whereas, with *Anacardium,* this is the time when the *suffering* is worst. I have cured many cases (some of them of quite long standing) of this description with *Anacardium,* and find almost as many of them as I do *Nux vomica* cases. I have found the 200th here more efficacious than the lower potencies. The potency here as well as elsewhere and with all remedies has more to do with success in curing than some imagine.

Case. In the fall of 1899 I was called to a lady, married, 35 years of age, mother of three children.

She was quite emaciated, with a yellowish cachectic look of the face. A couple of years before I treated her when she had an attack of vomiting, in which she vomited coffee-ground substances.

She was relieved at that time by a dose of *Arsenicum alb.*, 40m., but had more or less trouble with her digestion up to this time. This last attack was more persistent and did not yield to *Arsenicum* and some other remedies.

After awhile it appeared that the *pain* (which was very severe) *and vomiting came on when the stomach was empty.* She had to eat once or twice in the night for relief. The substance vomited was always black or brown looking like coffee grounds. Her sister had been operated for cancer of the breast, and of course she was very nervous and fearful of cancer of the stomach. *Anacardium* relieved promptly, and she has had no return of the trouble since then. Whether the cure is complete remains to be seen, but the benefit from the remedy was unquestionable.

Both these remedies have frequent ineffectual urging to stool, but *Nux vomica* is the result of irregular peristaltic action as observed by Carrol Dunham, while *Anacardium* has an insufficiency or paralytic state of the rectum which does not appear under *Nux vomica.* In other words, *Nux vomica* has desire, but with irregular or over-action. *Anacardium* has the desire, but with not sufficient action to carry it out. Then *Anacardium* has a sense of a lump or plug in the anus which ought to come away, which does not appear under *Nux vomica.*

Anacardium is also one of our leading remedies for

loss of memory, especially in old people of broken down constitutions. Of course, if the characteristic stomach or bowel symptoms were present, or had been suffered from, during former years as a concomitant, or the exciting cause of the mental trouble, the indication would be strengthened.

There are many remedies having **loss of memory** as a leading symptom, but none stronger than this one. Of course, the *whole case* must be taken into the account. This remedy has two other peculiar mind symptoms. First: "Irresistible desire to curse and swear." This symptom, queer as it may seem, is no more so than the other symptom found under *Stramonium,* and often verified, "patient wants to **pray** continually." Some of the most remarkable and convincing cures have been made on just such symptoms. Another symptom is, *"the patient feels as if he had two wills,"* each commanding or moving him to do opposite things, or one commanding him to do a thing and the other commanding him not to do it. Such symptoms are often found in dementia, and are valuable guides to the curative remedy. See my case reported under *Platina.* Then, again, *Anacardium* has two other peculiar symptoms. One as of a *hoop* around parts, and the other as of a *plug* in inner parts. This may be found in head, chest, abdomen or anus. The sensation of a hoop around parts may be found in spinal troubles and *Anacardium* will be the remedy. Other remedies have a general characteristic sensation, as *Anacardium* has the sensation of a **plug**; for instance, the feeling of fullness as if too full of blood of *Æsculus hippocastanum,* and the sensation of constriction of *Cactus* *grandiflorus*. *Anacardium* is also said to be a good antidote for *Rhus* poisoning. I have never used it for this.

ALUMINA.

Inactivity of the rectum; even the soft stool requires great straining.

Anæmia in women, who are hungry for starch, chalk, rags, charcoal, cloves and other ridiculous unnatural things; potatoes disagree; profuse leucorrhœa.

Great heaviness in lower limbs, weak, has to sit down; numbness of heels; sense of hot iron thrust through back.

* * * * *

The chief characteristic leading to the use of this remedy is found in its peculiar constipation. *"Inactivity of the rectum, even the soft stool requires great straining."*

Like *Bryonia,* there is no desire for stool and the constipation seems to depend upon dryness of the mucous follicles. Again it is adapted to dry, spare subjects. There are other points of resemblance between these two remedies and they complement each other well. They are both excellent in infantile constipation, which is often a very obstinate affection to treat. *Anacardium, Sepia, Silicea* and *Veratrum album* are nearest of kin in this lack of expulsive power in the rectum.

Alumina is one of our remedies in chlorotic conditions. The patient is pale, weak, tired, must sit down to rest. The menses are scanty, delayed, and are pale colored when they come, and after the menses the patient is exhausted and pale. *(Carbo an.* and *Cocculus.)* Then, again, there *is profuse leucorrhœa sometimes running down to the heels if she does not wear a cloth. (Syphilinum.)* It is as profuse as the menses ought to be. These anæmic patients are often hungry for *starch, chalk, rags, charcoal, cloves and other ridiculous and unnatural things. Alumina* is a great remedy in such cases. The *Natrum mur.* chlorotic couldn't eat bread, or had an aversion to it. The *Alumina* patient *can't eat potatoes;* they disagree. *Pulsatilla* can't eat *fat food,* pastries, etc. *Alumina* resembles *Pulsatilla* in chronic nasal catarrhs, and both are of tearful temperament, but the constitutions are different. *Alumina* being dry and thin, *Pulsatilla* phlegmatic. One thing I forgot to mention under stool and rectum, viz., *Alumina* is one of the best remedies for hæmorrhages of the bowels in typhoid fever. The blood comes in *large clots looking solid like liver.* This remedy is also very efficacious in chronic sore throats, like clergyman's sore throat. There is "soreness, rawness, hoarseness and dryness." This dryness excites a continual disposition to hawk, and after a long time the patient raises a little thick, tough phlegm. This kind of throat is temporarily relieved by *warm food and drinks.* The remedy nearest to this is *Argentum nitricum,* but in *Argentum* there are *wart-like excrescences or granulations in the throat.* Both remedies have a sensation of a splinter in the throat, as do also *Hepar sulphuricum, Dolichos* and *Nitric acid.*

Alumina has also a sensation of constriction in the throat and œsophagus. It hurts to swallow. *Alumina* is recommended for the following symptoms, which often appear in locomotor ataxia: *"Great heaviness in the lower limbs; can scarcely drag them; while walking staggers and has to sit down;* in the evening." "Inability to walk except with the eyes open and in the day time." *"Numbness* of the heel when stepping." *"Excessively faint and tired, must sit down."* "Pain in the back as if a hot iron were thrust through the vertebræ." I give these on the authority of others, for I have never verified them. I will add here the value of

ALUMEN

In typhoid hæmorrhages from the bowels. It is an excellent remedy and the stools are of dark clotted blood, in large quantities. It is also excellent for relaxed uvula in sore throat.

STICTA PULMONARIA.

Heavy full feeling, and pain and pressure in forehead and root of the nose > by discharge.

Secretions in the nose dry up and form crusts; constant inclination to blow the nose, without result, on account of the excessive dryness.

Dry night cough; can't sleep or lie down; must sit up; cough after measles *(Coff.)*.

* * * * *

This remedy, although never anywhere fully proven, has come to be a very useful one. In acute catarrh it is one of the best.

Its characteristic symptom here is *heavy pain and pressure in the forehead and root of the nose.* This is in the beginning of a cold; when the nose begins to discharge freely the pain ceases or becomes much less.

It is also of great value in the form of nasal catarrh, if when the discharges dry up there is this same pain in forehead and frontal sinuses. In these cases the nasal secretions incline to dry up and are hard to discharge, but the irritation is so great that there is a constant inclination to blow the nose, with little result. These secretions become so hard and dry as to form scabby concretions. This condition is next door to the plugs and clinkers of *Kali bichromicum,* which often go on to ulceration of the septum. I have relieved many cases of chronic catarrh with *Sticta;* some of years' standing.

You will remember that *Kali bichromicum* also has a severe frontal headache at the root of the nose, especially from suppressed catarrh, so that all the other symptoms must be considered in choosing between them. The other remedies that resemble *Sticta* in the acute form of catarrh are *Aconite, Ammonium carb., Camphor, Nux vomica* and *Sambucus,* and in the chronic form *Ammonium carb.* and *Lycopodium.*

There is never with *Sticta* the watery or fluent form of coryza, such as calls for *Euphrasia, Mercurius, Arsenicum* and *Kali hydroiodicum.* Nor have I ever found it of use in the thick, bland kind of discharge that calls for *Pulsatilla, Sepia* and *Kali sulphuricum. Sticta* is also one of our cough remedies, and one of the best indications for its use, especially in acute cough, is the aforementioned nasal catarrh attending it. The *Sticta* cough is also worse at night when lying down and keeps the patient awake, though I do not think the wakefulness is entirely owing to the cough, but that a nervous condition which also comes under the curative range of *Sticta* contributes to it.

This remedy is one of the best for the obstinacy of cough attending or following measles, and here we remember that sleeplessness is a frequent concomitant. In this respect *Sticta* is like *Coffea cruda,* which is wonderfully efficacious here. The cough of *Sticta* is at first dry, but later on may become loose; hence it is often found of use in the incessant, racking, wearing coughs of consumptives. In hay fever it is the remedy when the trouble centres in the head and frontal sinuses; the nose is completely *plugged* up, though there is continual sneezing.

I have found *Sticta* promptly curative in inflammatory rheumatism of the knee joint. It is very sudden in its attacks, and unless promptly relieved by *Sticta* will go on to the exudative stage and become chronic in character. In one case the pain was so severe that the patient, though a strong, resolute man, became delirious with the pain. *Sticta* relieved and completely cured him, so that he was able to attend to his business (teamster) within a week. *Sticta* deserves a thorough proving. There is a nervous symptom that has been several times verified, viz.—"legs felt as if floating in the air, or *she* felt light and airy as if not resting on the bed." See *Asarum* and *Valerian.* Such sensations are often found in hysterical conditions and are very distressing.

RUMEX CRISPUS.

Violent incessant dry cough; worse on inhaling the least cold air; covers the mouth to keep the cold air out, with relief.

Brownish diarrhœa, < in morning.

Intense itching of the skin when undressing to go to bed.

* * * * *

There are three localities in which this remedy acts very markedly, viz.: Respiratory organs, bowels and skin. "Violent, incessant cough, dry and fatiguing, with very little or no expectoration, aggravated by pressure, talking, and especially by *inspiring cold air,* and at night." (Dunham.) There is perhaps no remedy under which the sensibility of the mucous membranes of the larynx and trachea become more exalted than this one. The patient must cover up the head in bed in order to protect these membranes from contact with the air, which immediately excites cough. Several other remedies, like *Phosphorus* and *Spongia,* have cough aggravated by breathing cold air, but none so markedly as *Rumex.* Going from warm room into cool air and vice versa. *Bryonia* and *Natrum carbonicum* have the opposite. The tickling that excites the cough may locate in the throat-pit, supra-sternal fossa, or down behind the sternum to stomach, where is often added a sensation of soreness or rawness. *(Caust.)* Again we have found it efficacious in cough, with stitching pain *through left lung just below left nipple. (Natrum sulph.)*

The diarrhœa of *Rumex* is similar to that of *Natrum sulph., Sulphur* and *Podophyllum,* in that it occurs in the morning, but it is a *brown* diarrhœa and is apt to be accompanied with, or an accompaniment of, the cough. On the skin it cures an eruption which is characterized by intense itching *when undressing to go to bed.* This eruption may be vesicular, like army or prairie itch, or may look like simple urticaria. Itching on undressing is also found under *Natrum sulphuricum* and *Oleander,* but with *Natrum* this itching is apt to be found in connection with jaundice or malarial symptoms. If we should get intense itching over the body, which was aggravated by warmth, especially *warmth of the bed,* we would think of *Mercurius solubilis* or *protoiodide.*

ARUM TRIPHYLLUM.

Raw, red, bloody surface of lips, nose, buccal cavity; patients pick and bore into them incessantly, though they are so sore and painful.

Hoarseness, with changing voice when exciting it; from high to low and vice versa.

Discharges generally very acrid or corrosive; exceptionally bland.

* * * * *

This is a very unique remedy. I do not know of one that stands so far apart from any and all others, and its peculiar and characteristic symptoms are capable of such remarkable verification in different diseases as would, or ought to, convince the most skeptical of the truth of *Similia Similibus Curantur,* etc.

Hering's "Guiding Symptoms" gives it in the best rendering. Let us quote a few of the best symptoms: *"Appearance of raw, bloody surface, on lips, buccal cavity, nose, etc." "Patients often pick and bore into the raw surfaces, though doing so gives great pain, and they scream with it but keep up the boring." (Hellebor. nig.)* There is also one other symptom not so well expressed in Hering, viz.: That these raw surfaces are very **red,** like a piece of fresh beefsteak in appearance. Notice that in Hering these symptoms of mouth, tongue and nose are given in connection with *Scarlatina* mainly. I want to say that they are also found in typhoid and typhus fevers. Whenever, in any disease, this red, raw condition of the mouth, nose and lips, at which the patient bores and picks, continually appears, give *Arum triphyllum.* Another important use of this remedy is in affections of the larynx and bronchia. Hoarseness or loss of voice, or voice uncontrollable; it breaks when trying to sing or speak in a high tone or key. This is often found in clergyman's sore throat, or in operatic singers. Aggravation of hoarseness from singing is also found under *Argentum nitricum, Arnica, Selenium, Phosphorus* and *Causticum.*

ARNICA MONTANA.

Bruised, sore feeling all over; bed feels too hard.

Head, or head and face hot; body and extremities cold.

Ecchymoses; as from bruises.

Stupor; answers, then falls back into stupor (fevers).

Taste and eructations and stool like rotten eggs.

Recent and remote affections from injuries, especially contusions or blows.

Hæmorrhages, the result of mechanical injuries.

* * * * *

This is the leading remedy for **bruises** and the results therefrom, and the symptoms—"*Weakness, weariness, sensation as of being bruised.*" "Felt as if bruised over the whole body," as found in the provings, explain the reason and the many cures it has made, even in the high and highest potencies, of both acute and chronic affections. The result of trauma is another evidence of the truth of our law of cure. One of the best characteristics is *"Everything on which he lies* seems too hard" *(Pyrogen.)*; he must keep changing his position to get relief. This is because of the sensation of *soreness as if bruised all over.*

Baptisia has—"Feels as if lying on a board; changes position, bed feels so hard, makes him feel sore and bruised."

Phytolacca has—"Feels sore all over from head to foot; muscles sore and stiff, can hardly move without groaning."

Rhus toxicod. has—*"Soreness in every muscle, which passes off during exercise; feels stiff and sore on first beginning to move."*

Ruta has—"All parts of the body on which he lies are painful as if bruised."

Here are five remedies which seem much alike, and others might be added, like *Staphisagria,* which has—"All the limbs are *sore* as if bruised, and as if there were no strength in them," and

China—*"He is sore all over,* in the joints, the bones, and the periosteum, as if they had been sprained, like a drawing, tearing, especially in the spine, the sacrum, the knees and thighs." Now to know thus far of these remedies would be of little use for therapeutic purposes, for it would be senseless to prescribe all of these remedies mixed together, and full as much so to prescribe one of them to the exclusion of all the rest without a good reason for so doing. Fortunately there is always a possibility of making choice between them, but it is not always easy. Take, for instance, *Arnica* and *Baptisia.* Both have the symptom of *sore bruised feeling.* Both have feeling as if the bed were *too hard.* Both have *stupor,* from which they can be aroused, but fall quickly back into it again. Both have a dark streak running through the tongue.

Both have a *deep red face,* and all these similarities often occur in the course of a typhoid fever. How are we to choose between them? *Look further.* If in addition to these symptoms the patient "tosses about the bed, reaching here and there, and in his delirium complaining that he cannot *get himself together,*" *Baptisia* is the remedy, or if the stool, urine and sweat are *extremely offensive,* it is *Baptisia.* If the stool and urine are passed unconsciously and there appear suggillations under the skin, *Arnica* is the remedy. Now here are only a few of the characteristic differences. There are others, and we must "watch out" for them. It is no harder to choose between these two remedies than it is to choose sometimes between *Hyoscyamus* and *Opium* in the same disease. Here is the place where the old physician might exhort the young as Paul did Timothy. "Study to show thyself approved, * * * a workman that needed not to be ashamed, rightly dividing the truth, etc." Such close prescribing is business of course, and is also **successful.**

If I came to a case that had the bruised sensation very markedly in connection with a diphtheritic throat I would not give *Arnica,* because it does not have that kind of throat; but *Phytolacca* has, and it has one other symptom of *Arnica,* viz.: *heat and redness of head and face, while the body and limbs are cool or cold.*

I have met many such cases of diphtheria, and if prescribed early *Phytolacca* cures without the aid of any other remedy. Again if I found a patient with the sore, bruised sensation, who was brought into that condition by getting wet while perspiring, or by lying on damp ground, or between damp sheets, or from a strain of the muscles, *Rhus toxicodendron* would be the remedy.

If in cases of actual injury I should find the bruise in the periosteum or bone, I should expect more benefit from *Ruta,* which seems to be better also than *Rhus tox.* in one kind of muscular strain, viz., strain of the ciliary muscles. I have often relieved sewing girls or students of pains in the eyes from this cause and have sometimes enabled them to lay off the glasses that had been prescribed by the opticians. It is much better to use this remedy in a weakened power of accommodation than to try and compensate for it with artificial lenses. Of course where the impaired vision is purely optical this cannot be done.

So we might go on to draw the diagnostic symptoms between all the various remedies having a similar symptom if we had time and space. But it would not be the best thing to do, for every physician should get in the habit of doing this for himself.

In addition to all that has been said about the great value of the *sore as if* bruised sensation of this remedy, it should always be remembered in affections, acute or chronic, which are the *result of trauma.* Among these are concussion; fracture of the skull with compression of the brain; headaches of long standing; meningitis; apoplexy; inflammation of the eyes with suggillations, or even retinal hæmorrhages, where it expedites the absorption of the blood clots, deafness, epistaxis, newly filled teeth, affections from blows on stomach or other viscera. I once cured a man who had suffered from what he and his physician had called dyspepsia for several years. He had been obliged to give up his business because he could not eat enough to support his strength. He had been told by his physician that he would never be well again and had given up hopes himself. This condition was caused by the kick of a horse upon the region of the stomach. A few doses of *Arnica* 200th cured him in a short time and he resumed his business. Now I will conclude *Arnica* with a few characteristics that are genuine, and have been, with me, of inestimable value.

"Stupor with involuntary discharge of fæces and urine."

"Fears being struck or touched by those coming towards him."

"Putrid smell from the mouth."

"Offensive eructations or flatus, smelling like rotten eggs."

"Bruised sore feeling in uterine region, cannot walk erect."

"Soreness of parts after labor prevents hæmorrhages or pyæmia."

"Cough; child cries before paroxysms, as if sore."

"While answering falls into a deep stupor before finishing."

"Head alone, or face alone, hot, rest of body cool."

"Many small boils, painful, one after another, extremely sore."

"Prevents suppuration and septicæmia and promotes absorption."

Arnica, although an old remedy, is not so often used as it should be in general practice.

HAMAMELIS VIRGINICA.

Venous hæmorrhages (very dark and clotted); veins full, enlarged and *sore* to touch.

* * * * *

Hamamelis Virginica is another remedy having the symptom *"soreness as if bruised"* in a marked degree, and which I did not mention when writing of *Arnica*. This soreness is sometimes found in rheumatism and *Hamamelis* has cured when *Arnica* failed. But one of the chief distinctions between these two remedies is that *Arnica* acts more upon the capillaries, causing their relaxation, whereby suggillations take place, while *Hamamelis* acts more upon the veins, which are very full, enlarged and **sore.** One author says:

"It is the *Aconite* of the veins."

From clinical use we know enough of the remedy to value it highly in varicosities of almost all kinds. *(Fluoric acid.)* It is here a powerful rival of *Pulsatilla*, but except the soreness of the veins we do not know of guiding symptoms for its use.

It has produced, in provings, severe hæmorrhages, and clinical use has defined the bleeding to be of very dark clotted, venous blood. There is no doubt of its power over such hæmorrhages, whether occurring from the nose, bowels, uterus, lungs or bladder. I have used it in every place with satisfaction. It is not a powerful poison and can be used low without bad effects. One of its best uses is in orchitis and inflammation of the spermatic veins, the provings markedly indicating its homœopathicity here. In hæmorrhages from the anus, whether from piles or typhoid fever, if the blood is of the above described appearance, *Hamamelis* is excellent.

Like *Arnica* and *Calendula, Hamamelis* has often seemed to act well as a local application. I am not in favor, generally, of using remedies in this way, unless it be for external injuries, which *are not diseases.*

COLOCYNTHIS.

Disinclined to talk, to see friends, impatient, easily offended, anger with indignation; colic or other complaints as a consequence.

Colic, terrible; they seek relief by *bending double* or pressing something hard against the abdomen.

Dysentery-like diarrhœa; renewed after least food or drink, often with the characteristic colic pains.

Frequent urging to urinate, scanty; urine sometimes thick, fœtid, viscid, jelly-like.

Crampy pain in sciatic nerve, from hip down posterior portion of thigh; > from hard pressure and from heat; < in repose, driving patient desperate.

Tendency to painful cramps, with all pains.

Modalities: < evening, anger; after eating; > from coffee; *bending double* and *hard pressure.*

* * * * *

No remedy produces more severe colic than this one, and no remedy cures more promptly.

Dr. T. L. Brown once said to me in substance: If I was disposed to be skeptical as to the power of the small dose to cure, *Colocynthis* would convince me, for I have so promptly cured severe colic in many cases, from a child to adults, and even in horses. Of course, every true Homœopath can respond *amen* to that.

The colic of *Colocynthis* is terrible, and is only bearable by *bending double,* or *pressing something hard against the abdomen.* He leans over chairs, the table or bed posts to get relief. This colic is neuralgic in character, and is often attended with vomiting and diarrhœa, which seems to be a result of the great pain more than any particular derangement of the stomach or bowels. We often find it in connection with dysentery. My experience has been that it does not, as a rule, occur in the first stage of the disease, but later, when the disease has not been fully controlled by *Aconite, Mercurius, Nux vomica* and that class of remedies, but has extended upward to the small intestines. The pains are of a *crampy* nature. The remedy that comes nearest to *Colocynth* for colic is *Magnesia phosphorica,* especially in colic in children. They both have the cramping pains, but the pains of *Magnesia phos.* are most relieved by hot applications like *Arsenicum.* Both *Colocynth* and *Magnesia phos.* are also equally efficacious for neuralgic affections in other localities, for instance, in sciatica and prosopalgia, and even uterine colic of a neuralgic nature, though in this latter affection *Magnesia phos.* leads. Remember the modalities, for upon the individualization depends the choice between them. *Chamomilla* and *Colocynth* resemble each other, in that both have colic from a fit of anger or other neuralgic affections from the same cause. *Chamomilla* succeeds in the colic of children, if there is much wind which distends the abdomen; the child tosses about in agony, but does not double up like *Colocynth.* Other symptoms often come in of course and help to choose between them. If both fail I have succeeded with

Magnesia phos. Staphisagria is also a remedy for colicky children, with disposition like *Colocynth* and *Chamomilla.* In such children the teeth grow black and decay early. Again the *Staphisagria* child is often troubled with sore eyelids. In such a case there is chronic tendency to colic and *Staphisagria* is sometimes the only remedy. *Veratrum album* also has colic, bending the patient double, similar to *Colocynth,* but the patient walks about for relief, or is much prostrated and has cold sweats, especially on the **forehead.** *Bovista* has colic relieved by bending double, after eating.

Dioscorea is a good remedy for *wind* colic. The pain begins right at the umbilicus, and then radiates all over the abdomen, and even to extremities *(Plumbum,* with walls retracted), and, unlike *Colocynth,* the pain is aggravated by bending forward and relieved by straightening the body out. *Stannum* is a colic remedy, and the only way the child is relieved is by being carried with the abdomen on the mother's shoulder. I have cured a case of this kind. It was a very obstinate case of long standing in a weakly child. The usual remedies had signally failed. *Jalapa* cured one of the most obstinate cases of long standing that I ever saw, the child crying almost continually day and night for weeks. There was in this case diarrhœa all the time. Both colic and diarrhœa were very quickly cured. I have lengthened out these indications for colic remedies in connection with *Colocynth* because there is great temptation, especially with young physicians, to give "paregoric," soothing syrups, etc., because it is not always easy to find the homœopathic remedy. I never have to do it, and I cure my cases. Of course there are many other remedies for the same trouble, and all have their particular *guiding symptoms.*

Colocynth not only cures neuralgic affections originating in the abdominal region, but has been very efficacious in facial and sciatic neuralgia. The pains in these localities, like those in the abdomen, are of a decidedly crampy nature. Here also *Magnesia phos.* often disputes place with *Colocynth,* in the fact of its also having characteristically the same kind of pains. The relief from heat, although found under both remedies, is most marked under *Magnesia phos.* In sciatica, the pain of *Colocynth* extends from the hip down the posterior portion of the thigh into the popliteal fossa (>. lying on painful side, *Bryonia). Phytolacca,* the pains run down the *outer* side of the thigh. These two remedies, with *Gnaphalium,* are the leading remedies for the treatment of this most distressing malady. But of course other remedies often have to be given, and the indications are sometimes found outside of the local trouble, as they are in many other diseases. One of the worst cases of sciatica I ever saw was cured with *Arsenicum album,* on the indications, worse at midnight, especially from 1 to 3 o'clock; burning pains; and the only temporary relief during the paroxysms, was from bags of hot, dry salt applied to the painful part.

The lady was a sister of Charles Saunders, of New York, of school reader fame, who was himself a cripple from allopathically treated sciatica. She, after suffering indescribable agony for six weeks, was cured rapidly and permanently with a dose of Jenichen's 8m. of *Arsenicum album.* So we see again that no remedy and no particular set of remedies can be entirely relied upon, but the indicated *one* can. These are the chief uses of *Colocynth.*

PETROLEUM.

Eczemas, on scalp, behind ears, scrotum, anus, hands, feet, legs; hands chap and bleed; *all < in winter;* get better in summer.

Diarrhœa preceded by colic, *only in the day-time.*

Headache, or heaviness like lead in the occiput; sometimes with nausea on vomiting; < by motion, as in riding in boat or carriage.

* * * * *

One of our best anti-psoric remedies. The eruptions that it causes and cures are very similar in appearance to those of *Graphites.* They appear on different parts of the body, as scalp, behind ears, on scrotum, female genitals, hands, feet and legs, etc.

There is one very marked characteristic symptom that guides to this remedy out of a large list having similar eruptions, and that is that the eruption is worse during the winter season *(Aloe, Alumina, Psorinum).* There is no other remedy that has this so prominently. The hands chap, crack and bleed, and are all covered with *eczema during the winter and get well in summer.* I have cured a case of eczema of the lower legs of twenty years' standing, always worse in winter, with one prescription of the 200th. I have cured chapped hands the same way. I once had a very obstinate case of chronic diarrhœa, but as soon as the fact that he had eczema of the hands in winter came to light I cured him quickly of the whole trouble with *Petroleum* 200th. Chilblains *(Agaricus)*, which are moist, and itch and burn much in cold weather, are also cured by it. *Petroleum* also has a symptom similar to *Hepar sulphuris*, viz., the slightest scratch or abrasion of the skin suppurates. You remember that *Hepar sulphuris* is also worse in cold weather or cold air. *Petroleum* has headache in the *occiput, which is as heavy as lead,* also vertigo in the occiput.

Again, *Petroleum* is one of our best remedies for seasickness. In this it resembles *Cocculus.* Another curious symptom is cracking of the joints. This is like *Causticum.* Both of these remedies are valuable in chronic rheumatism, especially where this symptom is present. *Petroleum* has, with *Chelidonium* and *Anacardium,* a symptom, pain in stomach, *relieved* by eating. Again it is valuable in diarrhœa and dysentery, which is worse *during the day.* *Petroleum* deserves to be classed with the leading anti-psorics, such as *Sulphur, Graphites, Causticum* and *Lycopodium.*

HYDRASTIS CANADENSIS.

Pain and very *weak, faint, gone feeling* in stomach, which is sometimes actually sunken.

Affections of the mucous membranes, where there is a *viscid stringy discharge;* stomach, bronchi, uterus, etc.

Chronic constipation, that is remarkable for its absence of any other symptoms.

* * * * *

This is a more celebrated remedy with the eclectics than with us. They especially value it for what they call its *tonic* properties and its specific action in the way of healing ulcerations in mucous membranes. We have also found it useful in such cases, but we have more decided indications for its use. For instance, in stomach troubles, where they attribute its curative powers to its tonic properties, we find it especially valuable only when we have this symptom present: "Dull aching pain in stomach which causes a very *weak, faint, gone feeling* in the epigastrium." The stomach is sometimes actually sunken (objectively). There are two other remedies that have this symptom to a degree almost equal, viz., *Sepia* and *Ignatia,* but *Sepia* is generally in connection with uterine affections while *Ignatia* is purely nervous. *Hydrastis* is a good remedy for chronic constipation. E. M. Hale taught that it must be used in tincture or very low dilution. I have found it most efficacious in the 200th (B. & T.). I once cured a case that was of years' standing, had worn cathartics out, and all the way she could live (her words) was to swallow a spoonful of whole flaxseed with every meal. I have used it in infantile constipation successfully, and it is most useful when all other symptoms aside from the constipation are conspicuous for their *absence.* Again, *Hydrastis* is indicated in affections of mucous membranes where there is a *viscid* stringy discharge. This is like *Kali bichromicum,* but the other symptoms of these two remedies are not much alike. Chronic bronchitis of old debilitated people is sometimes greatly relieved by it; also leucorrhœa, with the stringy discharge as above described.

CAMPHOR.

Great coldness of the external surface, with sudden and complete prostration of the vital force; collapse.

The patient objects to being covered, notwithstanding the objective coldness; throws off all the covering.

Pains disappear when thinking of them; exceedingly sensitive to cold air.

* * * * *

The great characteristic around which the whole action of *Camphor* seems to revolve is: *"Great coldness of the external surface, with sudden and complete prostration of the vital forces."* It is no wonder Hahnemann headed his trio *(Camphor, Cuprum* and *Hellebore)* of cholera remedies with *Camphor.* If we were to sum up the same condition in one word it would be *collapse.* No remedy comes nearer to *Camphor* than the last of the trio, viz., *Veratrum album,* but *Camphor* has the collapse with painless stool or even no stool at all, while *Veratrum* has the collapse seemingly as a consequence of the very profuse evacuations of stomach and bowels. Both have great external coldness, but *Veratrum* has a very marked appearance of *cold sweat* upon the hippocratic face, especially **forehead.** *Cuprum* leads the trio, when the *cramp* in stomach and extremities is the most prominent symptom. These remedies are indicated when these characteristic symptoms appear, not only in cholera, but in any disease. There is one peculiarity in the coldness of *Camphor,* viz., *the patient will not be covered, or objects to it, no matter how objectively cold he is. Secale* coldness or collapse is exactly like this, and even in gangrena senilis it proves a great remedy on the same indications. The signal success of Dr. Rubini, of Naples, in treating five hundred and ninety-two cases of cholera with *Camphor* verified the prediction of Hahnemann beyond question.

Collapse with cold surface and aversion to heat may come on in retrocedent exanthema, or in the later stage of so-called cholera infantum, in pneumonia, or capillary bronchitis, from exposure to intense cold or traumatic shock. Indeed it does not matter from what cause except death. *Camphor* is the first remedy to be thought of, and according to susceptibility or strength of the patient the dose must be varied from tincture to highest potency.

THUJA OCCIDENTALIS.

Hahnemann's chief anti-sycotic.

Proliferations or pathological vegetations: condylomata, polypi, warts, sycotic excrescences, etc.

Bad effects following vaccination; never well since.

Especially suited to the treatment of ailments following suppressed gonorrhœa.

Urethritis in sycotic patients, which *Cannabis sat.* does not relieve; stream split, cutting after urination; discharge thick.

Sweat only on uncovered parts.

Modalities: < cold, damp air (hydrogenoid); after vaccination, excessive tea drinking, extension of limbs; > drawing up limbs.

* * * * *

Hahnemann recognized three miasms (as he called them) which complicated the treatment of all diseases. They were syphilis, psora and sycosis.

Sulphur was his chief anti-psoric, *Mercury* his anti-syphilitic and *Thuja* his anti-sycotic.

Whatever may be said against his theories along this line, certain it is that these three remedies do correct certain *states* of the system which seem to obstruct the curative action of other seemingly well-indicated remedies.

Thuja, for instance, cures or so changes the existing conditions that other remedies cure which could not do so before *Thuja* was given. Many diseases of various forms come under this rule. Whenever warts, condylomata, fig-warts, etc., which come in consequence of gonorrhœal affections, *especially suppressed gonorrhœa,* are found in any case we think of *Thuja.* For instance, a case of enuresis had resisted many seemingly indicated remedies, until the hands were discovered to be covered with warts, when a few drops of *Thuja* cured. Of course, the curative power of *Thuja* is not confined to sycosis, but can, like other remedies, cure when symptoms indicate it where no sycotic element in the case is apparent. Nevertheless, its chief power is manifested in those cases in which this miasm is unmistakably present. It is astonishing what widely different and varied forms of disease will be so modified by this miasm as to call for anti-sycotic treatment.

As *Sulphur* is not the only anti-psoric, or *Mercury* the only anti-syphilitic, so *Thuja* is not the only anti-sycotic; for *Nitric acid, Staphisagria, Sabina, Cinnabaris* and other remedies are sometimes called for, either before or after *Thuja,* or even when *Thuja* is not at all the remedy. But on the whole, *Thuja,* perhaps, as Hahnemann taught, stands at the head of the list. *Thuja, Agaricus* and *Lycopodium* have been called over-proven remedies; but when we realize the wide range of diseases which are complicated by the sycotic element in them we are not so sure of the over-proving of the *Thuja,* for it could not so benefit such a wide range of complaints if it could not produce a wide range of symptoms in its pathogenesis. This is also true of *Sulphur* and *Mercury*. *Thuja* has some very peculiar symptoms of the mind which have been verified.

"Fixed ideas, as if a strange person were at his side; as if the soul and body were separated; that the body and particularly the *limbs were made of glass, and will readily* break; as if a living animal were in the abdomen; tells about being under the influence of a superior power." Insane women will not be touched or approached. Aside from these curious mind symptoms we have: *"Headaches of sycotic origin, with various symptoms; white dandruff, hair falling out or grows slowly and splits; eyelids bear styes, chalazæ, tarsal tumors, or condylomata; ears inflame, discharge pus, or grow polypi. Nose discharges thick, green mucus like Pulsatilla, or scabs are formed in it; warts on the outside of the nose or eruptions on its wings; face has a greasy or shiny look; teeth begin to decay at the roots as soon as they come, the crowns remaining sound. Ranula under the tongue, or varicosities in the mouth or throat; a great deal of croaking, rumbling and grumbling in the abdomen, as if of an animal crying; abdomen puffed and big, protruding here and there as if from the arm of a fœtus, or of something alive; constipation of hard black balls; chronic; stools large; and stool recedes after being partially expelled (Sanic., Silic.); or diarrhœa forcibly expelled, copious gurgling like water from a bung hole of a barrel; diarrhœa, especially from the effects of vaccination; anus fissured or surrounded with condylomata* (see *Antim. crud., Graphites* and *Silicea*) ; *ovarian troubles; asthma; nails brittle, distorted, crumbling, misshapen or soft; warts, condylomata, bleeding fungous growths; nævi; epithelioma, and many other affections in sycotic subjects."* Finally don't forget to look for the three miasms in all obstinate cases, whether acute or chronic.

STAPHISAGRIA.

Cross, ugly, scrawny, pot-bellied children; subject to colic; < after food or drink. Extreme hunger even when stomach is full of food.

Styes, nodosities, chalazæ, on eyelids, one after another, sometimes ulcerating.

Burning in the urethra when *not* urinating; very sensitive to slightest mental impressions; least action or harmless word offends.

Bad effects from sexual abuse; mind dwelling continually on sexual subjects.

Teeth decay early in children; cannot be kept clean.

Sensation as if stomach and abdomen were hanging down, relaxed; craving for tobacco.

* * * * *

"Great indignation about things done by others or himself, grieving about the consequences, continual concern about the future."

"Throws tnings away indignantly, or pushes them away on the table."

"Children are ill humored and cry for things which after getting they petulantly throw away; worse in the morning."

"Very sensitive to the least impression, the least word that seems wrong hurts her very much."

"Hypochondriasis, apathy; weak memory; caused by unmerited insults, sexual excess, or by persistently dwelling on sexual subjects."

"Ailments from indignation and vexation or reserved displeasure; sleeplessness."

I quote all these symptoms in order to impress the reader with the value of *Staphisagria* as a mind remedy. *Chamomilla* is often used when Staphisagria would be better, especially for children, and *Nux vomica* is sometimes used for adults the same way.

Phosphoric acid is sometimes used for the results of onanism when *Staphisagria* would do better. You will also notice that this remedy may be indicated for the *effects* of anger instead of *Chamomilla* or *Colocynth.* Here are *Chamomilla, Nux vomica, Cina, Colocynth* and *Staphisagria* standing very close to each other for *cross, ugly, irritable subjects,* and there are few cases that one or the other will not fit. Then we have *Phosphoric acid, Natrum muriaticum, Anacardium, Aurum* and *Staphisagria* for the apathetic or hypochondriacal.

Staphisagria has a sensation as if the *stomach were hanging down relaxed. Ipecac* and *Tabacum* have the *same sensation.* Sometimes it is described as a sinking sensation. It also has the same sensation in the abdomen; feels as though it would drop, wants to support it with the hands. Colic, which might be styled *"habitual colic,"* in *scrawny, ugly, pot-bellied children,* and especially if they suffer much with their teeth, *which turn black, with tender, spongy gums,* which are sensitive and painful.

Now when we add dysentery to the foregoing, we see that *Staphisagria* acts along the whole intestinal tract. *Staphisagria* is one of the remedies which has a marked characteristic aggravation *after the least food or drink.*

This remedy has a very peculiar symptom, which appeared in the provings, and which I have verified, viz., "burning in the urethra when *not* urinating." While urinating the burning ceased. We have plenty of remedies for burning before, during and after urination, but *Staphisagria* is the only one having this burning all the time between the acts of urinating. In addition to being one of the best remedies for onanism, it is one of the best for affections of the prostate gland in old men, with frequent urination and dribbling of urine afterwards. A very common and troublesome symptom found in connection with troubles of the genital organs, both male and female, is *backache,* which is very peculiar, in that it is *always worse at night in bed and in the morning before rising.* It is a very efficacious remedy here. *Staphisagria* is a good skin remedy. It cures both dry and moist eruptions. The eczema of *Staphisagria* oozes an acrid moisture from under the scabs, and new vesicles form from the contact of the exudation. They generally itch very severely, and one peculiarity is, that when the itching is relieved by scratching in one place it immediately appears in another. The eczema is often on the head, on the sides around the ears, but the most marked action is in the eyelids. Hering's card expresses it thus: *"Styes, nodosities, chalazæ on eyelids, one after another, sometimes ulcerating."* There is only one remedy that can compare with this one in chronic blepharitis, and that is *Graphites* (see also *Borax).* It has some remarkable cures of cross, puny, sickly children, having the teeth and eyelid symptoms. Not only were the local troubles remedied, but the *patient was cured* every way.

I think of but two other uses of *Staphisagria,* which I wish to mention. First, its use in the cure of condylomata, figwarts, or cauliflower-like excrescences. In one case, with the 200th of this remedy, I removed an excrescence on the perineum of a lady in which the growth was an inch long and the appearance was exactly in appearance like cauliflower. It rapidly disappeared under the action of this remedy and never returned. *Second,* its use for *incised wounds.* It is the best remedy here, where there is a clean cut as after surgical operations. It is to such wounds what *Calendula* is to lacerations, *Arnica, Hamamelis, Ledum* and *Sulph. acid* for bruises, *Rhus tox., Calcarea ostrearum* and *Nux vomica* for strains, *Calcarea phosphorica* and *Symphytum* for fractures.

COLCHICUM AUTUMNALE.

The smell of food cooking nauseates to faintness.

Fall dysenteries when the days are warm and nights cold; stools shreddy and bloody, like scrapings.

Swelling of joints moving from one place to another; they are often *dropsical* and pit on pressure; < in extremes of wet and cold, or warm and dry (Kent).

* * * * *

This remedy has one of the most positive and reliable characteristic symptoms in the whole Materia Medica, and one which cannot be accounted for from any pathological standpoint that I know of. I mention this here because there is a seeming desire on the part of some to base all their prescriptions on pathological indications. I have no objections to their doing so if they can and succeed in curing their patients. But I claim full recognition for the value of those subjective, sensational symptoms and the modalities which cannot be accounted for. Indeed, I feel quite sure that the well-verified subjective symptoms are oftener to be relied upon in curing our patients than all the pathological conditions we know. Now for the symptom. *"The smell of food cooking nauseates to faintness."* To illustrate the value of this symptom I will give a case of my own practice; it was also my first experience with a potency as high as the 200th. Patient was a lady, seventy-five years of age, who was suddenly seized with sickness at the stomach and vomiting of blood in large quantities; then bloody stools followed, which were at first profuse, then became small and of bloody mucus. There was great tenesmus and pain in the bowels. *Aconite, Mercurius, Nux vomica, Ipecacuanha, Hamamelis* and *Sulphur,* all tried as well as I knew how to select them at that time, but no relief came, and at the end of twelve days my patient was rapidly going down and it looked to me as though she must die. She had become so weak that she could not lift her head from the pillow. By actual count the number of stools passed on cloths in the bed was sixty-five, in twenty-four hours, the pains, number of passages and all symptoms were aggravated from sundown to sunrise (this is another characteristic of *Colchicum).*

Now during all this sickness this patient had been so nauseated and faint at the smell of cooking food that they had been obliged to keep the doors closed between her bedroom and the kitchen, which was two large rooms away. I was not so well acquainted with Materia Medica then as now, and while I did not overlook the symptom did not know of any remedy that had it. But I had my Lippe text-book of Materia Medica in my carriage and I went out and got it and sat down by the bedside; determined to find that peculiar and persistent symptom and "fight it out on that line if it took all summer." I began at *Aconite,* and looked at the stomach symptoms of every remedy, until, the first time I remembered ever having noticed it, there it stood in plain English under *Colchicum.* Then I looked in my medicine case for the remedy. None there, and I was four miles from home. I had a box of Dunham's 200ths under my carriage seat that had been there for over a year, but which I had never used for want of confidence in high potencies. It was the best I could do for the present, so I dissolved a few pellets in a half-glass of cold water, and directed to give one teaspoonful after every passage of the bowels. On my way home I stopped my horse two or three times to turn around and go back and give that poor suffering woman some medicine. I felt guilty, but I said to myself this is Lippe's *Materia Medica,* and these are Carrol Dunham's potencies, and here is a clean cut indication for its administration, and the other symptoms do not counter-indicate. Well, I got home. But I started early the next morning to try and make amends for my rashness (if the patient was not dead) of yesterday. Imagine my surprise as I stepped into the sick-room when my patient slowly turned her head upon the pillow and said, with a smile, "Good morning, Doctor." I had been met with a groan several past mornings. I felt faint myself then. I dropped into a chair by the bedside and remarked, "You are feeling better." "Oh, yes, Doctor." "How much of that last medicine did you take?" "Two doses." "What!" "Two doses; I only had two more stools after you left." "Don't you have any more pain?" "Pain stopped like that" (putting her hands together) "and I feel well except weakness." She took no more medicine, quickly recovered, and was perfectly well for five years after, and finally died at eighty years of age. I never got over that surprise. Convinced against my will, but *not* of the same opinion still.

Now I fell to experimenting with the 200th in downright earnest. I have cured many cases since of autumnal dysentery with this remedy on the same indication, and with the same potency. I have also cured a very severe case of typhlitis (now called appendicitis, for which they so often operate with more deaths than were ever known before the operation became popular) on the same symptom, which was markedly present in the case. Bright's disease, a bad case, was also cured by it. Rheumatism, gout and dropsies have been cured, this symptom being present, and so I have been at length in giving my experience with this remedy in order to prove three things:

1st. That we should not be influenced by prejudice.

2d. That subjective symptoms are most valuable.

3d. That the 200ths do act and *cure*.

Of course, there are other valuable symptoms besides the one upon which we have laid such particular stress. For instance, *Colchicum* has two symptoms that are opposite one to the other, viz.: Violent *burning* and *icy coldness* in the stomach. These opposites are often found in the abdomen. Again, it is sometimes indicated in autumnal dysentery, the white or bloody mucous discharges having a *shreddy appearance,* looking as if the mucous membrane had been scraped off the intestines, with great tenesmus. *Cantharis* has these stools, looking like scrapings, as prominently as *Colchicum,* but with *Cantharis* the pain and tenesmus implicate the urinary organs at the same time. *Colocynth* also has such stools, but the doubling-up, colicky pains distinguish it from both the others. *Colchicum* has great meteoristic distention of the abdomen. It is in the 200th potency a good remedy for the bloating of cows that have eaten too much green clover. In dyspepsia, when there is complaint of burning or sensation of coldness in the stomach, and much gas in stomach or abdomen, or both, *Colchicum* is excellent, taking sometimes preference over *Carbo vegetabilis, China* or *Lycopodium.*

Colchicum is always set down in the text-books for rheumatism, articular, migrating and gouty, and I have often tried it, but never with anything like the success of our other rheumatic remedies. I have been greatly disappointed in it here. Perhaps I did not use it *low* enough. It is also said to be a good remedy for weakness or sudden prostration, but here I have no personal experience with it. However, if in any of these troubles, or others, I should find its prime characteristic present I should certainly give it and confidently expect good results.

CROCUS SATIVUS.

Spasmodic contractions and twitchings of single sets of muscles.

Hæmorrhages from different parts; blood black, viscid,

clotted, forming into long black strings, from the bleeding orifice.

Changeable disposition; laughs, sings, jumps, wants to kiss everybody, or again cries, gets mad, abuses everybody, etc.

Sensation as of something hopping or moving about in stomach, abdomen, uterus or chest.

* * * * *

This remedy has three different spheres of usefulness in homœopathic therapeutics.

1st. In hæmorrhages from different parts. The blood is *black, viscid, clotted, and forming itself into long black strings from the bleeding orifice.* It makes no difference whether from the nose, uterus, lungs or stomach, if the blood is of this nature *Crocus* must be given. *(Mercur. sol.,* the blood hangs from the nose like an icicle.)

2d. In hysterical conditions in which there is great changeableness of the mental symptoms.

The patient is alternately cheerful or depressed. In the former state she will sing, dance, jump, laugh and whistle, love and want to kiss everybody. In the latter she will cry, get into a rage, abuse her friends, and then repent it, etc.

Crocus, for these alternate mental states, resembles *Aconite, Ignatia* and *Nux moschata,* but with *Crocus* there is another peculiar and persistent symptom, viz., *sensation as of something moving, or hopping about in the stomach, abdomen, uterus or chest.* Often this sensation of movement is so positive that the patient mistakes it for the movement of a fœtus, and is sure she is in a family way. If the mind symptoms above described are present, don't be too ready to promise a baby, but give a dose of *Crocus* and await developments.

3d. *Crocus* is one of our remedies for chronic affections. *There are twitchings of single sets of muscles (Ignatia* and *Zinc.), twitchings of eyelids especially.* These twitchings are very common in hysterical subjects, and there are many remedies for them, so that one could not of course prescribe on that alone. There are, however, remedies which are suited to hysteria and also other nervous diseases, in which twitchings are very prominent and *Crocus* is one of them.

BORAX VENETA.

Dread of downward motion; child jumps and cringes or cries when laying it down; also very sensitive to noises.

Aphthous sore mouth; greenish stools day and night; mouth very hot.

Pain in right pectoral region; cough with expectoration of an *offensive, herby taste.*

* * * * *

This remedy, although an old one, is not universally appreciated. Its action upon the nervous system is very marked. In the first place it manifests itself in what is called nervousness in regard to *noises,* to which the patient is very sensitive. Almost any noise, as a cough, a sneeze, rustling of a newspaper, a cry, distant shot, etc. *Belladonna* is sometimes given for this starting at noises, when *Borax* would do better. Then there is another very peculiar nervous symptom, viz., *fear of falling, from downward motion (Gelsem., Sanicula).* The child cries out and clings to the nurse when she attempts to lay it down in the cradle. Carrying it down stairs has the same effect. It will scream and cling to the nurse as long as the downward motion continues. Adults get the same symptom. Will not sit in a rocking chair, or ride on horseback, or on the waves, or swing, or go coasting, because of this dread of downward motion. There is only one other remedy having this symptom that I know of, and that is *Gelsemium,* and so far I think that this has only appeared in intermittent fever.

A child may be sleeping quietly and awake suddenly screaming and holding on to the sides of the cradle, without an apparent cause for so doing, or it may start from sleep clinging to the nurse as if frightened. In such cases we might think of *Apis mellifica, Belladonna, Cina, Stramonium,* etc., but don't prescribe on the one symptom. Look at the child's mouth and if you should find an *aphthous sore mouth* it would settle it pretty surely for *Borax.* Then, again, *Borax* has a very strong action as a general remedy, even domestic, from "way back," and has been prescribed without rhyme or reason until the homœopaths took it and found its exact place. Now the choice has to be made between it and *Mercurius, Hydrastis, Sulphur* and *Sulphuric acid,* etc.

It is not necessary to draw the line between the different remedies here, but I will say that the sore mouth itself is only *one symptom* in every case. The rest are found outside the local affection and often have more to do with the final choice of the remedy. The nervous symptoms already mentioned are "pointers" for *Borax.* Not only upon the mucous membranes of the mouth is this action of *Borax* notable, but upon every other one. The *eye-*

lashes become gummy and stick together, or turn inward. The ears discharge. I cured a case of otorrhœa of fourteen years' standing with this remedy.

Dry crusts form in the nose and re-form if removed. *Greenish stools day and night, with aphthæ.* The infant cries when urinating or before, showing an inflamed condition of the urethra. If the crying spells before urinating should be followed with a deposit of sand in the diaper or vessel, *Lycopodium* or *Sarsaparilla* would be thought of.

The mucous membranes of the respiratory organs are also affected: There is cough, and expectoration of an *offensive herby taste.* Then we have decided pleuritis in the chest, in the right pectoral region.

Borax has also white, *albuminous, starchy leucorrhœa,* quite profuse, and with a sensation of warm water running down. These altogether show the action of *Borax* upon the mucous membranes. Like *Chamomilla, Hepar sulphuris* and *Silicea, Borax* has ulcerations of the skin from slight injuries, which suppurate.

EUPATORIUM PERFOLIATUM.

Painful soreness of eyeballs; coryza; aching in every bone; prostration in epidemic of influenza (La Grippe).

Deep hard achings as if in the *bones,* with sore, bruised feeling all over, back, arms, wrists, legs.

Vomiting of bile between chill and heat. Chill 7 to 9 A. M.

Hoarseness in the morning, with soreness in chest when coughing; holds it with his hands.

* * * * *

When writing upon *Arnica,* I there compared several remedies which have a sensation as if bruised. This remedy might also have been mentioned there, as it has *"Bruised feeling as if broken, all over the body." (Arnica, Bellis, Pyrogen.)* The bruised feeling of *Eupatorium* is accompanied with a *deep hard aching,* as if in the *bones.*

Let us quote some of the symptoms illustrating: *"Intense aching in the limbs and back as if the bones were broken." "Aching in the bones of the extremities, with soreness of the flesh; soreness of the bones." "Soreness and aching of the arms and forearms; painful soreness in both wrists as if broken or dislocated." "Soreness and aching of lower limbs; stiffness and general soreness when rising to walk." "Calves of the legs feel as if they had been beaten." "Aching pains as if in the bones, with moaning."* These symptoms are all characteristic and may be found in influenza, bilious or intermittent fever, bronchitis, especially of the aged, and many other diseases. This is what gave the popular name "bone-set" to *Eupatorium,* because on account of the severe aching, as if the bones were broken, that occurred in an epidemic of intermittent fever this was the remedy that cured, or "set the bones." The epidemic was called *break-bone fever.* Of course this curative property of the drug was then discovered by accident, but abundant proving and verification have demonstrated the homœopathicity of such cures. So with *Apis* in dropsies. If this remedy has no curative properties other than it has for intermittent it would still remain a priceless boon to Homœopathy. It cures a kind of intermittent for which the great anti-periodic (Quinine) of the old school can do little or nothing. Three characteristics stand out prominently, to indicate the cases in which it is appropriate:

1st. As to time of chill—7 to 9 A. M.

2d. The intense aching in the bones before the chill.

3d. Vomiting of bile between chill and heat.

There are, of course, other symptoms which may appear in a *Eupatorium* case, but these three are a sure guide, and many authentic cures corroborate the genuineness. This remedy is also very useful in diseases of the respiratory organs. In the so-called la grippe of recent years it has proven in my hands very valuable; the "aching all over as if in the bones" being the leading symptom.

It also has *hoarseness in the morning,* like *Causticum,* but while *Causticum* has more *burning* and rawness *Eupatorium* has more *soreness* in the *chest; Ranunculus bulb.* has pain in the chest when walking, turning, from touch, or weather changing; when coughing has to support the chest with the hands, it hurts so *(Bryonia, Drosera, Kreosot., Natrum sul., Sepia).* Both remedies have aching in the bones especially in influenza or la grippe, but *Eupatorium* the most. If either of these remedies fails to cure the hoarseness, *Sulphur* will often complement them. Altogether, *Eupatorium* is to be remembered in *many diseases* having these characteristic symptoms. *Eupatorium* is especially adapted to *worn* out constitutions of old people or inebriates. *Bryonia* is a near analogue, having *free sweat,* but pains keep patient quiet, while *Eupatorium* has scanty sweat, but pains make the patient restless.

EUPATORIUM PURPUREUM.

From the provings made by Dr. Dresser and his wife this remedy ought to be a good one for urinary diseases. And Dr. Hughes says: "The drug has become my favorite remedy for vesical irritability in women." I have not yet tried it in such cases; but I have done some good work with it in intermittents, when the chill *began in the small of the back and spread from there up and downward,* which is as near a keynote as any I know for its use. Like the *Eupatorium perfoliatum* there are *bone pains* present. A lady who had lived near a marsh or swamp for seven years never had any appearance of malarial symptoms while living there, but after she came away they developed and were unyielding to the usual Quinine treatment. In fact, it utterly failed to do more than suppress for a short time when it would return and in an intensified form. On the above indications she was quickly and permanently cured by *Eupatorium purpureum* 200th.

Capsicum seems to resemble this remedy, both in the chills beginning in the back and the vesical irritability, but the *Capsicum* chill begins exactly between the shoulders, while *Eupatorium* begins in the dorsal or lumbar region.

Capsicum has violent chill, with general coldness of the body. *Eupatorium purp.,* violent shaking with little coldness of the body. *Eupatorium purp., Eupatorium perf.* and *Capsicum* all have bone pains before the chill, but *Eupatorium perf.* the strongest.

CAPSICUM.

Burning pains, especially in mucous membranes, or *smarting,* as from red pepper, on the parts.

Cough with pains in distant parts as head, bladder, knees, legs, etc.

Chill or shuddering *after every drink;* begins between the shoulders and spreads all over.

* * * * *

Capsicum is also a good remedy for dysentery or the later stage of gonorrhœa, or in throat complaints, when there is great *burning* in the mucous membrane of the affected part. In short, it is a remedy to be remembered in all affections, accompanied with **burning** of mucous membranes in any locality. The characteristic burning is not like that of *Arsenicum,* but feels as if **red pepper** *had been applied to the parts;* nor is it relieved by heat applied, as is that of *Arsenic.* *Capsicum* has pain in head when coughing as if it would burst. I cured a very bad case of years' standing; the patient would cry out and grasp head with both hands at every cough. It finally became so bad that he had to lie in bed, because the hurt was so much < when sitting. *Capsicum* cured very quickly. Other remedies having similar < are *Bryonia, Natrum mur., Squilla, Sulphur.*

Capsicum also has pain in distant parts on coughing, such as bladder, knees, legs, etc.

Chilliness or shuddering *after every drink.*

Chill begins *between shoulders* and spreads.

Lack of reaction especially fat people.

SPONGIA TOSTA.

Croupy cough; sounds like a saw driven through a board; < on awakening out of sleep.

Awakens out of sleep with a sense of suffocation, with violent loud cough, great alarm, agitation, anxiety and difficult respiration.

Cough < talking, reading, singing, swallowing, lying with head low.

* * * * *

This is not a remedy of very wide range, so far as yet known, but is of such marked utility within its range that we could not afford to lose it. Its action upon the respiratory organs is first to be considered. It first attacks the larynx, extends from there to the trachea, bronchial tubes and into the air cells of the lungs themselves. Next to *Aconite* it is the remedy oftenest indicated in croup. The cough is dry and sibilant, or *sounds like a saw driven through a pine board,* each cough corresponding to a thrust of the saw. Croup often comes on after exposure to dry, cold winds. It generally comes on in the evening, with high fever, excitement and fearfulness. For this cause and these symptoms *Aconite* is the first remedy, and in the 30th or 200th cures a great majority of cases without the aid of any other remedy. But if after a few doses, or a reasonable time, it does not alleviate, and the case continues to grow worse, and the paroxysms of cough and suffocation come on oftener, and especially on *awakening out of sleep, Spongia* is generally the next remedy.

I live in a croupy climate and district, and after experimenting for thirty years, first with the low, then with the higher preparations, affirm that the 200th potency of this remedy does better work in croup than the lower preparations. I often give either of these remedies *(Aconite* or *Spongia)*, according to indications, as often as once in fifteen minutes in watery solutions until amelioration, and then lengthen the intervals between doses according to amelioration. After the croup becomes loose, but still retaining some of its croupy sound, *Hepar sulphuris* comes in, especially if inclined to get worse after midnight or in the morning hours. If the case inclines to relapse, or gets a little more croupy every evening, *Phosphorus* will often finish the cure. In the laryngitis or bronchitis of adults, *Spongia* is as useful as it is in the case of croup in children. There is a *great hoarseness, some soreness and burning, and the cough is worse on talking, reading, singing or swallowing.* I often find it particularly useful after *Belladonna* has improved the sore throat which often precedes the laryngeal or bronchial trouble, and which is generally brought on by colds so often contracted here in our northern climate.

In chronic affections of the respiratory organs, which may finally lead to consumption, *Spongia* vies with *Phosphorus, Sanguinaria* and *Sulphur.* There is soreness, burning, rawness and heaviness in the chest, while the cough is worse in the evening, from cold air, talking, singing or moving, and better from eating and drinking warm things. I will not attempt to give all the symptoms for its use in respiratory diseases, but proceed at once to its remarkable action upon the *heart.* I have never done better work with any remedy in valvular disease than with *Spongia.* *"Awakes out of sleep from a sense of suffoca-*

tion, with violent, loud cough, great alarm, agitation, anxiety and difficult respiration" is a key-note, and is frequently met in valvular affections. No remedy, not even *Lachesis,* can do better here. Not only are these paroxysms relieved or stopped, but valvular murmurs of years' standing have *disappeared* under the action of *Spongia. Cannot lie with head low* is characteristic, also *sleep into the paroxysm (Lachesis).*

The dry, chronic, sympathetic cough of organic heart disease is oftener and more permanently relieved by this remedy than by *Naja. Spongia* is also a good remedy for goitre, with sense of suffocation after sleep.

CHIMAPHILA UMBELLATA.

I have had some valuable experience with this remedy in cystitis. It has made some fine cures where there were *great quantities of ropy mucus in the urine.* There may be strangury or not in such cases. There is one symptom to which I wish to call attention, because it indicates that this remedy may become very useful in prostatic troubles, and is found under only one other remedy that I know of, viz., *Cannabis Indica.* These prostatic troubles are very serious ones, and anything that can contribute to their successful treatment is valuable. The symptom is—"Sensation of swelling in the perinæum or near the anus, as if sitting on a ball." We often have very large amounts of mucus in the urine in prostatic troubles, and if I found it coupled with this sensation would expect benefit from the remedy. I know of no other use for this remedy at present. While we are here upon a urinary remedy, we will call attention to another comparatively new but good one.

EQUISETUM HYEMALE.

This remedy is sometimes successful in cases which are not relieved by *Cantharis.* There is as much inclination to urinate as with *Cantharis,* and there is pain in the bladder, as if too full of urine, which must be voided in order to get relief from both pain and pressure, but urinating does not satisfy and he must soon go again. There is *burning* in the urethra when urinating, but there are larger quantities of urine discharged than with *Cantharis,* which has *characteristically* very small amounts, but often repeated, even but a few drops at a time. *Equisetum,* like *Chimaphila,* sometimes shows excess of mucus, and it is also very useful in enuresis. Both *Chimaphila* and *Equisetum* need further proving to draw out their characteristic. *Equisetum* sometimes has severe pain at the close of urination. (See *Berberis, Natrum mur., Sarsaparilla, Thuja.)*

LAPIS ALBUS.

This is the name given by Von Grauvogl to a species of gneiss that he found in the spring of Gastein. Goitre and cretinism abound among the people who drink this water. Grauvogl experimented with it, and found it to cause burning and shooting pains in the cardia and pylorus, and also in the uterus and mammæ. In practice he found it remarkably successful in scrofulous affections, but that it did harm in cases that had previously suffered from malaria. He treated five cases of uterine carcinoma, pronounced true and incurable by allopaths, and cured them all. I have a case now under my care, to which I was called a year ago. She has a very large uterine fibroid. Under various remedies she grew worse, having hæmorrhages, frequently repeated, so profuse that it seemed as if she would bleed to death. The tumor, which involved the whole body of the womb, laid across the pelvis, the upper part, in the left sacro-iliac fossa, and the os, of course, exactly opposite in the other side of the pelvic cavity so far up on the other side that it was impossible with the speculum to get the least view of it. After the bleeding had gone on for months in this way the discharges became black and horribly offensive, and the os had a decidedly rough feel to the finger. Finally she began to complain of intense burning pains all through the diseased parts. *Arsenicum album* effecting nothing for her, I put her upon *Lapis albus* as an experiment, for I had no hope she could live more than two weeks at the longest. Under the action of this remedy she began to improve immediately, and from the half dead wreck that could not turn in bed without help, a skeleton, white as a ghost, she has steadily improved until she is now doing her own housework, the discharges having all ceased except her natural menses at her regular periods. The tumor grows smaller, and it seems as though she might get well. She takes a dose of *Lapis albus* 30th once a week.

MEDORRHINUM.

The gonorrhœal virus, is undoubtedly a great remedy. Any one who has had much to do with gonorrhœa well knows the severe form of rheumatism, which is often the consequence of the introduction of this disease product into the system. I have seen some remarkable results from the use of this remedy in chronic forms of rheumatism. One case (a middle-aged lady) was not able to attend church, a few rods from her residence, for a long time, the trouble being in her feet and ankles and soles of the feet. The ankles were so sore and stiff and soles so tender that she could not walk on them. *Antimonium crud.*, which had cured some bad cases with similar symptoms for me, was without any beneficial effect, but *Medorrhinum* c.m., one dose, so benefited her that she could walk where she pleased. In the *Organon* (journal), Vol. 3, Dr. J. A. Biegler, of Rochester, N. Y., reports a remarkable cure of chronic rheumatism in a man 60 years of age. No history of previous gonorrhœa appears in the case, and I have never found any such history in the cases which I have been able to benefit with this remedy. In Vol. 1, of the same journal, is a remarkable cure reported by Dr. Skinner, of Liverpool, England. It is a cure of caries of the spine of long standing by *Syphilinum* (high). I had a very similar case, for which I had been prescribing for over a year without success, when I first read the report of this case. In my case, as in his, the patient had severe pains in the diseased part *during the night*. Every one acquainted with syphilitic troubles, especially of the bones, knows of these (terrible, sometimes) nightly bone pains. Three doses of Swan's *Syphilinum* c.m. cured this case in the remarkably short space of forty days. I could not find any reliable history of syphilis in this case. Then the question arises, is Swan's nosode theory true, or are disease products homœopathically curative only in those cases resembling them, not having a disease product history? Let others answer, I am not able to as yet.

Since writing the above I have experimented more with

the so-called nosodes and have had seemingly very good results from this remedy as well as *Syphilinum* in intractable cases of chronic rheumatism. The most characteristic difference between them is that with *Medorrhinum* the pains are worse in the *day-time,* and with *Syphilinum* in the *night.*

There are, no doubt, great curative powers residing in these two disease poisons and they should not be discarded simply because they are the products of disease.

In regard to the other nosodes, I have, within two years past, seen some remarkable effects from them.

TUBERCULINUM.

Cosmopolitan; never satisfied to remain in one place long; wants to travel.

Wandering pains in limbs and joints; stiff when beginning to move; < standing, > continued motion.

Longs for open air, wants doors and windows open, or to ride in strong wind.

Takes fresh cold on least exposure, can't get rid of one before another comes.

Emaciation, even while being well, and so hungry must get up nights to eat.

Pain through left upper lung to back. Tubercular deposit begins there.

Persons with a history of tuberculosis in the family.

Symptoms ever changing, begin suddenly, ceasing suddenly.

* * * * *

One case of retarded menstruation in a young girl who had greatly enlarged tonsils and who began to grow tired and weak, pale and short breathed on any exercise. The menses appeared twice under the action of *Pulsatilla,* but at intervals of several months, and finally not at all. After the failure of several other remedies to give her any benefit, she took one dose of *Tuberculinum* 1m. with prompt, easy and natural appearance of the menses and corresponding improvement in other respects, and is now attending school in apparent good health. I forgot to state that her sister, older, died of consumption a few years before.

Again, while on a visit to my daughter in Athens, Pa., I called upon one of the homœopathic physicians of the place, whom I had never met before. He had read "Leaders," and after we had talked books a while he asked me if I would not like to see a curious case, and there was no *money* in it, but it had come into his hands from the allopaths who had given it up to die. Of course, there being no *money* in it, I readily consented to go. Found a child of seven months, with "head on him" larger than a man's head, with eyes pushed out and turned upwards, only movable a little from side to side. It looked idiotic. The fontanelles could not be felt, because of the hydrocephalic condition which filled the whole scalp, distending it as above described.

I could not see that that child recognized anything, except that its whining, moaning (almost constant) seemed to increase if it was spoken to or moved.

Inquiry into its family history discovered that several of the mother's sisters had died with tuberculosis. She was the only one left of the family, I think. I gave, with the doctor's consent, a powder of *Tuberculinum* 1m. and advised to let it act. This was on the Monday following Easter Sunday.

May 24th, 1900, I received the following letter:

"Dr. E. B. Nash,
"Cortland, N. Y.

"Dear Doctor:—You will doubtless remember the case of hydrocephalus you saw with me while in Athens, and for which you prescribed *Tuberculinum*. Well, from that day, the head ceased to increase in size and (though it has taken no medicine at all, since taking that) has begun to gradually *decrease*. They measure it in the same place every Sunday, and last Sunday it was half an inch smaller than a week before. Will you kindly send me a graft at once of *Tuberculinum* high, that I may continue the remedy at intervals, etc., etc."

I received one letter since, reporting further improvement. I can hardly expect a *cure* in such a case, but the effects of the remedy, so far, seem to be quite remarkable. A case of lung trouble brought to me over a year ago from Seneca Falls, N. Y., had been under allopathic treatment for four years and had been every summer up in the Adirondacks at Saranac, at a Sanitarium established by Dr. Loomis, of New York, lung specialist. She continued to grow worse until I took her case in hand. Under the action of two doses of *Sulphur* c.m. followed by *Tuberc.* c.m. she is so improved that I think it would be hard to convince any one that she ever suffered from such conditions.

The trouble located in the upper left lung, where there was a distinct cavity, which as far as I can discover, is now healed, though there is a little dullness of respiratory murmur remaining.

One result of the action of these remedies was to restore a granular surface to the eyelids which had been cured (?) with local applications. I am sure that many incurable chronic diseases have had their beginning in just such tampering with local manifestations of *Psora*.

One more case.—L. D. G., a man sixty years of age, whose brothers and sisters had several of them died of consumption, had been troubled at times with a spasmodic gagging cough for twenty-five years. He was operated for a stricture of the urethra, and a few weeks after was attacked with chills resembling fever and ague. It was in the winter season, and chills and fever are not common here at any time of the year, unless imported He had several of these chills daily, until there developed a strong *Rhus toxicod.* condition, when a dose of that remedy put an end to them. But here followed frequent attacks of great pain from the back all through the abdomen, especially the hypogastric region. When I would get these pains in the bowels relieved in a measure he would have what appeared to be neuralgic pains in different parts all over him, first in one place, then in another. When these would seem to subside, he would begin to cough more, and so the thing travelled from pillar to post, for months.

Dr. Sheldon, of Syracuse, a man of large experience, was called in consultation. After careful examination, he decided, in view of the family history and (as he expressed it) a peculiar doughy feeling in the abdominal walls, that the case was tubercular in character, and advised *Verat. album* at present, because the patient was so weak and reduced and cold, especially the extremities.

It was given, but with little or no effect, and things went on as usual until on his theory of *Tuberculosis* one evening I dropped a dose of *Tuberculinum* upon his tongue. The effect was that he slept that night as quietly as if under the influence of an anodyne, and every symptom was alleviated, and he improved in every way for weeks until he was able to be out on the street every day. It was very cold weather and he caught cold and came down to the bed again. After a few doses of *Aconite* for symptoms following his exposure, he received another dose of *Tuberculinum* as before, with similar effect, and in a short time he had so far improved as to be able to go on a visit to his friends in Troy, N. Y.

How he will come out is still a question, but repeated effects of the remedy were so apparent in so grave a case that I have deemed them worthy of narration.

If you turn to H. C. Allen's "Key-Notes of Leading Remedies," page 297, you will find recorded: *"Symptoms ever changing,* ailments affecting one organ, then another, the lungs, brain, kidneys, liver, stomach, nervous system —beginning suddenly, ceasing suddenly."

This seemed to be the case with this patient.

In conclusion, I have seen apparent benefit follow the exhibition of this remedy in both incipient as well as advanced cases of Phthisis, always giving the high preparations in the latter and letting it act a long time without repetition. In view of what Dr. Burnett has written, and my own limited experience lately, I am confident that *Tuberculinum* is destined to rank with *Psorinum* in the treatment of chronic diseases.

I will add now, Dec. 17th, 1900, that the case of L. D. G. has continued to improve until he seems as well as he has during the last ten years and weighs more.

Another case.—Maude Porter, age 27, unmarried; sanguine, nervous temperament; short, and stout when in health; blue eyes, brown hair.

Has had bad occasional epileptic fits for eleven years. Have been less frequent for past two years under the influence of a specialist's medicine that she got by letter from New York. Her mother had just died of tubercular consumption. Maude cared for her and was continually over her for the last month of her sickness.

After her mother died, on May 28, 1900, she came to me bringing symptoms as follows:

Can't eat anything.

Mouth tastes very badly; in the morning <.

Smell of cooking food nauseates.

Coughs badly, especially nights.

Soreness middle of chest, behind sternum, worse when coughing or ascending hill or stairs.

Has lost 22 lbs. of flesh since May 1st.

Backache when tired.

Feels cold and shivery, < morning and evening.

Feels very weak, can't walk without fatigue.

Passed her last period without menses.

Greatly depressed and cries easily.

Has had a cough since la grippe last December.

Has had a diarrhœa for past four weeks.

Pulse from 100 to 120 all the time.

Sweaty nights.

On that date I prescribed *Pulsatilla* 200th and later 10m. with no perceptible change for the better.

After *Pulsatilla* failed I prescribed for her *Tuberculinum* 1m., and for the next four months she got about once in two weeks the same, once or twice changing to *Bacillinum* 200, under which treatment she made a perfect recovery, and is doing her usual housework, looking as well as ever at this date, December 17, 1900.

I believe that she would have gone with quick consumption but for this remedy. What do you think, my reader?

PYROGEN.

Diseases originating in ptomaine or sewer gas infection.

The *bed feels hard,* parts lain on sore and bruised, must move to relieve the soreness.

Tongue: large, flabby, clean, *smooth as if varnished; fiery red,* cracked, difficult articulation; vomiting, persistent, brownish coffee ground, offensive, stercoraceous.

Diarrhœa; horribly offensive, brown or black; painless, involuntary.

Distinct consciousness of a heart; it feels tired; as if enlarged; purring, throbbing, pulsating, constant in ears, preventing sleep.

* * * * *

I have not used this remedy myself, but (if Allen's "Keynotes" are reliable) it must be of great value in affections of the most serious nature. A remedy recommended so highly, by such authority, for septicæmia, puerperal and surgical, and for diseases originating in ptomaine or sewer gas infection should not be passed lightly over. Let me quote: **"The bed feels hard** *(Arnica), parts laid on feel sore and bruised (Baptisia),* rapid decubitus *(Carbol. acid)." "Great restlessness,* must move constantly to > the soreness of the parts *(Arnica, Eupator. perf.)."* "Tongue: large, flabby;

clean, smooth as if varnished; fiery red; dry, cracked, articulation difficult."

Diarrhœa; horribly offensive *(Psorin.)*, brown or black *(Leptand.)*, painless, involuntary, uncertain when passing flatus *(Aloe, Oleander)*.

Did you ever meet such an array of symptoms in typhoid? I have, and when we remember that typhoid is often traced to defective drains, sewer gas, etc., as its cause, this remedy, if these symptoms are reliable, ought to be invaluable. The other symptoms given by Allen are just as valuable if true, and if not true the sooner they are proven to be untrue the better.

So far as prejudice against using such remedies is concerned, we should be as honest as was James B. Bell when he said of *Psorinum*—"Whether derived from purest gold or purest filth, our gratitude for its excellent services forbids us to enquire or care." As might be expected, *Anthracinum* is more like this than any other remedy. In all cases simulating septic fever or poisoning *Arsenicum, Anthracinum* and *Pyrogen* should be remembered. The horrible **burning pains** of the first two are prominent.

CHENOPODIUM.

I have the 30th potency marked *Chenopodium glauci,* with which I cured one case of pain under the left shoulder-blade. This case was of several years' standing, the pain at times becoming very severe. I have also used it in other cases with benefit. I always think of this remedy where I find such a pain and of *Chelidonium* where it is under the right shoulder-blade. According to Dr.

Jacob Jeanes, *Chenopodium anthelminticum* cures a pain under the *right* shoulder-blade similar to that of *Chelidonium*. The pain in both seems to depend upon some hepatic derangement. Having succeeded with the *Chelidonium* so well, I have never used it. *Chelidonium* is well proven, and a full proving of the *Chenopodium* may enable us to distinguish between them. Between the two *Chenopodiums* and *Chelidonium,* we have an important trio for infra-scapular pains which ought to be better understood. Such single symptoms are, of course, small guides to follow, but are sometimes the only ones we have, and when, after full proving, the drug having them is developed, we often find that they were reliable though we could not at first give their pathological significance. I would, I think, as often follow such a guide, as speculations and theories. For instance, here are some such single symptoms which have often been verified. Inframammary pains at climacteric, *Actæa racemosa.* Pain drawing through from nipple to back when child nurses, *Croton tiglium. (Silicea.)* Pain in upper left chest through to scapula, *Myrtus com., Pix liquida, Theridion* and *Sulphur.* Pain through lower right chest, *Chelidonium, Mercurius vivus* and *Kali carbonicum.* Pain through upper right chest, *Calcarea ostrearum* and *Arsenicum album.* Pain through lower left chest, *Natrum sulphuricum.* We might add many more such to this list, and they are very valuable.

AMMONIUM CARBONICUM.

Nose-bleed when washing the face in the morning.

Weak, anæmic, flabby women. Weak, no reaction. Addicted to the smelling bottle.

Tendency to gangrenous degeneration of glands, as in scarlatina; the parotids.

* * * * *

Guernsey says: This remedy seems particularly useful in constitutionally delicate women who faint easily and want some kind of smelling salts around them most of the time. They are weak, with deficient reaction and generally of the lymphatic temperament. Such patients want stimulants, especially such stimulants as act through the olfactory nerves, like spirits of Ammonia, Camphor, Musk, Alcohol, etc. In the first onset of such a suddenly prostrating disease as cerebro-spinal meningitis this has been found a good remedy to excite reaction and place the patient in a condition for the choice of the next remedy indicated by the now aroused vital force in conflict with the disease (so called). One thing *Ammonium carb.* is good for is dry or stuffed coryza, acute or chronic. The patient is worse at night, has to breathe with the mouth open. *Sambucus, Lycopodium, Nux vomica* and *Sticta pulmonaria* may be compared with it.

Another frequently verified symptom of the nose is epistaxis *while washing the face. (Kali carbonicum.)* I don't know why it comes on then, but it does, and this remedy cures it. The only other affection in which I have found it very useful is scarlatina. The body is very red, almost bluish-red, and the throat seems to be the center where the force of the disease seems to be expended in malignant intensity. The eruption is faintly developed, or has seemed to disappear, from sheer inability from weakness of the patient's vitality to keep it on the surface. (*Zinc.* has convulsions from the same cause.) Erysipelas of old, debilitated persons comes under the same head. Cerebral symptoms, simulating a drunken stupor, are present in both cases. The whole system seems to be overpowered by the toxic effect of the disease poison. (See also *Ailanthus.*) *Ammonium carb.* will sometimes help us out in such cases.

AMMONIUM MURIATICUM.

One symptom of this remedy that has proved to be a valuable keynote for its administration is: "*Sensation of coldness in the back, between the shoulders.*" It is generally found in chest affections, such as cough or pains in the chest without cough. I have found it as reliable a keynote as is the *burning* between the shoulders of *Lycopodium* or *Phosphorus.* It is also a remedy for constipation, the stool being *hard, dry and crumbling and also very difficult to expel.* Sometimes the stool is covered with mucus, something like *Causticum,* which has stool covered with mucus, shining, as if greased. There is also a resemblance between these two remedies affecting the muscles and ligaments. *Ammonium mur.* has pain with a *sensation* as if the muscles were contracted or too short, while *Causticum* goes a step further and has *actual* contraction of these parts, producing what is known as arthritis deformans. *(Cimex, Nat. m.)*

There are two remedies that have menses, or flow of blood from the uterus, *at night.* They are *Ammonium mur.* and *Bovista,* the other symptoms, of course, deciding the choice between them. *(Kreosot. menses flow only on lying down,* cease when sitting or walking about; *Lilium tig. flows only when moving about,* ceased to flow when she ceased to walk; *Magnesia carb. flows only at night or when lying,* ceases when walking.) This remedy is also sometimes useful in sciatica. Here we have the sense of contraction in the tendons and the patient is worse while sitting, some better when walking and entirely relieved when lying down. It also has pains in the heels as if ulcerated. For pains in the heels see also *Phytolacca, Cyclamen, Manganum, Ledum* and *Causticum.* I once cured a case, very severe and long lasting, with *Valeriana.*

ÆTHUSA CYNAPIUM

Is one of our best remedies for vomiting in children. The milk comes up as soon as swallowed, by a great effort, after which the child becomes greatly relaxed and drowsy; or if the milk stays down longer it finally comes up in *very sour curds, so large that it would seem almost impossible the child could have ejected them.* If this condition of the stomach is not cured the case will go on to cholera infantum, with green watery or slimy stool, colic and convulsions. The convulsions of this remedy are peculiar, in that the eyes *turn downward* instead of up or sidewise. If the case still progresses unfavorably there is an appearance of sunkenness in the face with *linea nasalis,* which is a surface of pearly whiteness on the upper lip, bounded by a distinct line from the outer nasal orifice to the angles of the mouth.

This last symptom is more characteristic of *Æthusa than any other remedy. Æthusa* has complete absence of thirst. The *prostration and anxiety* are very marked, but the absence of thirst rules for *Æthusa* instead of *Arsenicum album.*

Vomiting of large curds (sour) is also found under *Calcarea ostrearum,* but with this remedy we have at the same time sour stools, and then sweaty head, and open fontanelles as well as *Calcarea* temperament would generally be found in the case.

There is another very peculiar symptom of *Æthusa* that has been cured twice to my knowledge by this remedy, viz.: Imagined she saw a rat or mouse run across the room. In both these cases the symptom occurred in hard worked, nervous women, but the symptom was very persistent and annoying. *Æthusa* not only cured the aberration but improved the general health. I always use it in the 200th potency.

JALAPA.

"Child 'good' all day; screaming, restless and very troublesome at night" (frequently verified). I once had a case of entero-colitis that for more than eight weeks baffled my best efforts to cure. The case went from bad to worse, until it was reduced almost to a skeleton. Instead of screaming all night it screamed day and night, all the time (so the mother said), and certain it was, it was always screaming when I saw it. With the screaming there were constant contortions of the body, bending forward, backward and sidewise alternately. I cannot tell how many different remedies I tried, but finally, in the course of human events, I gave it some *Jalapa* 12th, run up from some of the crude drug which I procured from an ordinary drug store. The child went to sleep, and from that nap, which was a good, long one, recovery was rapid and perfect. The only indication I had was that it caused colic and diarrhœa.

RHEUM

Is another remedy which, like *Jalapa,* has been abused by the old school, but is very valuable when used homœopathically. The leading indication is *sour stools.* They may be brown mixed with mucus, or thin and pasty. There is often much *pain before the stool,* of a colicky nature, and there may be tenesmus after stool. It is most useful in colicky diarrhœa of children. There is another very characteristic symptom, viz.: "Not only the stools are sour; *the whole child smells sour,* no matter how much it is bathed." In colic and diarrhœa during dentition a choice will sometimes have to be made between this remedy and *Magnesia carb.*

COLLINSONIA CANADENSIS.

This remedy has not been thoroughly proven, but enough has been learned from what we have, and clinical experience, to indicate that it is a very valuable one. As a remedy for hæmorrhoids or rectal trouble it may be compared with *Æsculus hippocastanum,* for both have a *sensation as if the rectum was filled with sticks.* From this one symptom we could not know which one to prescribe. But let us note some of the differences:

Æsculus has also a prominent *sense of fullness* in rectum, *Collinsonia* has not.

Æsculus piles do not, as a rule, bleed.

Collinsonia piles often bleed persistently.

Æsculus has great pain, soreness and *aching in the back.*

Collinsonia does not as yet develop that symptom.

Æsculus sometimes has constipation, sometimes not.

Collinsonia is greatly constipated, with colic on account of it.

This comparison is carried far enough to show that a choice between these remedies is not generally difficult. With *Collinsonia* I once cured a very severe colic which had been of frequent occurrence in a lady for several years and had completely baffled the old school efforts to cure. I was led to choose the remedy on account of the obstinate constipation, the great flatulence and the hæmorrhoidal condition present.

I also cured one of the most obstinate cases of chronic constipation I ever met. The patient for two years had only averaged a movement of the bowels once in two weeks, and then only under the action of powerful cathartics, after which he would be almost sick two or three days in bed. *Collinsonia* cured him within a month so perfectly that his bowels moved naturally every day and the trouble never returned so long as I knew him, for years afterwards.

CORALLIUM RUBRUM

Is useful for spasmodic cough, like whooping cough. It is continual, short, hawking through the day, so constant and frequent as to have merited the description given it of *"Minute gun"* cough. This is during the day and there is not much whooping, but at night there is more whooping. The night paroxysms are sometimes very severe.

I have found *Coral.* one of the very best remedies for post nasal catarrh, with *much dropping of mucus* into the throat. *(Natrum carb.)* I do not know any other remedy so efficacious in the majority of cases, and generally prescribe it, unless I have strong indications for some other remedy. I seldom fail to hear a good report from it.

Coral. has also been found useful in *chancre.* The ulcer is red (coral red), flat and exceedingly sensitive, sometimes painful. Chancroids or soft chancre, for which the old school cauterize, may find a swift and sure cure in *Coral.*

COCCUS CACTI

Is another animal remedy often found valuable in whooping cough. With this remedy the aggravations generally come on in the after part of the night or in the morning when the child awakens. The paroxysms are not confined to this time, but the worst one comes then. The paroxysm ends in vomiting of clear *ropy mucus* in large quantities, hanging in long strings from the mouth. For such a cough *Coccus cacti* is *excellent.*

CLEMATIS ERECTA.

This is a good remedy for gonorrhœa when there are on account of slow or intermittent flow of urine indications of formation of a stricture, and will, if given early (high), often prevent it. So much pain and suffering often necessitating operation for the relief of stricture has been experienced that everything possible should be done to avert it. In the first place the cauterization method, or fashionable local treatment, is responsible for nearly, if not quite, all strictures. I know that such practice is neither scientific nor curative in the remotest sense, and on the other hand I know that constitutional treatment alone is adequate to cure (not simply suppress) the worst cases, and that in the shortest possible time. Another use for *Clematis* is for curing the orchitis arising from the suppression of gonorrhœa, or when it may have extended to the testicles without such suppression, which latter condition seldom occurs. The testicle becomes greatly swollen, and if not promptly relieved becomes indurated and hard as a stone. I have cured this very promptly with *Clematis*. *Pulsatilla* is undoubtedly the remedy oftenest indicated in orchitis from suppressed gonorrhœa, but if after it has reduced the pain and restored the discharge it fails to reduce the swelling or induration, *Clematis* will do the rest. It has not disappointed me. *Clematis* has a symptom similar to *Coffea,* viz.: "Toothache relieved by holding cold water in the mouth."

COPAIVA.

This remedy acts strongly upon mucous membranes. It has, like many other remedies, been so abused by the old school that it has fallen into disrepute, and the tendency even with our own school under such circumstances is to underrate its virtues or to fail to investigate as they ought to. It is, however, an excellent remedy in the form of chronic bronchial catarrh, with profuse expectoration of greenish or gray purulent matter. (*Stannum, Lycopodium, Sulphur, Phosphorus,* etc.) Among remedies not yet well understood we have

Copaiva, profuse greenish-gray, disgusting smelling sputa.

Illicium anisatum, pus, with pain at third cartilage, right or left.

Pix liquida, purulent sputa, pain at left third costal cartilage.

Myosotis, copious sputa, emaciation, night sweats.

Balsam Peru., catarrhal phthisis, copious purulent expectoration.

Yerba santa, accumulation of mucus causing asthmatic breathing.

I mention these remedies in order to call attention to them for trial in case we cannot find the curative among the better proven ones. All the old remedies had to have their *beginnings.*

Copaiva is a valuable remedy in gonorrhœa. There is great irritation in the urethra and at the neck of the bladder. It may be indicated in the beginning, when the discharge is thin or milky, and later, especially when the disease has extended to the bladder, with discharge of a large amount of viscid mucus or blood and mucus in the urine. Although not so violent in its action on the urinary tract as *Cantharis,* it stands very close to it.

CUBEBA.

This remedy, also fallen into disrepute from its empirical use in the old school, has an important place in the therapeutics of gonorrhœa, if after the first or inflammatory stage is passed under the usual remedies for that stage there still remains burning in the urethra after urination and the discharge remains thick, yellow or puslike. Notwithstanding *Mercurius* or *Pulsatilla,* we may find our remedy in *Cubeba.* I have made some fine cures myself in such cases. With *Pulsatilla* the discharge, while thick, or yellow, or green, is more likely to be *bland,* as it is on mucous membranes elsewhere. *Mercury* has a similar discharge, but all the symptoms are *worse at night.* When the discharge becomes thin (gleety) neither of these remedies are, as a rule, appropriate.

Right here let us call attention to another remedy which ought to be mentioned in connection with the treatment of gonorrhœa.

PETROSELINUM.

It has a very characteristic indication for its administration, viz.: "Great and **sudden** desire to urinate," children stand and jump right up and down from pain and urging. This is mostly found in chronic cases (especially after gonorrhœa) after the inflammation has extended backward to the neck of the bladder. Another very troublesome symptom found under *Petroselinum* is **itching** in the urethra; feels as if he must run a stick or something in there and *scratch* it. Burning, tingling, from perinæum throughout whole urethra. Children are sometimes troubled with such sudden and intense desire to urinate that they will jump right up and down, trying to hold on until their clothes are unbuttoned. It is like the sudden desire for stool of *Aloe—"must git thar."*

ALLIUM CEPA.

Coryza with frequent sneezing and profuse acrid discharge, corroding upper lip and nose. Lachrymation also profuse but bland. *(Euph.* reverse.)

Cold extends to the bronchi, with profuse secretion of mucus; coughing and much rattling *(Chelidon.)*.

Modalities: < in the evening, and in warm room, > in open air (the coryza).

* * * * *

Anyone who has cut up raw onions for cooking knows

what is the effect upon the eyes and nose—irritation, which causes violent sneezing and lachrymation. Then, if the homœopathic law of cure is true, it ought to be a good remedy for coryza, and so it is; but, like every other remedy, it cures its own peculiar and characteristic form of the disease.

It has constant and frequent sneezing, with profuse acrid discharge, which burns and corrodes the nose and upper lip, and it is worse in the evening and indoors and better in open air. It has also profuse lachrymation, with burning, biting and smarting of the eyes, but the discharge is bland; that is, it does not make the eyes sore afterwards. There may or may not be headache; if there is it is, like the coryza, worse in warm room or evening and better in open air. I have found it particularly useful in children when the profuse coryza or cold extended downward to the bronchi, with a like profuse secretion in the bronchial tubes, with much coughing and rattling of mucus. Before *Cepa* came into homœopathic use we used to give *Euphrasia* when there was profuse coryza and lachrymation. The difference between the two remedies is, that with *Cepa* the nasal discharge is acrid and the lachyrmal bland, while exactly the reverse is true of *Euphrasia.* The action of the remedy seems to be primarily in the nose with the one and in the eyes with the other, and thus we must learn to differentiate between all remedies.

EUPHRASIA.

The action of this remedy seems to *center* in the eyes. If you read the symptoms as laid down in "Hering's Guiding Symptoms," you would think that it would cure almost all possible affections of the eyes, acute or chronic conjunctivitis, iritis, kerato-iritis, spots, vesicles, pannus, etc., and so it will if indicated by the symptoms.

In colds with cough and severe fluent coryza it will sometimes cure, but here the choice must be made between it and *Arsenicum, Cepa* and *Mercurius.* (See *Cepa* for comparison.)

In measles with watery eyes and fluent coryza it is sometimes the best remedy. I remember Dr. C. W. Boyce, of Auburn, N. Y., reporting great success with it in an epidemic in that city. He cured all his cases with it. So I went for the next epidemic in my vicinity with *Euphrasia,* and my failure was as marked as his success. It was *not* the remedy for *my* epidemic. But I know enough not to "go it blind" that way very long, and hunted up my simillimum. Then I succeeded, too. Look out, young man, for the remedy that is recommended for *all cases* of any disease, or you'll "come down hard" some time.

One very prominent characteristic in eye troubles for this remedy is a *tendency to an accumulation of sticky mucus* on the cornea, which is removed by winking. All cases of any kind attended with photophobia and lachrymation, with or without coryza, should suggest this remedy, or at least call it to mind. In the eye affections of *Euphrasia* the lids are often involved. Of course this is so with other remedies, such as *Arsenicum, Apis, Rhus toxic.,* etc. *Study up.* One more symptom: Cough, sometimes dry, but generally loose, *worse during the day,* not troublesome at night. This is important, as more coughs are $<$ at night.

PHYTOLACCA DECANDRA.

Tonsils red, swollen, with white spots, which sometimes coalesce and form patches; pains run up into the ears, and aching, bruised, sore feeling in head, back and limbs; < on motion, but must move; he aches and is so sore.

Irresistible inclination to bite the teeth or gums together. (Dentition.)

Breasts very hard, swollen, hot and painful; pain radiates all over the back when the child nurses.

* * * * *

Phytolacca decandra is one of our most valuable remedies for sore throat, and the indications are plain. The throat becomes generally inflamed; the tonsils swell and become very red at the first, and then white spots appear which (unless checked) soon spread and coalesce and form patches of a diphtheritic appearance. *There are sharp pains often running up into one or both ears.* These are the local throat symptoms, and the constitutional symptoms are:

Intense head and backache, and a sore, aching, bruised feeling all over the body, causing the patient to groan, and while, like *Rhus toxicodendron,* he feels as if he *must move,* the act of moving greatly aggravates all his pains and soreness. The patient is also greatly prostrated, and sitting upright makes him faint and dizzy like *Bryonia.* There is high fever, for the pulse is very quick; but the heat, like that of *Arnica,* is mostly in the head and face while the body and limbs are cool. Now these symptoms present, it makes no difference whether the case is called tonsilitis, diphtheria or scarlatina. Abundant experience in my own person and observation with my patients has proven *Phytolacca* to be a remedy of inestimable value. Nor is it necessary to give it in twenty drop doses of the mother tincture, and gargle in addition, as some advise, but it will in the potentized dose do much better, the same as other homœopathic remedies. I have done some good work with this remedy in follicular pharyngitis, especially when in public speakers the voice gave out from overwork and there was much *burning* in the throat, as of a hot substance there. In this kind of sore throat I have the best success with the remedy very high.

Now let me call attention to a symptom of this remedy that has been of great value to me: "Irresistible inclination to bite the teeth or gums together." On this indication I have often relieved the complaints of various kinds incident to the period of dentition. I once had a case that was sent up to the country from New York City. The child had been sick a long time, with cholera infantum (entero-colitis), and its physicians said it must leave the city or die. But country air and change of diet brought no relief. The little fellow was greatly emaciated, having frequent loose stools of dark brown color, mixed with slime or mucus of the same color. After trying various remedies I discovered that the child wanted to bite its gums together, or to bite on everything that it could get into its mouth, and the mother then told me that this had been the case all through its sickness. *Phytolacca* produced immediate relief of the symptoms and rapid recovery followed. I have since verified this symptom several times. *Phytolacca* is also one of our best remedies for mastitis. The breasts are very hard, greatly swollen, hot and painful. When the child nurses the pain *radiates all over the body.* There is fever, great pain in the head and back, and if it is a bad case, unless checked, is very liable to go on to suppuration. Every time the child nurses the pains spread all over the body.

The choice often lies between this remedy and *Bryonia,* and they complement each other. Almost every case of swollen breasts with the milk fever, when the breasts fill for the first time after confinement, may be speedily relieved with one or the other of these two remedies. If the case should have gone on to suppuration, with large fistulous, gaping and angry ulcers discharging a watery or fœtid pus, *Phytolacca* is still the remedy, and will often do more good than *Hepar sulphur.* and *Silicea.* But the choice sometimes has to be made between other remedies, such as

Croton tiglium. The pain runs through to the back when child nurses. (**Silicea,** *Pulsatilla.)*

Phellandrium. Pain runs along the milk ducts *between* the acts of nursing.

Lac caninum. The breasts are greatly filled and so **sore** that their own weight hurts the patient, who wants to *hold them up* and shrinks from the *least jar.* Of course *Aconite, Apis* and *Belladonna* must not be forgotten, and have as positive indications for their use as any of the above remedies. (See also *Castor equorum.)*

I have removed a great many suspicious lumps or tumors in the breasts, some of them of years' standing, by giving a dose of *Phytolacca* c.m., once a month, *during the wane of the moon.* What has the moon to do with it? I do not know. I cure goitre the same way (but not with *Phytolacca),* and was led to that way of administration by a suggestion of Jahr. That some diseases have their aggravations in certain times of the moon I *know,* and that certain remedies act better then, I know just as well. Do not forget that the bruised, sore feeling of *Phytolacca* that we noticed at length when writing of *Arnica* is sometimes markedly present in sciatica, for which it is one of our successful remedies. The characteristic symptom for *Phytolacca* in this painful affection is, that the pain *runs* down the *outer side of the limb.* Sciatica is one of the complaints in which Homœopathy has scored some of its most brilliant victories over the anodyne treatment of the old school. Periosteal rheumatism, where the pains are especially worse in wet weather, sometimes finds a remedy in *Phytolacca.* This drug seems to resemble in its action on the periosteum, glands, bones and skin *Kali hydroiodicum,* and the two remedies complement each other, of course, with indications, or the choice may sometimes lie between them. H. C. Allen says: *Phytolacca* occupies a place midway between *Bryonia* and *Rhus tox.,* and will often help when these seem indicated but fail. It is curious to note that almost every chemical remedy has a closely resembling relative from the vegetable kingdom. *Kali hydroiodicum* and *Phytolacca, Aloes* and *Sulphur, Cepa* and *Phosphorus, Chamomilla* and *Magnesia carb., China* and *Ferrum, Belladonna* and *Calcarea ost., Ipecac* and *Cuprum, Bryonia* and *Alumina, Mezereum* and *Mercury, Pulsatilla* and *Kali sulphuricum.* This has been before mentioned by Hering.

GLONOINE.

Sudden local congestion, especially to head and chest; bursting headache rising up from neck, with great throbbing and sense of expansion as if to burst; cannot bear the least jar.

Can't bear anything on the head, especially hat; or pressure as of a hat.

Over-heating in the sun, or sunstroke.

* * * * *

This is, in the first place, one of our great head remedies. It has intense pain in the head, with great throbbing and sensation of fullness and constriction of the vessels of the neck. There are so many symptoms attending this condition of congestion that it is not wise to try to give them all here. I used, in my early practice, to carry a small vial of the 1st dilution in my case on purpose for those who were inclined to sneer at the young doctor and his sweet medicine, and many a disbeliever have I convinced, in about five or ten minutes, that there might be power in small doses of sweet medicine, by dropping on the tongue a drop of this preparation, for it seldom failed to produce its characteristic throbbing headache within that time. One lady, not willing to acknowledge that it affected her, rose to leave the room, and fainted and would have fallen to the floor if I had not caught her. No one ever asked after that experiment for any more proof of the power of homœopathic medicine. This throbbing headache, *seeming to arise from the neck,* is very characteristic, and the throbbing is not a mere sensation but is visible in the carotid arteries. The vessels are full to bursting, and if their walls were not healthy there is danger of apoplexy. No remedy equals this one for producing sudden and severe congestion of the head, and none can cure it quicker when indicated by the symptoms. The remedies that stand nearest *Glonoine* in their effect on the head I believe to be *Belladonna* and *Melilotus*. *Belladonna* and *Glonoine* both have the fullness, pain and throbbing, but that of *Glonoine* is more intense and sudden in its onset, and, on the other hand, subsides more rapidly when relieved. Again, *Glonoine* is better adapted to the first or congestive stage of inflammatory diseases of the brain, while *Belladonna* goes further and may still be the appropriate remedy after the inflammatory stage is fully initiated. *Belladonna* is better by bending the head backward; *Glonoine* worse. *Belladonna* is made worse by having the head uncovered, and suffers from having the hair cut; *Glonoine must have* the head uncovered, can't bear to wear his hat, or wants the hair cut. *Belladonna* is *worse lying* down, even if he keeps still; *Glonoine,* though sometimes worse *after* lying down, is also sometimes *better* when *lying still.* One symptom *very* characteristic *of Glonoine* is, that the patient carries the head very carefully, for the **least jar** or shaking of it greatly aggravates the pain. Another peculiar symptom is, it seems to the patient that there is not only throbbing, but there is an undulating sensation as if the brain were *moving in waves* synchronous with the pulse. There is more disturbance of the heart action with *Glonoine* than with *Belladonna,* though both have it strongly. *Glonoine* has a *sensation* of rush of blood to the heart or chest.

Melilotus also has great congestion to the head, with

pain and sense of fullness. Not being so thoroughly proven as *Belladonna* and *Glonoine,* we cannot so clearly indicate the exact place for it, but there is one very prominent symptom which always makes one think of it, viz.: "*Glowing redness of the face.*" No remedy that I know of has it more strongly. *Glonoine* and *Belladonna* may both have very red face; on the other hand, a pale face, with the other congestive symptoms, does not contraindicate them, but does *Melilotus.* Then, again, with *Melilotus* the head symptoms are often relieved by a profuse epistaxis, which is also another very prominent symptom of this remedy. I cured a very bad case of typhus cerebralis, and also a case of insanity of long standing, with this remedy, being guided to it by these symptoms.

"Loses his way in well-known streets" is a symptom of *Glonoine* that has several times been confirmed. The local congestions of *Glonoine* are often found in different diseases; for instance, climacteric flushings are often most felt in the head. *Glonoine* cures such cases. It is also useful in puerperal convulsions. And another symptom often present in these cases is, a sense as if the head were expanding from fullness. Now look out for convulsions and give *Glonoine,* especially if there be albumen in the urine. Congestion to the head from suppressed or retarded menses sometimes finds a remedy here; also, different pathological conditions of the heart, but the *symptoms* must be present.

For sunstroke it is probably oftener indicated than any other remedy; also for the after-sufferings therefrom. Not only from sunstroke, but from other bad effects of *radiate heat;* for instance, children get sick in the night after sitting too long or falling asleep before an open coal fire.

Then, again, warm room increases the headache and warm bed the faceache.

"Burning between the shoulders" is another symptom of this remedy, like *Lycopodium* and *Phosphorus*. *Ammonium muriaticum* and *Lachnanthes* have the opposite. While we are here now I will call attention to another remedy, which, for flushings and congestions to head and face, resembles *Glonoine,* that is, *Amyl. nit.*

MELILOTUS ALBA (Sweet Clover).

Here is a remedy of undoubted great value. The best rendering of it is given by Dr. H. C. Allen in the transactions of the I. H. A., page 104, year 1887, although a very fair one is found in the "Guiding Symptoms" (Hering). The provers all had fearful headaches and hæmorrhages except myself (Bowen).

The congestion to the brain is equal to that of *Belladonna* and *Glonoine,* and the most characteristic symptom of such congestion is *intense redness of the face, with throbbing carotids,* which is often > by a *profuse epistaxis.* Several years ago I cured a very bad case of mania of the religious form with the 6th potency. This lady had had one similar attack a few years before, when, after she had been given up by two allopaths, who said she must go to the asylum, I relieved her with *Stramonium.* She was *very loquacious* at that time.

This time *Stramonium* failed, but on indication of the *intensely red face* I gave her *Melilotus* with a rapid and permanent cure. The first cause of these attacks was *overheating in the sun.*

One more case will illustrate the action of this truly great remedy.

During a run of typhoid fever in a young lady she had frequent attacks of profuse epistaxis. One attack followed another, sometimes twice or three times in twenty-four hours, until I became alarmed on account of the great loss of blood.

She had been subject to frequent attacks of nosebleed since childhood, from the time she was injured in the nasal passage by a button she pushed up the nose, and which a "regular" claimed, after much violence, to have pushed down her throat, but which in reality remained in her nose a long time—several months—when it was ejected in a fit of coughing and sneezing. Two years before I carried her through a very severe attack of diphtheria, which was also attended by severe nosebleed, occurring at night, the blood *hanging in clots* from the nose like icicles.

Mercurius sol. 30th then stopped it very nicely. Now the blood clotted some, but not so markedly. *Mercurius* did no good. Every attack was preceded by the most *intense redness and flushing* of the face and throbbing of the carotids I ever witnessed. The nosebleed would invariably follow within a few hours this apparent rush of blood to head and face. *Belladonna did no good.* Neither did *Erigeron,* which, in Hering, "has congestion of the head, red face, nosebleed and febrile action."

Melilotus 30th relieved promptly not only these attacks of congestion to head and nosebleed, but the whole case afterward progressed without an untoward symptom to perfect recovery.

F. A. Waddell, M. D., reports a case of pneumonic congestion, in which the characteristic *red face and epistaxis* were present, as cured with this remedy.

Dr. Bowen, to whom belongs the credit of first introducing this remedy to the profession, reports many cases of headaches, colic, cramps in the stomach and spasms relieved and cured by it. It seems to me that this remedy should be classed with *Belladonna* and *Glonoine,* and never forgotten in comparison with remedies having strong head symptoms.

AMYLIS NITRIS.

It has quite a reputation for arresting paroxysms of epilepsy and resuscitating patients sinking under *anæsthetics.* It is given here by olfaction. There are various speculations as to how it does this; the most important thing, after all, is that it does it.

We know that it causes and cures tumultuous heart action very similar in appearance to that of *Glonoine.* I have cured a very bad case of chronic blushing or flushing of blood to the face on the least excitement, either mental or physical. It was in a young married woman, not near the climacteric, and she had suffered very much for a long time. The cure is permanent and the patient is very grateful, for, as she said, she supposed it was natural and medicine could not help it. Those who *cannot blush* don't need it. This is all the experience I have had with this remedy and I always use it in the 30th.

KALI BROMATUM.

I do not know much about this remedy from a homœopathic standpoint. It first gained a reputation with the old school profession for its sleep-producing qualities and its power over epileptic seizures. As usual, it was pushed for these things until they found it was a dangerous remedy in the large doses which they had to use to produce the desired effect.

They discovered that it produced sleep, not by increasing the blood in the brain to stupefaction, like *Opium,* but by decreasing the amount of blood, thus resembling more nearly natural sleep. Then they exclaimed, Eureka! But, alas! too great and long-continued *anœmia* resulted in lack of nutriment to the brain tissue, and as a consequence there developed depression, melancholia, insanity and signs of brain softening until Hammond, its chief advocate, admitted that it put more patients into the insane asylum than any other remedy.

Well, for what can we safely use the remedy? For the symptoms arising from cases simulating the effects of *Kali bromatum,* just as we do any other homœopathic remedy. I do not understand the remedy well enough to give characteristic indications for its homœopathic uses. There is one symptom which I think is valuable as a "guiding symptom," viz.: "fidgety hands." The patient must be working or playing with them continually; even the sleeplessness is somewhat relieved by moving the fingers over the bed clothes; or he plays with his watch chain or the head of his cane, anything to work off this excess of nervousness. *Zincum* has "fidgety feet," and *Phosphorus* a general fidgetiness or uneasiness; can't sit still, but changes position continually; not like *Rhus toxicodendron,* because he is relieved of pain by moving, but because he is simply *nervous.* The homœopathic uses of *Kali bromatum* ought to be better understood.

MOSCHUS; CASTOREUM; ASAFŒTIDA; VALERIAN; AMBRA GRISEA.

Here are five so-called hysterical remedies. They have many nervous symptoms that are similar, and I will only give a few characteristic symptoms of each and leave their study to those who love to study.

Moschus. "Hysterical spasms of the chest, nervous suffocative constrictions, especially on becoming cold." Palpitation (hysteric) with dyspnœa, prostration, fainting, exclaiming, "I shall die! I shall die!" etc., greatly excited. Laughs immoderately, or cries or scolds until her lips turn blue, eyes stare and she falls down fainting or unconscious.

Castoreum. "Exhausted, pains better from pressure, menstrual colic, with pallor and cold sweat."

Asafœtida. Enormous accumulation of flatulence all pressing upward; ball rising in throat.

Great suffering, especially hysterical, from suppression of discharges. Discharges fœtid.

Great sensitiveness to contact; in ulcers, especially periosteal.

"Full of wind; flatulence with eructations all *pressing upward,* but none downward. Seems as if she would burst with the upward pressure, reverse peristalsis." "Especially useful if its nervous symptoms come on after the suppression of leucorrhœal or other habitual discharges." All discharges offensive, even of ulcers, and great sensitiveness to contact or touch. Osteitis or caries with this same exceeding sensitiveness to contact *(Hepar).*

Valerian. General nervous irritation, cannot keep still, tearing pains and cramps in different places. Feels as if *floating in the air (Sticta pulm.* as if legs were floating in the air). Over-sensitiveness of all the senses. Sensation as of a thread hanging down throat. With this remedy I once cured a severe case of sciatica in a pregnant woman on the symptom, pain worse when standing and letting the foot rest on the floor. She could stand with that foot resting on a chair, or could lie down in comfort.

Ambra grisea. Convulsive cough, with frequent eructations of gas.

Discharge of blood between the periods; after a hard stool; or walk.

Very nervous women, cannot void stool or urinate when others are in the room.

Discharge of blood between periods; any little exertion or straining at stool causes it. Nervous cough followed by eructations of wind. It is particularly adapted to nervous affections of old people and spare subjects nervously "worn out."

These five remedies should be studied together.

CANNABIS INDICA.

A lady with dropsy, consequent on valvular heart disease, after being relieved of the bloating, was suddenly unable to talk. In answer to a question she could begin a sentence, but could not finish it, because she could not remember what she intended to say. She was very impatient about it and would cry, but could not finish the sentence, but could signify her assent if it was finished by some one else for her. This continued for several days, or until she received *Cannabis Indica,* when she rapidly recovered her power to express herself. This is all the experience I have had with this remedy that is worth relating.

AGARICUS.

Ears, face, nose and skin in general, red and itch as if from *chilblains.*

Twitching in eyelids (especially), face, extremities, even choreaic jerkings, which cease during sleep.

Spinal column painful and sensitive to touch, aching extending into the lower limbs.

* * * * *

Agaricus has some very characteristic skin symptoms. "*Ears, face, nose, toes and skin in general are affected* with *a redness, itching and burning as if from being frozen.*" This is a very valuable symptom and may lead to the choice of this drug in many very different diseases. I have used the remedy a good many years with very gratifying results for *chilblains.* I always use it internally in the 200th. It is also a remedy of first importance for *twitchings,* from simple twitching *in face, eyelids* (especially) and *extremities, to severe cases of chorea.* In the latter disease the twitchings cease during sleep. Again it has been found useful in spinal irritation. The symptoms indicating it here are best given in Allen's *Encyclopædia.* No doubt this remedy has been over-proven, and as a consequence many of its recorded symptoms are unreliable. The best work that can be done with it now is to separate them, if possible, "proving all things and holding fast that which is true."

LITHIUM CARBONICUM.

Chronic rheumatism connected with valvular heart troubles should call our attention to this remedy, for it has done good service in such cases. Symptoms: *"Rheumatic soreness in the cardiac region." "Violent pains in the heart when bending over." "Pains in heart when urinating or at menstrual period." "Fluttering of the heart with mental agitation,"* are all valuable guides to its selection. Then if we have the rheumatic symptoms, swelling and redness with great tenderness of the small joints, the indications are very positive for its use.

There are often heavy *deposits in the urine of mucus,* uric acid or pus. I have done some excellent work with it in such cases.

SAMBUCUS NIGRA

Is a prime remedy for *"snuffles"* in small children. It is of the dry variety, completely obstructing the nose, child must breathe through the mouth. It is also one of the best remedies for asthma millari. The attacks come on suddenly in the night; *child turns blue, gasps for breath* and seems as if almost dying. Then it goes to sleep and wakens with another attack again and again. I once relieved a very bad case of chronic asthma in an old lady having similar attacks of suffocation with the 200th of this remedy. The relief was followed, or rather accompanied, by a profuse flow of urine which carried off a large amount of dropsical effusion in her legs and abdomen. She has remained much better of all her symptoms since and is now *very* old. One very peculiar characteristic which should never be forgotten is *"dry heat"* while asleep and *"profuse sweat when awake."* No other remedy has it, and it has been confirmed many times. *Conium* has "sweats as soon as he closes his eyes to sleep." *Thuja* has sweats on uncovered parts. (*Belladonna* on covered.) *Pulsatilla,* one sided sweats, and many of our best characteristics are found under the so-called fever symptoms, including chill, heat and sweat, and as we are apt to have one or the other, or all of these three conditions in most diseases, it is well to have a ready understanding of them. It will save much time sometimes in hunting after the simillimum.

SQUILLA

Has been found useful in cough, with sneezing; watering of the eyes, and involuntary micturition. There may also be pleuritic stitches in the chest, with or without effusion. The cough is generally loose and rattling, with expectoration of much mucus, and the loose cough in the morning is more fatiguing than the dry one in the evening.

Verbascum thapsus. Cough, deep, hollow, hoarse, with sound like a trumpet. I have cured many cases and always used it low. I have never used the remedy for anything else.

Senega. Cough with great accumulation of mucus, which seems to fill the chest, with much rattling, wheezing and difficult breathing; especially valuable with old people, but works well with others. Have also cured many cases of this kind and always use it low; no success with the high.

Illustrations.—Several years ago I was called to an old asthmatic, who was having a terrible paroxysm. After several days of intense suffering, which ordinary remedies did not relieve in the least, I gave him *Senega* three or four drops of tincture in one-half glass cold water, dessertspoonful doses once in two hours until relieved, with a promise to call again in the evening. Imagine my surprise when I called as he ushered me in with a smile and bow, for he was perfectly free from hard breathing and cough, and remained so for a long time after.

During September, 1900, I was called again to a lady 50 years of age, suffering the same way. She had been suffering for over a month, at times very severely, but this paroxysm was worst of all. The dyspnœa was very great; had to sit propped up in bed; chest rattling and wheezing; filled with mucus which she could not raise; face and hands purple from unoxygenized blood. *Ipecac.*, *Arsenic* and *Antimonium tart.* were of no benefit. One evening after their failure I dropped seven drops of the tincture of *Senega* into one-half glass water, with directions to give teaspoonful once an hour until relieved, then at longer intervals. The next A. M. as soon as she saw me exclaimed, "Oh, Doctor, I wish you could just realize how I slept. In one-half hour after the first dose I went right to sleep, and I have had a beautiful night." I give these two cases to impress the value of this remedy upon the reader. I have used it many years in obstinate coughs with dyspnœa and difficult expectoration of mucus which seemed to fill the bronchial tubes.

Myrtus communis. Obstinate cough, mostly dry, with *pain in upper portion of left chest, right through to left shoulder-blade.* This is a gem and has, I believe, cured more than one case of incipient consumption for me. *Sulphur, Pix liquida, Anisum, Arum tri.,* and *Theridion* have a similar symptom, but *Myrtus* leads, unless there is decided psoric taint, when *Pix liquida* or *Sulphur* would lead.

Drosera rotundifolia has a deep sounding, hoarse, barking or *trumpet-toned cough,* something like that of *Verbascum,* but there is more laryngeal trouble with *Drosera,* for the voice in talking has a *deep base sound. Drosera* is also one of our leading remedies in spasmodic coughs, whooping cough. With the cough there is *great constriction of the chest and abdominal muscles,* so that the patient holds them with the hands. The cough is worse after midnight.

GAMBOGIA

Is a very valuable remedy for diarrhœa, though not so often used, I think, as it should be. It resembles *Croton tiglium* in the suddenness of the desire for stool, and in the all coming out at one gush. Again, it resembles it, in that it is sometimes watery and yellow, but *Croton tig.* is aggravated by the least food or drink, which is not the case with *Gambogia.* Again, *Gambogia* has all the way from yellow, watery, to almost formed stools, and in each case, the stool comes all at once in one prolonged effort, and there is a feeling of great relief after stool, as if an irritating substance were removed. Sometimes there is burning of the anus after the stool, similar to *Arsenicum, Iris versicolor* and *Capsicum.* It is curative in both acute and chronic forms of diarrhœa. There is often much rumbling in the bowels.

Gratiola officinalis is another remedy that has the yellow, watery diarrhœa, gushing out with great force. It is sometimes especially useful in the summer complaints of children, especially where they have been drinking too much cold water, which frequently happens. *Gratiola* resembles *Aloes* in some points, but has not the hæmorrhoids.

Oleander is one of our best remedies for diarrhœa of undigested food, and the best indication for it is *involuntary stool when emitting flatus.* The least passage of flatus is always accompanied with stool, so that the clothes are always liable to be soiled. I cured with the 200th of this remedy a case of three years' duration in a child. It was my own child, and I had tried many remedies (it was in the beginning of my practice) and was almost despairing that she would ever be well or strong, but after taking the *Oleander* she was cured, not only of the diarrhœa, but became perfectly strong and well and has always remained so, not having the slightest tendency to a return of the trouble.

CONVALLARIA MAJALIS.

I believe the lily of the valley is to become one of our very valuable remedies. It ought to receive a Hahnemannian proving. I have used it with much satisfaction in women who complained of great *soreness in the uterine region and sympathetic palpitation of the heart.* It has also served me well in dropsies of cardiac origin, especially in women who have at the same time the above-mentioned soreness in uterine region. I once checked the progress of a very bad case of cardiac dropsy after the effusion in the chest had so increased that the patient could not breathe when lying down, and there was much bloody expectoration. I used the 30th potency in this case, though many times very fine results follow the use of the remedy in much lower preparations. The dropsy all disappeared and she was able to be around and enjoy life very well, though the organic heart trouble was not removed.

Bovista has been of use to me in only one affection, but in that it is invaluable—menorrhagia. The *flow is always worse,* or sometimes *flows only in the night in bed.* I do not know of a more reliable symptom. It has helped and cured many cases, both acute and chronic.

It has also sometimes a flow *between* the periods like, *Ambra grisea,* but the latter remedy has more nervous or hysterical symptoms.

Ustilago maydis is also a remedy that is very useful in menorrhagia or metrorrhagia, and I think I have observed that it is best adapted to those cases where the flow is of a passive nature. *(Thlaspi bursa pastoris.)* There is apt to be more or less pain and irritation, at the same time, in one or both ovaries. It is especially useful in these cases at the climacteric. I have cured some very bad cases, and always use both this remedy and *Bovista* in the 200th potency.

CARDUUS MARIANUS

Is a so-called liver remedy, and I have seen good results from it in liver troubles, yet I do not know of any *special* indications for its use. I have known cases of habitual colic from gall stones checked and the further formation of the stones prevented by this remedy. One of them was a very bad case, for which old Dr. Pulte, of Cincinnati, prescribed *Carduus.* Her daughter inherited the trouble, and I saw her, in consultation with another physician, at one of these terrible attacks of gall stone colic. She could not lie down, but sat in her chair, bent over forward, for forty-eight hours, and during this time she passed two hundred gall stones, very hard and nearly the size and shape of a beech-nut, which were found by washing the fæces. I have a dozen or so now in a little vial in my office. *Carduus* was also a help to her, but she takes, right along for years at a time, olive oil, thinking that it dissolves the stones or keeps them from forming.

When other remedies fail for pain in the region of the liver, with dizziness, bad-tasting mouth, jaundiced skin and the usual symptoms called "bilious," if I have no special indications for other remedies, I have given *Carduus,* and several times with good results. But, as I said before, I can give no special indications for its use. I can do better for

PTELEA TRIFOLIATA

Another liver remedy, for it has one very characteristic symptom, viz.: Aching and heaviness in the region of the liver, *greatly aggravated* by lying on the *left side;* turning to the left causes a *dragging sensation.* (See *Bryonia,* which is also < lying on left side and has the dragging sensation. Remember, *Bryonia* is generally > lying on *painful side.)* *Magnesia mur.,* you will remember, has all these symptoms, termed "bilious," but like *Mercurius,* it is worse when lying on the *right* side. Then

Mercurius is apt to have loose stools, while *Magnesia mur.* is greatly constipated. *Ptelea* may have either constipation or diarrhœa, or, like *Nux vomica,* constipation and diarrhœa alternately. I cured one bad case of liver trouble with *Ptelea* after œdema of the feet and legs had set in; she had the symptoms, could not lie comfortably on the left side; her breathing was becoming oppressed, and I thought the case looked as if it would not be very likely to be much better. I used the 30th in this case. The trouble rapidly disappeared and never returned. I considered it a brilliant cure.

MARUM VERUM TEUCRIUM.

I have found this remedy one of the best for ascarides. Have cured many cases who had *"tried everything"* (so they said) without avail. I have noticed that people troubled with ascarides often have a great deal of tickling, tingling, etc., in the nose, which they are frequently rubbing. (Children troubled with ascarides have this symptom.) And it is notable that *Teucrium* is one of the best remedies for polypus of the nose; will cure it, and that never to return. I have a preparation of the remedy, made on the Santee potentizer, 50m., which does the best of any preparation I ever used.

MEZEREUM.

Pains in the long bones, especially tibia.

Facial neuralgia or toothache, when the pains are greatly < by eating or motions of the jaws, > by radiate heat.

Nose; vesicular eruptions, with excoriations, formation of thick scabs, < at night; zona.

* * * * *

Pains in the *long bones,* especially the *tibia,* are sometimes greatly relieved by this remedy. I once cured a very obstinate case of facial neuralgia with it. The pains were brought on, or greatly aggravated, by *eating,* and the only relief he could get was to hold that side of his face as near as he could to a hot stove. Hot cloths, wet or dry, or any other heat applied did *not* relieve.

Zona. Skin diseases, etc. See Materia Medica.

TELLURIUM.

With this remedy I have had the pleasure of curing several cases of otorrhœa of long standing, generally following scarlatina in childhood. I used the 6th in these cases. The high failed.

EPIPHEGUS (Beech Drops)

Cures headaches coming on after a hard day's work, over-fatigue from work or excitement, what is often called "tired headache." Such cases are very frequent, and the patients volunteered to mention the fact that they always came on when they were "tired out." Of course one swallow does not make a summer, neither does one symptom always make unfailing indication for a remedy, but a symptom often verified is always a valuable leader to the totality of symptoms.

Epiphegus needs further proving.

LAUROCERASUS.

Suffocative spells about the heart, < sitting up, > lying down; cardiac cough; gasping, twitching and jerks.

Lack of re-active power, low vitality, with blueness or cyanoses, especially in heart troubles.

Drink rolls audibly down through the œsophagus and intestines; very low pulse.

* * * * *

"Want of energy, of vital power; want of reaction, especially in chest and heart affections." And there is another characteristic symptom under this remedy in *heart* troubles: "The cyanosis, dyspnœa, etc., are worse when sitting up." Only one other remedy has this aggravation, and that is *Psorinum.* "Want of nervous reaction; the well-chosen remedy does not act."

"*Capsicum,* lack of reaction in persons of lax fibre."

Opium, in patients where there is no pain; stupidity and drowsiness.

Valerian and *Ambra* in nervous affections, well chosen remedies fail.

Carbo vegetabilis, collapse, coldness of knees, breath; perfect indifference.

Sulphur and *Psorinum,* where Psora complicates and hinders reaction.

Each one of these remedies may be called for in defective reaction, and there may be many more, and in each case, as with all remedies elsewhere, symptoms must decide **which** one.

LACTIC ACID

Is a great remedy for diabetes mellitus. It is especially indicated if in addition to the thirst, voracious hunger and profuse urine loaded with sugar there are *rheumatic pains* in the joints. It is generally given low, but abundant experience has taught me that the high is much better, and it does not need frequent repetition.

Oxalic acid has a very peculiar symptom which has

often been verified by myself. Palpitation and dyspnœa in organic heart disease, *worse* when thinking of it, a very peculiar modality, but *genuine*.

HYPERICUM

Is the remedy "*par excellence*" for wounded or injured nerves; from simple punctures from nails, splinters, pins, rat bites, etc., to severe concussions of the spine and brain, and especially to parts rich in centient nerves. It is to this kind of injuries what *Arnica, Hamamelis, Ruta,* etc., are to bruises, and *Calendula* to lacerated muscular tissue, and *Staphisagria* to cuts with sharp instruments.

ABIES NIGRA.

Severe pain in stomach after eating. Sensation of an undigested hard-boiled egg in stomach.

MANGANUM ACET.

Cough better lying down.

APOCYNUM CANN.

Great thirst, but water disagrees, causing pain, or is immediately thrown off; sinking feeling at pit of stomach. (Dropsy.)

APOMORPHIA.

Easy vomiting without previous nausea.

DIOSCOREA VILL.

Colic pain begins at umbilicus and radiates to all parts of the body, even extremities.

DOLICHOS PRUR.

Violent itching over the body, without any visible eruption; jaundice; white stools.

EQUISETUM HYEM.

Frequent inclination to urinate, with pain in bladder as if too full, which must be relieved; normal quantity at a time, sometimes excess of urine.

KALI NITRICUM.

Great difficulty in drinking on account of short breathing; drinks in sips.

LACHNANTHES TINC.

Stiffness of neck, head drawn to one side; torticollis.

GNAPHALIUM.

Intense pain along the sciatic nerve, alternating with numbness.

GUAIACUM.

Cough with expectoration of fœtid pus.

GRINDELIA ROB.

When dropping off to sleep the breath stops, the patient awakens catching for it, with a gasp, cannot get to sleep on this account.

LOBELIA INFLATA.

Nausea and vomiting with great relaxation of muscular system and profuse accumulation of saliva.

OLEANDER.

Chronic diarrhœa, stools undigested; passes stool with the least emission of flatus.

OXALIC ACID.

Complaints < when thinking of them. *(Helon., Calc. phos.)*

OCIMUM CANUM.

Great pain in renal region, with much red sand in urine. *(Lycopodium.)*

MENYANTHES.

Icy coldness of hands and feet with warmth of the rest of the body (intermittents).

PAREIRA.

Constant urging to urinate; goes down on his knees with straining; pain runs down thighs.

ABROTANUM.

Marasmus most pronounced in lower extremities, from malnutrition; diarrhœa; diarrhœa alternating with rheumatism.

ROBINIA PSEUDACACIA.

Excessive acidity of the stomach; vomits substance that sets teeth on edge.

ARALIA.

Loud wheezing breathing, with cough, < in evening or night, after the first sleep (asthma).

CALCAREA FLUOR.

Indurated swellings, of a stony hardness; in glands, or fasciæ, or ligaments.

GRINDELIA ROB.

Stops breathing when falling asleep; wakens with a start.

NATRUM PHOS.

Excess of acidity; yellow, creamy coating at the back part of the roof of the mouth; sour eructations and vomiting.

RANUNCULUS BULB.

Blister-like eruptions (eczema) in the palms of the hands.

VIOLA ODORATA.

Eczema capitis, cracks, exudes and wets the hair, strong urine like cat's urine.

ZINGIBER.

Diarrhœa from drinking impure water.

MERCURIUS DULC.

Catarrhal inflammation of the Eustachian tube and middle ear. *(Kali mur.)*

CYCLAMEN.

Violent headache, with flickering before the eyes, or spots and various colors, < in the morning and at the menses.

STILLINGIA.

Extreme torture from bone pains and periosteal affections, especially in the "tibia," syphilitic eruptions, etc.

ASARUM EUROP.

Remarkable over-sensitiveness of the nerves; scratching linen or silk or even thinking of it is unbearable.

TARAXACUM.

Tongue coated white, which peels off in patches, leaving dark, red, tender, sensitive spots; mapped tongue.

BADIAGA.

Spasmodic cough, which ejects viscid mucus, which flies out of the mouth.

FLUORIC ACID.

Diseases of the bones, especially the long bones, > from cold. *Silicea,* > by warmth.

CARBOLIC ACID.

Vesicular eruption all over the body, which itches excessively; better after rubbing, but leaving a burning pain.

CEDRON.

Clock-like periodicity of complaints, in low, deep, marshy districts.

CEANOTHUS.

Deep-seated or cutting pains and fullness in region of spleen.

PHELLANDRIUM.

Sticking pains through right breast, near sternum, extending to back under shoulders. Cough with profuse fœtid expectoration, compels to sit up.

RAPHANUS.

Abdomen tympanitic; hard; no flatus up or down. (Dunham.)

INDEX TO REMEDIES.

The black faced numbers indicate the page where the remedy may be found as treated in the text. By comparing this with the first edition it will be seen that a number of new and imporant remedies have been added, but the chief improvement is in the numerous comparisons which have been added.

Abrotanum, 136, 316, 331, 333, 353, 472.

Abies, 470.

Acetic acid, 126, 146, 190, 250, 331.

Aconitum nap., 19, 32, 51, 59, 67, **82**, 83, 84, 85, 86, 87, 88, 95, 96, 100, 101, 142, 157, 158, 159, 162, 164, 165, 166, 167, 187, 194, 197, 220, 225, 228, 232, 256, 273, 278, 343, 351, 382, 393, 408, 411, 419, 428, 449.

Actæa race., 209, **214**, 215, 216, 227, 339, 433.

Æsculus hip., 21, **179**, 180, 181, 224, 295, 342, 378, 438.

Æthusa cynap., 75, **436**, 437.

Agaricus, 144, 166, 183, 324, 397, 401, **459**.

Agnus cast., 61, 63, 67.

Ailanthus gland., 98.

Aletris far., 219.

Aloe socc., 31, 135, 180, **319**, 320, 321, 322, 323, 324, 364, 396, 432, 449.

Alumen, 184, 333, 381.

Alumina, 251, 281, 332, **379**, 449.

Ambra gris., 458, 465, 469.

Ammonium carb. 62, 382, **433**, 434, 435.

Ammonium mur., 332, 333, **339**, 435.

Amyl. nit., 400, 453, **455**.

Anacardium orient., 18, 63, 134, 195, 331, 343, 350, 351, **375**, 376, 377, 378, 379, 397, 404.

Angustura, 292.

Anisum stell., 154.

Antimonium crud., 14, **35**, 36, 37, 39, 40, 122, 182, 198, 206, 229, 349, 358, 367, 402, 424.

Antimonium tart., 100, 230, 231, 234, **235**, 236, 237, 351, 357.

Anthracinum, 123, 152, 432.

Apis mel., 28, 53, 67, 98, **143**, 144, 145, 146, 149, 150, 177, 180, 192, 193, 206, 265, 275, 295, 296, 312, 322, 334, 335, 350, 351, 358, 413, 415, 445, 448.

Apocynum can., 146, **470**.

Apomorphia, 230, **470**.

Aralia, **472**.

Aranea diad., 153.

Argentum met., 186, 197, 363.

Argentum nit., 28, 131, 179, 209, 251, 280, **293**, 294, 295, 296, 297, 298, 299, 316, 324, 328, 333, 386.

Arnica Mont., 97, 214, 221, 232, 242, 250, 267, 274, 343, 364, 367,

386, 387, 388, 390, 391, 392, 415, 432, 437, 446, 449.
Arsenicum alb., 28, 40, 50, 51, 53, 65, 67, 71, 82, 85, 87, 88, 89, 90, 91, 92, 93, 94, 95, 144, 146, 150, 152, 158, 161, 181, 191, 194, 231, 234, 320, 334, 341, 342, 354, 369, 377, 382, 393, 395, 418, 423, 432, 433, 436, 445, 463.
Arum tri., **385**, 386.
Asafœtida, 52, 293, 343, 457.
Asarum Europ., 154, 383, **474**.
Asterias rub., 177.
Aurum met., 16, 134, **291**, 292, 293, **308**, 363, 404.
Aurum mur., 125, 343.

Badiaga, **474**.
Balsam Peru., 442.
Baptisia tinct., 97, 168, 242, 256, 257, 258, 343, 387, 388, 431.
Baryta carb., 38, 63, 95, 279, 281, 352, 354, 357, 361.
Belladonna, 19, 31, 32, 59, 67, 83, 84, 97, 98, **99**, 100, 101, 102, 103, 104, 105, 106, 107, 110, 111, 135, 140, 142, 161, 166, 179, 180, 188, 210, 227, 232, 249, 256, 280, 293, 302, 328, 330, 341, 342, 343, 354, 412, 413, 420, 448, 449, 451, 454, 455, 461.
Bellis peren., 415.
Benzoic acid, 248, **314**.
Berberis vulg., **310**, 311, 312, 314, 315, 422.
Bismuth, **368**, 369.
Borax, 61, 179, 186, 255, 297, 357, 405, 412, 413, 414.
Bovista, 465.
Bromine, 61, **356**.
Bryonia alb., 16, 20, 25, **29**, **30**, 31, 32, 33, 34, 35, 37, 38, 68, 87, 95, 96, 108, 118, 127, 128, 131, 139, 157, 158, 159, 173, 178, 179, 186, 227, 249, 324, 325, 333, 343, 351, 353, 358, 384, 395, 416, 418, 446, 448, 466.

Cactus grand., 35, 114, 209, 210, **224**, 225, 226, 227, 343, 379.
Calcarea fluor., **473**.
Calcarea hypophos., **282**.
Calcarea ost., 18, 19, 55, 71, 72, 73, 74, 75, 76, 77, 79, 161, 178, 179, 186, 199, 219, 242, 252, 277, 281, 287, 314, 322, 330, 335, 342, 343, 352, 406, 433, 449, 457.
Calcarea phos., 49, 77, 78, 172, 199, 242, 297, 298, 301, 328, 363, 368, 406.
Calcarea sulph., 80, **282**.
Caladium, 61.
Calendula, 382.
Camphora, 212, 263, 264, 266, 351, 382, **398**, 399, 400.
Cannabis Ind., 312, 421, **458**.
Cannabis sat., **313**, 351, 440.
Cantharis, 44, 67, 98, **147**, 148, 149, 159, 208, 272, 312, 335, 342, 384, 400, 410, 421, 442.
Capsicum, 44, 50, 52, 67, 167, **170**, 203, 208, 234, 257, 313, 342, 343, 417, **418**, 463, 469.
Carbo an., 67, 174, 177, **251**, 356.
Carbo veg., 26, 48, **52**, 53, 54, 55, 56, 58, 59, 64, 90, 92, 127, 131, 232, 245, 291, 297, 301, 330, 379, 410, 469.
Carbolic acid, **474**.
Carduus m., **465**, 466.

Castoreum, 448, **457**.
Caulophyllum, 209, 210, **213**, 214, 216, 217, 340, 342.
Causticum, 53, 56, 58, 65, 66, 70, 87, 175, 177, 204, 206, 253, **268**, 269, 272, 273, 274, 275, 276, 285, 298, 330, 357, 386, 397, 416, 435, 436.
Ceanothus, **474**.
Cedron, **474**.
Cepa, 89, **443**, 444, 445, 449.
Chamomilla, 15, 23, 37, 71, 84, 102, 120, **156**, 157, 158, 159, 161, 162, 163, 164, 165, 166, 187, 188, 209, 226, 338, 340, 343, 358, 359, 393, 394, 404, 414, 449.
Chelidonium maj., 40, 46, 179, 185, 195, **306**, 307, 308, 323, 331, 432, 433, 443.
Chimaphila umb., **421**, 422.
Chenopodium, **432**, 433.
China off., **46**, 48, 49, 51, 52, 53, 56, 59, 60, 131, 146, 219, 227, 233, 243, 277, 285, 290, 297, 301, 302, 303, 322, 324, 327, 328, 331, 342, 343, 387, 410, 448.
Cicuta vir., 108, **267**, 268.
Cimex lect., **155**, 335, 435.
Cimicifuga, 342, 347.
Cina, 49, 102, 267, **357**, 358, 359, 360, 404, 413.
Cinnabaris, 401.
Clematis erect., 178, 363, **440**, 441.
Cobalt, 183.
Cocculus Ind., 20, **170**, 172, 173, 174, 175, 179, 210, 267, 342, 379.
Coccus cact., 148, **154**, **440**.
Coffea crud., 84, **161**, 162, 163, 164, 165, 166, 318, 323, 324, 343, 347, 381, 383, 441.
Colchicum aut., 173, 205, 312, **400**, 407, 408, 409.
Collinsonia, **438**, 439.
Colocynth., 63, 95, 157, 175, 185, 186, 338, 340, 342, 343, **392**, 393, 394, 396, 404, 410.
Commocladia, 226.
Condurango, 329.
Conium mac., 154, **175**, 176, 177 178, 179, 356.
Convallaria maj., **464**.
Copaiva, **441**, 442.
Corallium rub., 336, **439**, 464.
Crocus sat., 187, 216, 233, 351, **410**, 411, 412.
Crotalus horr., 47, 52, 119, **126**, 233, 249, 312, 343.
Croton tig., 303, **322**, 433, 448, 463.
Cubeba, **442**.
Cuprum met., 20, 66, 175, 182, 210, 236, 263, **265**, 266, 299, 342, 399.
Cyclamen, 179, 216, 301, 436, **473**.

Digitalis purp., 122, **221**, 222, 223, 224, 226, 227, 261.
Dioscorea vill., 305, 394, 463, **470**.
Dolichos prur., 131, 298, 381, **471**.
Drosera rotun., 191, 272, 416.
Dulcamara, 153, 279, 324, **360**, 362, 363.

Elaps cor., 233, 343.
Epiphegus, **468**.
Equisetum hyem., 315, **422**, 471.
Erigeron Can., **219**.
Eupatorium per., 49, 50, 170, 234, 334, 343, **414**, 415, 416, 417, 432.
Eupatorium purp., 257, 273, 363.
Euphrasia, 382, 443, **444**, 445.

Ferrum met., 28, 47, 52, 129, 154, 159, 179, 216, 233, 264, **299**, 304, 337, 449.
Ferrum phos., 32, 47, 51, 142, 259, 343.
Fluoric acid, 182, 292, 294, 391, **474**.

Gambogia, 317, 463.
Gelsemium, 38, 115, 121, 122, 123, 167, 177, 179, 184, 204, 223, 244, 251, **252**, 254, 255, 256, 257, 258, 269, 270, 294, 295, 343, 412.
Glonoinum, 38, 100, 105, 110, 114, 122, 182, 224, 255, 302, 336, 343, **450**, 451, 455.
Gnaphalium, 228, **471**.
Graphites, 38, 66, 72, 82, 278, **283**, 284, 285, 286, 287, 290, 291, 297, 329, 343, 357, 396, 397, 402, 405.
Gratiola off., 179, 322, 464.
Grindelia rob., 122, 223, **471**.
Guaiacum, 333, **471**.

Hamamelis Vir., 343, **391**, 392, 406, 407.
Helleborus niger, 63, **264**, 265, 312, 385, 399.
Heloderma horr., 74, 342.
Helonias dio., 78, 207, 217, 218, 342.
Hepar sulph., 23, 51, 52, 62, 67, 73, 87, 95, 100, 101, 131, 137, 141, 146, 160, 154, 247, 249, **270**, 276, 277, 278, 279, 280, 281, 282, 290, 298, 335, 343, 357, 380, 399, 414, 420, 448.
Hydrastis Can., 93, 132, 148, 168, 196, 205, **397**, 398, 413.
Hyoscyamus niger, 97, 100, **105**, 106, 107, 108, 110, 166, 194, 233, 243, 322, 346, 386.
Hypericum perf., 368, **470**.

Ignatia amara, 15, 24, 35, 50, 86, 93, 157, 161, **163**, 164, 165, 166, 167, 168, 169, 175, 180, 183, 187, 196, 205, 234, 241, 244, 246, 270, 333, 351, 364, 398, 411, 412.
Illicium anis., 441.
Indicum met., 20, 33.
Indigo, 231.
Iodium, 195, 224, 273, 282, 316, 331, 333, 343, 350, **354**, 355, 356.
Ipecacuanha, 49, 51, 168, **228**, 229, 230, 231, 232, 233, 234, 236, 319, 343, 404, 407, 449.
Iris vers., 132, 135, **237**, 238, 249, 256, 463.

Jalapa, 394, **437**.
Jatropha, 322.

Kali bich., 14, 19, 20, 24, **131**, 132, 133, 134, 135, 136, 137, 145, 148, 152, 193, 204, 238, 320, 329, 350, 398.
Kali brom., 46, **456**, 457.
Kali carb., 6, 27, 31, 32, 43, **127**, 128, 129, 130, 131, 137, 146, 178, 192, 298, 325, 327, 343, 433, 434.
Kali iod., 26, 51, 63, **136**, 138, 141, 142, 186, 203, 239, 313, 343, 449.
Kali mur., 68, **142**.
Kali nit., 216, **471**.
Kali sulph., 26, 136, **374**, 382, 449.
Kalmia lat. 24, **227**, 228, 366.
Kobalt, 21.
Kreosote, 119, 120, 351 **369**, 370, 371, 416, 435.

Lac caninum, 24, 61, 136, 280, 343, 357, 372, 373, 374, 448.
Lac defloratum, 256.
Lachesis, 18, 19, 29, 45, 52, 58, 61, 82, 97, 98, 110, 111, 112, 113, 114, 115, 116, 117, 120, 121, 122, 123, 124, 125, 126, 153, 168, 179, 182, 194, 223, 224, 233, 240, 241, 251, 255, 257, 269, 280, 312, 330, 335, 336, 343, 346, 350, 353, 371, 421.
Lachnanthes, 453, 471.
Lactic acid, 469.
Lapis alb., 422, 423.
Laurocerasus, 347, 350, 468.
Ledum pal., 38, 42, 182, 225, 227, 250, 364, 365, 366, 367, 406, 436.
Leptandra Vir., 308, 309, 310, 432.
Lilium tig., 17, 100, 104, 205, 207, 208, 209, 219, 224, 294, 319, 342, 435.
Lithium carb., 292, 314, 460.
Lobelia inflat., 223, 230, 235, 338, 471.
Lycopodium clav., 19, 26, 38, 46, 48, 53, 57, 58, 59, 60, 61, 62, 63, 66, 72, 73, 82, 119, 124, 131, 157, 198, 209, 280, 281, 285, 292, 297, 307, 308, 309, 314, 315, 316, 319, 331, 334, 342, 343, 350, 351, 353, 357, 365, 382, 397, 401, 414, 434, 435, 441, 455.
Lyssin, 104, 132, 207, 255, 336.

Magnesia carb., 77, 281, 337, 338, 339, 438, 449.
Magnesia mur., 81, 249, 332, 338, 340.
Magnesia phos., 28, 209, 219, 340, 341, 342, 393, 394, 395.
Manganum acet., 24, 136, 436, 470.
Marum verum teuc., 467.
Medorrhinum, 71, 288, 315, 343, 423, 424, 425.
Melilotus alba, 100, 219, 243, 451, 452, 453, 454.
Menyanthes, 114, 472.
Mercurius corr., 43, 208, 312.
Mercurius cyan., 44.
Mercurius dulc., 473.
Mercurius protoiod., 45, 46, 61, 135, 280.
Mercurius sol., 289, 313, 385, 411, 454.
Mercurius viv., 16, 25, 28, 32, 39, 40, 41, 42, 43, 45, 51, 59, 89, 91, 100, 101, 115, 128, 136, 142, 206, 247, 248, 278, 280, 281, 282, 292, 293, 308, 313, 330, 338, 340, 343, 351, 364, 382, 393, 400, 401, 407, 413, 433, 442, 445, 449, 466, 467.
Mezereum, 49, 467.
Millefolium, 219, 220, 221.
Moschus, 457.
Murex pur., 205, 207, 246.
Muriatic acid, 53, 90, 92, 245, 320, 321, 330, 364.
Mygale lasi., 1, 53.
Myosotis, 442.
Myrtus com., 151, 433, 463.

Naja tripudians, 124, 125, 126, 226, 292, 420.
Natrum carb., 18, 35, 38, 110, 114, 122, 252, 255, 336, 337, 362, 439.
Natrum mur., 18, 32, 41, 49, 50, 51, 78, 122, 135, 179, 187, 196, 226, 227, 242, 257, 270, 299, 301, 302, 316, 325, 328, 329, 330, 331, 332, 334, 335, 345, 351, 353, 380, 404, 418, 422, 435.

Natrum phos., 46, 135, **473**.
Natrum sulph., 31, 35, 87, 153, 279, 322, 323, 324, 325, 362, 363, 384, 416, 433.
Nitric acid, 20, 51, 131, 169, 175, 233, **247**, 248, 280, 298, 314, 329, 330, 332, 333, 343, 380, 401.
Nuphar lutea, 324.
Nux mosch., 14, 19, 20, 24, 87, 97, 134, 153, 165, 187, 243, **348**, 350, 357, 363, 411.
Nux vom., **13**, 14, 15, 16, 17, 18, 20, 23, 25, 33, 34, 44, 60, 61, 87, 108, 118, 125, 134, 159, 160, 161, 164, 166, 168, 169, 178, 179, 185, 208, 219, 234, 248, 267, 271, 272, 277, 292, 328, 349, 350, 376, 377, 382, 393, 404, 406, 409, 434, 467.

Oleander, 320, 384, 432, 463, 472.
Opium, 31, 63, 84, 86, 97, 105, 106, 109, 111, 165, 237, 243, 254, 261, 317, 333, **344**, 345, 346, 347, 348, 349, 350, 351, 388, 456, 469.
Origanum, 207.
Oxalic acid, 70.

Pareira, **472**.
Paris quad., 26.
Petroleum, 179, 195, 278, 285, 331, **396**, 397.
Petroselinum, 37, **443**.
Phellandrium aquat., 448, **475**.
Phosphoric acid, 5, 7, 93, 97, **240**, 242, 243, 244, 257, 270, 327, 343.
Phosphorus, 26, 30, 52, 63, 66, 67, 77, 82, 93, 139, 146, 152, 179, 185, **190**, 192, 193, 194, 195, 196, 197, 198, 199, 206, 226, 233, 250, 251, 259, 327, 342, 343, 362, 370, 384, 386, 420, 435, 441, 449, 453, 456.
Phytolacca decand., 61, 318, 353, 371, 387, 388, **446**, 447, 448, 449.
Picric acid, 63, 67, 253, 343, 404.
Pix liquida, 154, 441.
Platinum, 136, **187**, 188, 189, 207, 210, 228, 233, 304, 343, 357, 378.
Plumbum, 52, 281, **305**, 306, 394.
Podophyllum pelt., 31, 40, 180, 234, 309, **316**, 317, 318, 319, 320, 321, 322, 324, 364, 384.
Psorinum, 41, 55, 66, 82, 138, 161, 167, 277, 285, **287**, 288, 289, 290, 291, 343, 347, 350, 353, 396, 428, 429, 432, 469.
Ptelea trif., 340, **466**, 467.
Pulsatilla nig., 17, 20, 21, **22**, 23, 24, 25, 26, 27, 28, 30, 33, 34, 38, 51, 80, 81, 129, 136, 154, 158, 160, 178, 179, 183, 187, 195, 204, 209, 210, 216, 227, 229, 233, 287, 295, 301, 303, 313, 315, 323, 327, 329, 333, 338, 343, 363, 372, 374, 375, 380, 382, 391, 402, 430, 431, 441, 442, 448, 449, 461.
Pyrogen, 218, 257, 312, 343, 387, 415, **431**, 432.

Quinine, 90, 233, 234, 299, 302, 304, 326, 365, 415, 417.

Ranunculus bulb., 416, **473**.
Raphanus, **475**.
Ratanhia, 247, 248, 338.
Rheum, 249, 338, **438**.
Rhododendron cry., 153, 324, **362**, 363.
Rhus. tox., 18, 21, 28, 29, 34, 39, 40, 55, 83, 84, 85, 87, **94**, 95, 96, 97, 98, 99, 106, 108, 145, 153, 158,

159, 183, 206, 225, 227, 234, 243, 249, 273, 274, 279, 288, 296, 297, 311, 319, 333, 343, 362, 370, 387, 389, 406, 445, 446, 457.
Robinia pseud., 249, 472.
Rumex crisp., 324, 383, 384.
Ruta grav., 169, 246, 250, 328, 343, 363, 364, 368, 387, 389.

Sabadilla, 104, 116, 336.
Sabina, 214, 216, 217, 401.
Sambucus nig., 62, 282, 434, 460.
Sanguinaria Can., 137, 239, 240, 420.
Sanicula, 24, 61, 79, 80, 82, 190, 316, 331, 402, 412.
Sarsaparilla, 61, 190, 286, 315, 316, 333, 343, 414, 422.
Secale corn., 88, 94, 210, 211, 212, 213, 214, 216, 220, 233, 319, 343, 399.
Selenium, 61, 189, 190, 386.
Senega, 364, 461.
Sepia, 17, 26, 82, 93, 100, 104, 116, 138, 168, 169, 177, 185, 186, 187, 196, 199, 201, 202, 203, 204, 205, 206, 207, 208, 228, 248, 253, 257, 269, 289, 313, 333, 342, 372, 379, 382, 398, 416.
Silicea, 18, 23, 38, 63, 64, 77, 78, 79, 80, 81, 82, 105, 154, 167, 177, 178, 179, 206, 226, 250, 251, 252, 277, 281, 316, 329, 332, 338, 339, 353, 354, 362, 367, 379, 402, 414, 433, 448, 458.
Spigelia, 178, 225, 226, 227, 239, 249, 334.
Spongia tost., 125, 197, 273, 279, 363, 384, 419, 420, 421.
Squilla, 32, 343, 418, 461.
Stannum, 26, 57, 93, 103, 137, 138, 179, 185, 186, 187, 188, 189, 191, 205, 244, 304, 378, 394, 441.
Staphisagria, 15, 147, 248, 297, 358, 387, 394, 401, 403, 404, 405, 406.
Sticta, 133, 381, 382, 383, 434.
Stillingia, 474.
Stramonium, 40, 84, 97, 100, 105, 109, 110, 263, 369, 413, 453, 458.
Sulphuric acid, 47, 52, 116, 233, 248, 249, 250, 342, 367, 413.
Sulphur, 21, 26, 33, 38, 43, 57, 58, 63, 64, 65, 66, 67, 68, 69, 70, 71, 72, 73, 74, 75, 76, 88, 93, 114, 139, 144, 154, 160, 179, 182, 191, 198, 202, 206, 209, 213, 214, 233, 237, 240, 244, 250, 251, 270, 271, 274, 275, 276, 277, 284, 285, 286, 287, 289, 298, 313, 314, 320, 324, 326, 343, 347, 350, 351, 353, 355, 370, 384, 397, 400, 401, 402, 407, 413, 416, 418, 420, 424, 433, 441, 449, 469.
Symphytum, 78, 368, 406.
Syphilinum, 288, 343, 380, 424, 425.

Tabacum, 153, 173, 226, 264, 404.
Tarantula Cub., 29, 101, 123, 152, 251.
Tarantula Hisp., 151, 343.
Taraxacum, 154, 330, 473.
Tellurium, 468.
Terebinthina, 311, 312.
Theridion cur., 153, 179.
Thlaspi bur. pas., 250.
Thuja occ., 23, 38, 43, 79, 80, 141, 153, 248, 270, 315, 323, 343, 400, 401, 402, 422, 461.
Tilia Europ., 42.
Trillium pend., 219.

Tuberculinum, 27, 71, 277, 278, 331, 343, 425, 426, 427, 429, 431.

Ustilago, 465.

Valeriana off., 383, 436, 458, 469.
Veratrum alb., 23, 86, 159, 165, 167, 172, 209, 262, 263, 264, 266, 281, 332, 369, 379, 394, 399, 429.
Veratrum vir., 166, 256, 260, 262, 271.
Verbascum thaps., 461, 463.
Veronica off., 309.
Viburnum op., 209, 217.
Viola odorata, 473.

Yerba santa, 442.

Zincum met., 166, 181, 182, 183, 185, 189, 192, 198, 207, 250, 304, 333, 372, 412.
Zincum sulph., 21, 166, 203, 230, 266, 434, 456.
Zingiber, 473.

PREFACE TO THERAPEUTIC INDEX.

A few words of explanation in regard to this index seem necessary.

There is no case in which all the remedies liable to be indicated in any disease are mentioned; for instance, in scarlatina only twelve are mentioned, while in Johnson's Therapeutic Key there are twenty-four, and even this list does not by any means cover the possible number. So in diphtheria there are eleven by myself and eighteen by Johnson.

One of the main objects of this work is to give that knowledge (or the beginning of it) of the genius of each remedy which will enable us to prescribe for THE PATIENT, even if pathology has never yet coined a name for his malady. This is Homœopathy.

No remedy ever yet produced a case of scarlatina; but several remedies have produced a condition and symptoms similar to that found in different cases of this disease, and are, therefore, homœopathically curative for it.

When names of diseases are mentioned it is always to be understood that the name counts for *nothing* unless the *symptoms* are covered with the remedy. If there were no names there would be no *routinism,* which so often stands in the place of good *prescribing.*

E. B. NASH.

THERAPEUTIC INDEX.

Abortion.—Vib., 209; Acon., 86; Sabina, 185.
Abscesses.—Merc., 42; Tarant. Cub., 152; Calc. hyp., 283; Hepar, 277; Graph., 283.
Albuminuria.—Tereb., 312; Merc. corr., 44; Helon., 218; Canth., 147.
Anæmia.—Carbo v., 53; Lach., 114; Kali car., 127, 128; Hell., 218; Ferr. met., 299; Nat. m., 325, 327; Alumi., 379; Amm. c., 433; Kali brom., 456; Phos., 190.
Aphthæ.—Sul. ac., 249; Merc., 39; Borax, 412.
Apoplexy.—Opi., 346; Bar. c., 352; Arn., 389; Glon., 450.
Asthenopia.—Nat. m., 328.
Asthma.—Carbo v., 55, 56; Lach., 120; Kali c., 127; Kali b., 135; Zinc., 182; Ip., 228, 231; Ant. t., 236; Sul., 279; Ferr., 304; Nat. sul., 324; Dulc., 361; Samb., 460; Squilla, 462; Aralia, 472.

Backache.—Nux v., 20, 21; Rhus t., 95; Kali c., 127; Zinc., 183; Ip., 228; Dulc., 360.
Blepharitis.—Arg. nit., 297; Staph., 405; Borax, 414.
Boils.—Sul., 67; Lach., 124; Tarant. Cub., 152; Sul., 282; Arn., 390.
Bright's Disease.—Merc. corr., 44; Sul., 282; Colch., 409.
Bronchitis.—Carbo v., 56; Acon., 82; Kali b., 135; Canth., 148; Phos., 192, 197; Ant. t., 36; Sang., 240; Verat. a., 264; Hep. sul., 279; Hydras., 398; Cam., 400; Eup. perf., 415; Spong., 420; Copai., 441; Allium c., 444.
Burns.—Caust., 286.

Cancer.—Bell., 103; Lach., 119, 120, 123; Con., 177; Phos., 193; Sepia, 202; Iod., 355; Bism., 369; Kreos., 370; Lapis, 422; Carbo an., 251; Sepia, 199.
Caries.—Therid., 154; Aur. met., 291; Syph., 434; Asaf., 458; Phos., 190.
Catarrh.—Kali b., 133, 134; Aur. met., 292; Nat. car., 336; Dulc., 360; Kali sul., 374; Stict., 381; Merc. dulc., 473; Cepa, 443; Hepar sulph., 276; Sepia, 199.
Chancre.—Merc. prot., 46; Corall., 440.
Chilblains.—Puls., 28; Apis m., 144; Agar., 460; Pet., 397; Agar., 459.
Chlorosis.—Alumi., 379.
Cholera.—Secale, 212; Verat. a., 264; Cup., 265; Camp., 399.
Cholera Infantum.—Puls., 24; Calc. ost., 74; Sepia, 206; Sec. 212; Ant. t., 237; Iris, 238; Psori., 290; Arg. nit., 298; Pod., 318; Nat. m., 333; Bism., 369; Kreos., 371; Cam., 400; Æthusa, 436; Jalap., 437.
Cholera Morbus.—Ant. t., 236, 237; Cup., 265.
Chorea.—Tarant., 152; My. las., 153; Cup., 266; Agari., 459; Ign., 163; Caust., 268.

Colic.—Puls., 28; Cocc. Ind., 170, 174; Plumb., 305; Mag. phos., 340; Dulc., 360; Melil., 455; Carbo, 457; Card. m., 466; Dioscor., 470; Coloc., 392; Lyc., 57; Cham., 156.
Congestion.—Ferr. p., 25; Sulph., 283; Phos., 190; Sepia, 199; Verat. v., 260; Bell., 99; Acon., 82.
Constipation.—Nux v., 16; Bry., 29; Ant. c., 36; Sil., 78, 80; Lach., 122; Plat., 186; Phos., 196; Sepia, 205; Caust., 271; Graph., 283; Plumb., 305; Pod., 317; Aloes, 32; Nat. m., 332; Mag. m., 339; Alumni., 379; Hydras., 398; Thuja, 402; Amm. mur., 435; Collin., 438; Ptelea, 467.
Convulsions or Spasms.—Nux vom., 13; Calc. ost., 74; Sil., 81; Bell., 99, 104; Stra., 109; Ign., 165; Actæa, 214; Gels., 254; Ver. vir., 263; Cup., 265; Cicut., 267; Caust., 269; Arg. nit., 299; Mag. m., 339; Cina, 359; Æthusa, 436; Glon., 452; Melil., 455; Mosch., 457.
Corns.—Ant. c., 36.
Cough.—Ant. c., 38; Calc. ost., 77; Ars., 91; Hyos., 108; Lach., 120; Kali c., 130; Kali b., 135; Kali hy., 136; Cham., 161; Coffea, 163; Ign., 164; Stann., 185; Sang., 239; Caust., 273; Psori., 287; Ferr., 304; Chel., 307; Nat. sil., 325; Stict., 381; Rum., 383; Cap., 418; Amb. g., 458; Squilla, 461; Lauroc., 468; Manganum, 470; Badiaga, 474; Phel., 475.
Coryza (see Catarrh).—Ars., 89, 91; Allium c., 443; Euph., 445.
Croup.—Acon., 82; Kali b., 135; Phos., 192, 197; Hep. sul., 278; Iod., 355; Cap., 419; Kali sul., 374; Spong., 419.
Curvature.—Calc. ost., 73.
Cyanosis.—Lauroc., 468; Ant. t., 235; Dig., 221.
Cystitis.—Caust., 272; Chin., 421; Equis., 422; Dulc., 360.

Deafness.—Kali m., 142; Phos., 195; Caust., 270; Arn., 389; Phos., 190.
Debility.—China, 46, 47; Ars., 92; Phos. ac., 244; Sul. ac., 249; Pic. ac., 251; Carbo an., 251; Gels., 252; Caust., 268; Psori., 287; Ferr., 303; Nat. m., 335.
Dentition.—Calc. ost., 74; Cham., 156; Zinc., 184; Pod., 318.
Diabetes.—Nat. m., 332; Lact. a., 469.
Diarrhœa.—Bry., 29; Ant. c., 36, 39; China, 47; Sul., 71; Calc. ost., 75; Calc. phos., 72; Ars., 91; Kali bi., 6, 132; Cham., 157; Ip., 229; Iris, 237; Phos. ac., 241, 243; Mur. ac., 345; Nit. ac., 248; Gels., 255; Hep. sul., 281; Graph., 283; Arg. nit., 244; Ferr., 303; Chel., 301; Aurum m., 308; Benz. ac., 314; Pod., 317; Aloe, 319; Crot. t., 322; Nat. sul., 324; Mag. car., 337; Nux m., 350; Dulc., 360; Bism., 368; Rum., 383, 384; Coloc., 393; Pet., 397; Pyro., 432; Jalap., 437; Rheum, 438; Gamb., 463, 464; Grat. off., 464; Olean., 464; Ptelea, 467; Zingi., 473.
Diphtheria.—Merc. cyan., 44, 46; Lyc., 61; Lach., 116; Naja, 124; Crotal., 126; Kali b., 132, 134; Ign., 167; Brom., 357; Arn., 388; Phyt., 446; Melil., 454.
Dropsy.—China, 47; Kali c., 130; Kali b., 134; Apis m., 143, 146; Dig., 223; Hell., 265; Hep. sul., 278; Tereb., 312; Benz. ac., 314; Canna., 458; Con. maj., 464, 465; Apocy., 470.

Dysentery.—Nux v., 16; Merc., 40; Rhus t., 96; Kali b., 132, 135; Canth., 127; Phos., 196; Nit. ac., 248; Ferr. phos., 259; Aloes, 321; Coloc., 393; Pet., 397; Staph., 404; Colch., 406; Cap., 418.
Dysmenorrhœa.—Coffea, 163; Cocc. Ind., 174; Vib., 209; Caul., 214; Cup., 266; Mag. phos., 341; Brom., 357.
Dyspepsia.—Carbo v., 56; Kali b., 134; Hep. sul., 281; Arg. nit., 297; Anac., 376; Puls., 25; Bry., 33; Ant. c., 35; Arn., 390; Colch., 410.

Eczema.—Calc. ost., 75; Ars. 89; Rhus t., 99; Cicut., 268; Caust., 275; Graph., 284; Psori., 289; Cro. tig., 323; Nat. m., 325, 335; Pet., 396; Staph., 405; Ranun. bulb., 473; Viola od., 473; Carbol. ac., 474.
Emissions.—Selen., 189; Phos. acid, 240; Cina, 46.
Emphysema.—Ip., 231.
Enuresis.—Sepia, 199, 200; Thuja, 401; Kreos., 369; Sulph., 64; Cina, 357.
Epilepsy.—Hyos., 108; Lach., 121; Cup., 266; Caust., 269; Amyl. nit., 455; Arg. n., 293; Kali brom., 456.
Epistaxis.—Erig., 219; Cact., 224; Arn., 389; Amm. c., 434; Glon., 451; Melil., 454; Crotalus, 126.
Erysipelas.—Rhus t., 94, 98; Lach., 124; Apis m., 146; Canth., 147; Graph., 284; Amm. c., 435; Verat. v., 260; Bell., 99.
Exostosis.—Merc., 39.

Felon.—Sul., 67; Apis m., 143; Tarant. Cub., 152.
Fever, Gastric.—Ant. c., 37; Rhus t., 96.
Intermittent.—China, 50; Ars., 90; Rhus t., 96; Apis m., 143, 146; Cimex, 155; Ip., 233; Ant. t., 237; Verat. a., 264; Ferr., 304; Pod., 319; Nat. m., 334; Eupa. perf., 415, 417; Meny., 472; Cedron, 474; Ign., 163; Phos. ac., 240; Pod., 316.
Inflammatory.—Nux v., 19; Merc., 41; Acon., 82; Bell., 101; Ferr. phos., 259; Ver. vir., 261.
Puerperal.—Ign., 165; Glon., 452; Kali c., 127.
Typhoid.—Carbo v., 54; Rhus t., 96; Hyos., 106; Lach., 117; Crotal., 126; Apis m., 144; Zinc., 184; Sel., 189; Phos. ac., 192, 241; Mur. ac., 245; Gels., 257; Bap., 258; Verat. a., 264; Psori., 290; Lept., 310; Tereb., 311; Ip., 346; Nux m., 350; Alumi., 380; Arum t., 386; Ham., 391; Pyro., 432; Melil., 454.
Yellow.—Carbo v., 53; Crotal., 126.
Fibroid.—Phos., 193.
Fissure ani.—Graph., 286; Nit. ac., 247; Nat. m., 325.
Fungus.—Lach., 111; Phos., 190.

Gall stone.—Chel., 308; Carduus, 466.
Gangrene.—Sec., 212; Ars., 87.
Gastralgia.—Ars., 89; Cham., 160; Ign., 168; Stann., 186; Iris, 238; Arg. nit., 297; Bism., 369; Kreos., 371; Nux v., 13.

Gastric ulcer.—Ant. c., 39; Arg. nit., 293; Kali bich., 131.
Goitre.—Iod., 356; Spong., 421; Lap. alb., 422.
Gonorrhœa.—Puls., 26; Merc. corr., 44; Sab., 215; Cinn., 313; Sars., 316; Nat. sulph., 323; Nat. m., 333; Rhod., 363; Thuja, 401; Cap., 418; Medorrh., 423; Clema., 440; Copaiv., 442; Cubeb., 442; Petros., 443.
Glandular troubles.—Merc., 39; Kali hyd., 140; Con., 177; Baryt. c., 352; Iod., 354; Dulc., 361; Phyt., 449; Calc. fluor., 473; Brom., 356.
Gravel.—Sars., 315; Lyc., 60.

Hay fever.—Lach., 115; Stict., 383.
Headache.—Nux v., 20; Bry., 34; Ant. c., 36, 39; Calc. phos., 78; Sil., 81; Bell., 103; Lach., 114; Kali bi., 132, 135; Coff., 161, 163; Ign., 166; Cocc. ind., 173; Sepia, 202, 204; Spig., 226; Ip., 228; Iris, 238; Sang., 239; Phos. ac., 341, 342; Gels., 255; Arg. nit., 295; Benz. ac., 314; Sars., 316; Nat. m., 327, 328; Nat. car., 336; Mag. m., 339; Arn., 389; Pet., 397; Thuja, 402; Glon., 450; Melil., 453; Epigea, 468; Cycla., 473.
Hæmorrhages.—Puls., 22; Ant. c., 39; China, 46; Carbo v., 52; Lach., 111, 118, 119; Crotal., 126; Phos., 197; Sec., 210; Caul., 214; Mill., 219; Cact., 224, 225; Ip., 228, 232; Nit. ac., 247; Sul. ac., 248, 249; Ferr. phos., 259; Ferr., 299; Tereb., 312; Iod., 355; Kreos., 370; Alumen, 381; Arnica, 386; Ham., 391; Crocus, 411.
Hæmorrhoids.—Nux v., 20; Sul., 66; Ars., 91; Lach., 118; Apis m., 143, 144; Ign., 164; Æcs., 180; Mill., 219; Muria. ac., 245; Nit. ac., 248; Caust., 271; Ham., 391; Collin., 438; Melil., 453; Gamb., 464; Aloes, 321.
Hernia.—Lyc., 60.
Herpes cir.—Nat. m., 330; Sepia, 109.
Herpes zost.—Rhus t., 94; Mez., 467.
Hoarseness.—Carbo v., 56; Phos., 190; Spong., 419; Caust., 268; Arum, 385.
Hydrocephalus.—Apis m., 144; Arg. nit., 298; Ip., 228.
Hydrothorax.—Kali c., 130.
Hypochondriasis.—Nux v., 15; Arg. nit., 294; Chel., 306; Nat. m., 333; Staph., 403.
Hysteria.—Platina, 189; Nux m., 341; Ign., 165; Puls., 25; Tarant., 151; Crocus, 411; Asaf., 457; Cimic., 215; Mag. m., 339; Stict., 383; Mosch., 457.

Impotence.—Lyc., 61; Phos., 196.
Influenza.—Caust., 273; Eupa. perf., 415; Rhus t., 94; Gels., 252.
Injuries.—Ruta, 363; Led., 364; Rhus t., 94; Calc. ph., 77; Arn., 389; Hyper., 470.
Insanity.—Kali brom., 456; Hyos., 105; Plat., 187; Verat. alb., 262; Verat. vir., 260
Itch.—Sepia, 206; Sulph., 64; Psorin., 287.

Jaundice.—Acon., 86; Crotal., 126; Dig., 222; Plumb., 305; Chel., 307; Aurum m. nat., 308; Card. m., 466; Dolich., 471; China, 46.

Kidney trouble.—Phos., 193; Berb., 310; Benz. ac., 314; Tereb., 311.

La Grippe.—Gels., 253; Eupa. perf., 414; Caust., 268; Rhus t., 94.
Labor pains.—Nux v., 13; Cham., 156; Puls. 22; Caul., 213.
Laryngitis.—Apis m., 145; Canth., 251; Caust., 271; Hep. sul., 279; Spong., 420.
Leucorrhœa.—Puls., 26; Merc., 41; China, 48; Kali b., 135; Æsc., 180; Stann., 186; Sab., 215; Iod., 355; Kreos., 370; Alum., 379; Hydras., 398; Borax, 414; Asaf., 457; Sep., 202.
Liver.—Merc., 46; China, 51; Lyc., 59; Phos., 193; Chel., 307, 308; Aurum m. n., 308; Pod., 317; Nat. sul., 324; Nat. m., 330; Mag. m., 340; Card. m., 466; Ptel. t., 466, 467.
Locomotor ataxia.—Sil., 82; Lach., 121; Con., 175; Phos., 192; Caust., 296; Psori., 290; Arg. nit., 295; Alumni., 380.
Lumbago.—Rhus t., 98; Dulc., 360; Calc. c., 71; Fluor. ac., 474.

Mania.—Melil., 453.
Marasmus.—Calc. ost., 74; Calc. phos., 78; Hep. sul., 287; Sars., 315; Baryt. c., 352; Iod., 355; Nat. mur., 325.
Mastitis.—Bry., 35; Apis m., 143; Cro. tig., 323; Lac can., 372; Phyt., 447.
Masturbation.—Phos. acid., 240.
Measles.—Puls., 28; Bry., 35; Lach., 124; Apis m., 143; Stict., 382; Euph., 445; Bell., 99; Coff. crud., 161.
Meningitis.—Bry., 32; Lyc., 63; Apis m., 144, 146; Hell., 264; Cup., 265; Cicut., 267; Arn., 389; Amm. c., 434.
Menorrhagia.—Nux v., 17; Puls., 27; Sec., 211; Actæa, 216; Sab., 216; Carbo an., 252; Bor., 465; Ustil. m., 465.
Menses suppressed.—Puls., 27; Ant. c., 39; Calc. ost., 76; Bry., 29; Acon., 82.
Metrorrhagia.—Stra., 111; Cham., 160; Sec., 211; Caul., 214; Sab., 214; Plumb., 305; Ip., 228.
Mumps.—Puls., 29.
Myelitis.—Rhus t., 98.

Neuralgia.—Cham., 158; Coff., 162; Stan., 186; Actæa, 214; Spig., 225, 226; Kalmia, 227; Gels., 254; Caust., 274; Chel., 307; Sars., 315; Mag. phos., 348; Coloc., 392; Mez., 467.
Night sweats.—Calc. c., 71; China, 46; Mercurius, 39.
Nymphomania.—Plat., 189; Murex, 207.

Obesity.—Calc. ost., 73; Graph., 283; Caps., 418.
Œdema.—Kali hyd., 138, 140; Canth., 149; Cact., 225; Apis mel., 143.
Ophthalmia.—Con., 176; Arg. nit., 296; Euph., 445.
Orchitis.—Rhod., 363; Ham., 391; Clema., 441; Puls., 22; Cham., 156.
Otalgia.—Cham., 156; Puls., 22.
Otorrhœa.—Tell., 468; Hepar s., 270; Psori., 287.
Ovaries.—Lach., 111; Apis m., 143, 144; Canth., 151; Tarant., 152; Pod., 319; Ustila. m., 465.

Paralysis.—China, 52; Stra., 111; Lach., 120; Cham., 158; Ign., 164; Cocc. ind., 171; Plumb., 305; Nat. m., 330; Op., 346; Phos., 192; Sec., 213; Gels., 253; Caust., 269; Arg. nit., 298.
Pericarditis.—Bry., 32; Spong., 420.
Peritonitis.—Bry., 32; Merc., 42; Rhus t., 96; Canth., 151; Sulph., 64.
Pharyngitis.—Kali c., 131; Æsc., 181; Nat. m., 330; Phyt., 447.
Phthisis.—Calc. ost., 76; Kali c., 129; Kali hyd., 137; Therid., 134; Phos., 198; Iod., 356; Brom., 356; Stict., 388; Spong., 420; Tuberc., 429; Puls., 22; Stann., 109.
Pleuritis.—Bry., 32; Merc., 42; Acon., 82, 86; Kali c., 129; Phos., 198; Borax, 414; Kali iod., 136; Squilla, 461; Sulph., 64.
Pneumonia.—Merc., 42; Carbo v., 57; Lyc., 62; Acon., 82, 86; Ars., 92; Rhus t., 96; Hyos., 107, 108; Lach., 117; Kali c., 127, 129; Kali hy., 137, 139; Phos., 197; Ip., 231; Ant. t., 236; Sang., 240; Verat. a., 264; Chel., 307; Nat. sul., 325; Op., 346; Cam., 400; Melil., 455.
Polypus.—Calc. ost., 73; Thuja, 402; Mar. ver. teuc., 467.
Prolapsus Ani.—Ign., 164, 168; Mur. ac., 246; Pod., 317; Ruta, 364.
Uteri.—Murex, 207; Benz. ac., 315; Pod., 316; Aloes, 321; Puls., 27; Thuja, 403; Staph., 405.
Prostatic disease.—Benz. ac., 314; Staph., 405; Chin., 421.
Pruritus.—Sepia, 206; Chim., 421; Tarant. Hisp., 151.
Psora.—Bry., 29; Sulph., 64; Psorin., 287; Caust., 268; Graph., 283.
Purpura.—Lach., 123; Phos., 193; Terb., 312; Glon., 452.

Rachitis.—Calc. ost., 74; Therid., 154.
Rheumatism.—Puls., 24; Nux v., 19; Bry., 29, 30; Ant. c., 38; Merc., 42; China, 49; Sul., 68; Calc. phos., 77; Acon., 82, 86; Rhus t., 96; Kali b., 132, 140; Cham., 157, 158; Actæa, 214; Cact., 224, 225; Kalmia, 227; Sang., 240; Verat. a., 264; Caust., 270, 274; Hep. sul., 281; Berb., 311; Benz. ac., 314; Mag. phos., 342; Dulc., 361; Led., 364; Lac can., 372; Kali sul., 375; Stict., 383; Hama., 391; Colch., 409; Medorrh., 423; Phyt., 449; Lith. c., 460; Lact. a., 469.

Scarlatina.—Bell., 99; Rhus t., 94, 96; Hyos., 107, 108; Lach., 117, 124; Apis m., 143, 147; Zinc., 182; Cup., 265; Tereb., 312; Arum t., 385; Amm. c., 434; Phyt., 446; Tellu., 468.
Sciatica.—Puls., 28; Lyc., 62; Iris, 239; Amm. m., 436; Phyt., 449; Valer., 458; Gnaph., 471.
Scrofula.—Sulph., 64; Kali iod., 136.
Stomatitis.—Merc., 46; Nit. ac., 247; Sul. ac., 249; Hep. sul., 280; Abies nig., 470.
Strangury.—Tereb., 311; Cantharis, 147.
Sunstroke.—Glon., 452; Melil., 453; Lach., 111.
Sweat.—China, 48; Merc., 39.
Sycosis.—Nit. ac., 247; Thuja, 400.
Syphilis.—Kali hyd., 136, 138; Aur. met., 291; Sars., 316; **Merc., 39**; Nit. acid., 247.

Throat, sore.—Nux v., 19; Merc., 42; **Merc. cyan., 45**; Sul., 66; Apis m., 143, 145; Æsc., 181.

Tonsilitis.—Lyc., 61; Bell., 104; Lach., 116; Kali m., 142; Ign., 165; Psori., 287; Benz. ac., 314; Baryt. c., 353, 354; Lac can., 373; Alumni., 380; Arum t., 386; Phyt., 446; Still., 474.
Toothache.—Puls., 28; Ant. c., 39; Cham., 158, 160; Coff., 161; Mag. car., 337; China, 440; Mez., 467.
Typhoid (see Fevers).—Lyc., 63; Ars., 87; Lach., 115; Phos., 194.
Tumors.—Lach., 119; Con., 177; Lapis, 422.

Ulcers.—Puls., 25, 28; Ars., 94; Lach., 112, 113; Kali bi., 132; Calc. hyp., 285; Arg. nit., 297; Hyd., 398; Asaf., 457.
Urticaria.—Apis m., 143; Nat. m., 335; Rum., 384; Hep., 220.

Variola.—Rhus t., 99; Lach., 111.
Vertigo.—Nux v., 18; Puls., 28; Bry., 29; Sil., 79, 81; Lach., 114; Therid., 153; Phos., 194; Dig., 223; Arg. nit., 295; Nat. car., 336; Cocc. ind., 171; Con., 175.
Vomiting.—Ip., 228; Ant. t., 235; Iris, 237; Sang., 239; Chel., 307; Bism., 368; Æthusa, 437; Apomor., 470; Lobelia, 471; Robinia, 472; Nat. phos., 473; Verat. vir., 260; Verat. alb., 262.

Warts.—Caust., 276; Nat. m., 326; Thuja, 401.
Wens.—Grap., 286.
Whooping cough.—Carbo v., 55; Cocc., 155; Ip., 231; Ant. t., 236; Cup., 265; Mag. phos., 340; Cina, 359; Corall., 439; Coccus, 440; Squilla, 463.
Worms.—Cina, 358; Bell., 102; Cicuta, 267; Mar. ver. teuc., 467.

Grouping and Classification

of

The Leaders in Homoeopathic

Theraputics

(Dr. E. B. NASH)

BY

PROF. MUHAMMAD FAIQ

GROUPING OF REMEDIES

Pages

1. **Digestion Remedies**
   1. Nux Vomica 13
   2. Pul Satilla 22
   3. Bryonia Alba 29
   4. Antimonium Crudum 35
2. **Mouth Remedies**
   1. Mercurius 39
   2. Merc. Sol 43
      Merc. Vivus 43
   3. Merc. Corrosivous 43
   4. Merc. Cyanatus 44
   5. Merc. Protoiodide 45
3. **Flatulence Remedies**
   1. Cinchona Officinalis 46
   2. Carbo. Vegetabilis 52
   3. Lycopodium 57
4. **Anti-psoric Constitutional Remedies**
   1. Sulphur 64
   2. Calcarea Ost 71
   3. Calcarea Phos 77
   4. Silicea 78
5. **Restless Remedies**
   1. Aconitum Napelus 82

Pages

2. Arsenicum Album 87
3. Rhus Tox 94

6. Delirium Remedies

1. Belladonna 99
2. Hyoscymus 105
3. Stramonium 109

7. Snake Poisons

1. Lachesis 111
2. Naja Tripudians 124
3. Crotalus Horr 126

8. Kalis

1. Kali Carb 127
2. Kali Bichrom 131
3. Kali Hydroiod 136
4. Kali Muriaticum 142

9. Burning Remedies

1. Apis Mellifica 143
2. Cantharis Vesic 147

10. Spider Poisons

1. Tarantula Hispania 151
2. Tarantula Cubensis 152
3. Mygale Lasiodora 153
4. Aranea Diadema 153
5. Theridion Curassanvicum 153

11. Bug Family

1. Coccus Cacti 154
2. Cimex Lectularius 155

Pages

12. Mental States Remedies

1. Chamomilla 156
2. Coffea Cruda 161
3. Ignatia 163

13. Spinal Remedies

1. Cocculus Indicus 170
2. Conium Maculatum 175

(Lower back) 3. Aesculus Hippoc 179

14. The Metals

Nerves 1. Zincum 181
Chest 2. Stannum 185
Superiority 3. Platina 187
Male-sex 4. Selenium

15. Burning Bleeding Remedy

Phosphorus 193

16. Bearing Down Remedies

1. Sepia 199
2. Murex 207
3. Lilium Tigrinum 207

17. Women Remedies

1. Viburnum Opulus 209
2. Secale Cor 210
3. Caulophyllum 213
4. Actaea Racemosa 214
5. Sabina 216
6. Helonias 217

18. Haemorrhage Control Remedies

1. Erigeron 219

Pages

2. Trillium 219
3. Millefolium 219

19. Heart Remedies

1. Digitalis 221
2. Cactus Grand 224
3. Spigelia 225
4. Kalmia Latif 227

20 Emetic Remedies (Nausea)

Haemorrhage 1. Ipecacuanha 228
Rattling 2. Antimonium Tart 235
Headache 3. Iris Versicolor 237
4. Sanguinaria 239

21. Acids

1. Phosphoric Acid 2-0
2. Muriatic Acid 245
3. Nitric Acid 247
4. Sulphuric Acid 248
5. Picric Acid 250

22. Prostration Remedies

1. Carbo Animals 251
2. Gelsemium Nit 252
Fevers after 2 3. Baptisia Tinc 257

23. Inflammatory Diseases

1. Ferrum Phos 259
2. Veratrumviride 260

24. Collapse Remedy

1. Veratrum Album 262

Pages

25. Brain Troubles

Helleborus Niger 264

26. Convulsions Remedies

1. Cuprum Met 265
2. Cicuta Virosa 267

(Unique A.P.) 3. Causticum 268

27. Calcareas

1. Hepar Sulphuris Calcareum 276
2. Calcarea Sulph 282
3. Calcarea Hypophosphorica 282

Hepar Sulph is in between Calc and Sulphur and its strongest characteristic is Hyper Sensitiveness.

28. Skin Leaders

1. Graphites 283
2. Psorinum 287

29. Metals

1. Aurum Met 291
2. Argentum Nit 293
3. Ferrum Met 299
4. Plumbum Met 305

30. Liver Remedies

1. Chelidonium Majus 306
2. Aurum Muriaticum 308
3. Leptandra Virginica 309

31. Renal Remedies

1. Berberis Vulgaris 310
2. Terebinthina 311
3. Cannabis Sativa 313

Pages

4. Benzonic Acid 314
5. Sarsaparilla 315

32. Cathartics

1. Podophyllum Peltatum 316
2. Aloe Socotrina 319
3. Croton Tiglium 322

33. Natrums

1. Natrum Sulphuricum 323
2. Natrum Muriaticum 325
3. Natrum Carb 336

34. Magnesia

1. Magnesia Carb 337
2. Magnesia Mur 338
3. Magnesia Phos 340

35. Stupor Remedies

(Painlessness) 1. Opium 344
(Insensibility) 2. Nux Moschata 348

36. Anti-Scrofulous Remedies

1. Baryta Carb 352
2. Iodium 354
3. Bromine 356

37. Lumbricoides Remedy

Cina 357

38. Weather Remedies

(Wet and Cold) 1. Dulcamara 360
(Before Storm) 2. Rhododendron 362

			Pages
39.	**Periosteum Remedy**		
		Ruta	363
40.	**Rheumatic Remedy**		
		Ledum Pal	365
41.	**Cholera Infantum**		
		1. Bismuth	368
		2. Kreosotum	369
42.	**Alternating Sides**		
		Lac Caninum	372
43.	**Chronic of Pulsatilla**		
		Kali Sulph	374
44.	**Dyspepsia and Stools**		
		1. Anacardium	375
	(Constipation)	2. Alumina	379
		3. Alumen	381
45.	**Catarrh and Cough (Dry)**		
		1. Sticta Pulmonaria	381
		2. Rumex Crispus	383
46.	**Raw Bruise and Sore Remedies**		
		1. Arum Triphyllum	385
		2. Arnica Montana	386
		3. Hamamelis Virginica	391
47.	**Colic Remedy**		
		Colosynthis	392
48.	**The Etcs**		
	(Anti Psoric)	1. Petroleum	396
	(Tonic Remedy)	2. Hydrastis	397
	(External Coldness)	3. Camphor	398

		Pages
(Anti-Sycotic)	4. Thuja	400
(Mind Remedy)	5. Staphisagria	403
(Smell of food faints)	6. Colchicum	407
(Haemorrhages, Hysteria-Twitchings)	7. Corocus Sativus	410
(Nervous System)	8. Borax Veneta	412
(Deep System Deep Aching Lower)	9. Eupatorium Perf	415
(Intermittents)	10. Eupatorium Purp	417
(Red Pepper burnning)	11. Capsicum	418
(Cough, Saw Driven sound)	12. Spongiatosta	419
(Cystitis)	13. Chimaphila	421
(Indication to Urinate)	14. Eouisetum Hyemale	422
(Antigonorr hoea)	15. Medorrhinum	423
(History of Tuberculosis)	16. Tuberculinum	425
(Septicaemia)	17. Pyrogen	431
(Left shoulder-blade pain)	18. Chenopodium	432
(Nose bleed when washing the face)	19. Ammonium Carb	433
(Coldness between shoulders)	20. Ammonium Mur	435
(Vomiting child)	21. Aethusa	436

		Pages
(Screaming at night) Colic and Diarrhoea	22. Jalapa	347
(Sour Stool)	23. Rheum	438
(Rectal trouble)	24. Collinsonia Canad	438
(Spasmodic cough) like whooping	25. Corallium Rub	439
(Whooping cough)	26. Coccus Cacti	440
(Gonorrhoea)	27. Clematis Erecta	440
(Chronic Bronchial) Catarrh	28. Copavia	441
(Gonorrhoea)	29. Cubeba	442
(Sudden Urination)	30. Petroselinum	443
(Acrid Coryza)	31. Allium Cepa	443
(Fluent Coryza)	32. Euphrasia	445
(Sore throat)	33. Phytolacca	446
(Head Remedies)	34. Glowoine	450
	35. Melilotous Alba	453
	36. Amylisnitris	455
(Fidgety)	37. Kali Bromatum	456

49. Hysterical Remedies

	Pages
1. Moschus	457
2. Castoreum	
3. Asafoetida	
4. Valerian	458
5. Ambra Grisea	

50. Valvular Heart Disease

	Pages
1. Cannabis Indica	458

			Pages
51.	**Twitchings Remedy**		
		1. Agaricus	459
52.	**Cardiac Rheumitism**		
		1. Lithium Carb	460
53.	**Gough Remedies**		
		1. Squilla	461
		2. Verbascum	
		3. Senega	to
		4. Myrtus Comm	
		5. Drosera	463
54.	**Diarrhoea**		
		1. Gambogia	463
		2. Gratiola	464
		3. Oleander	
55.	**Uterine Soreness**		
		1. Convallaria Maj	464
		2. Bovista	
		3. Ustilago	465
56.	**Liver Remedies**		
		1. Cardus Mar	465
		2. Patelea	466
57.	**Nasal Polypus**		
		1. Teucrium (Marum Ver)	467
58.	**Pain Long Bones**		
		1. Mezereum	467

		Pages
59. Otorrhoea		
	1. Tellurium	468
60. Tired Headache		
	1. Epiphegus	468
61. Cardiac Cough		
	1. Laurocerasus	469
62. Diabetes		
	1. Lactic Acid	469
63. Injured Nerves		
	1. Hypericum	470

CLASSIFICATION OF REMEDIES

1. Analogus Remedies

	(Chemicals)	(Vegetables)
1.	Kal Hydroiodicum	Phytolacca
2.	Sulphur	Aloes
3.	Phosphorus	Cepa
4.	Magnesia Carb	Chamomilla
5.	Ferrum Met	China
6.	Calcarea Ost	Belladonna
7.	Cuprum Met	Ipecacuanha
8.	Alumina	Bryonia
9.	Mercury	Mezereum
10.	Kali Sulph	Pulsatilla

2. Alimentation Disorders Remedies

Nux Vomica, Pulsatilla, Bryonia, Antimonium Crudum

3. Anger Remedies

Chamomilla, Aconite, Bryonia, Colosynth Ignatia, Lycopodium, Nux Vomica, Staphys

4. Bearing Down

Belladonna, Lilium Tig, Sepia

5. Bruised Feeling

Arnica, Bellis, Pyrogen, Eupatorium Perf (Deepaching) Baptisia, Ruta

6. **Burnning Remedies**
Arsenicum, Sulphur, Phosphorus, Acid Sulph, Cantharis, Capsicum

7. **Coldness Objectives**
Camphor, Secale, Veratrum Alb, Heloderma

8. **Colic Remedies**
Colocynthis, Magnesia Phos, Chamomilla, Staphisagria, Veratrum Album, Bovista, Dioscorea (Straightening) Stannum, Jalapa

9. **Constipation Remedies**
Alumina, Bryonia, Anacardium, Sepia, Veratrum Alb

10. **Delirium Trio**
Belladonna, Hyoscyamus, Stramonium

11. **Falling of the Eye-lids**
Gelsemium, Causticum, Sepia, Conium

12. **Fedgety Remedies**
Kali, Bromatum (Hands), Zincum (Feet), Phosphorus (General)

13. **Flatulent Remedies**
Carbo Veg, Lycopodium, China

14. **Fluent Coryza Remedies**
Arsenicum Album, Allium Cepa, Mercurius, Euphrasia

15. **Fright Remedies**
Aconite, Opium, Ignatia, Veratrum Album

16. **Haemorrhages Remedies**

1. Passive

Hamamelis, Secale, Crotal, Elaps

2. *Active*
   Ferrum Phos, Ipecacuanha, Phosphorus
3. *Bright Red, Profuse, Active*
   Ipecacuanha. Nitric Acid
4. *Bright with Fear and Anxiety*
   Aconitum Nap
5. *From Injuries*
   Arnica
6. *Congestion to Head and Throbbing*
   Belladonna
7. *Wants to be Fanned*
   Carbo Vegetabilis
8. *Great Loss of Blood*
   China
9. *Dark Strings and Longclots*
   Crocus
10. *Partly Fluid, Partly Solid*
    Ferrum Met
11. *Delirium and Jerking*
    Hyoscyamus
12. *Blood Decompossed*
    Lachesis
13. *From all Outlets, Black*
    Crotalus, Elaps, Acid Sulph
14. *Profuse and President*
    Phosphorus
15. *Partly Fluid, Partly Hard Black Clots*
    Platinum